ETIOLOGY, PATHOGENESIS AND PATHOPHYSIOLOGY OF AORTIC ANEURYSMS AND ANEURYSM RUPTURE

Edited by **Reinhart T. Grundmann**

Etiology, Pathogenesis and Pathophysiology of Aortic Aneurysms and Aneurysm Rupture
Edited by Reinhart T. Grundmann

Published by InTech
Janeza Trdine 9, 51000 Rijeka, Croatia

Publishing Process Manager Mirna Cvijic

Technical Editor Teodora Smiljanic

Cover Designer InTech Design Team

Additional hard copies can be obtained from orders@intechopen.com

Etiology, Pathogenesis and Pathophysiology of Aortic Aneurysms and Aneurysm Rupture,
Edited by Reinhart T. Grundmann
p. cm.
ISBN 978-953-307-523-5

For EU product safety concerns:
IN TECH d.o.o., Prolaz Marije Krucifikse Kozulić 3, 51000 Rijeka, Croatia,
info@intechopen.com or visit our website at intechopen.com.

Meet the editor

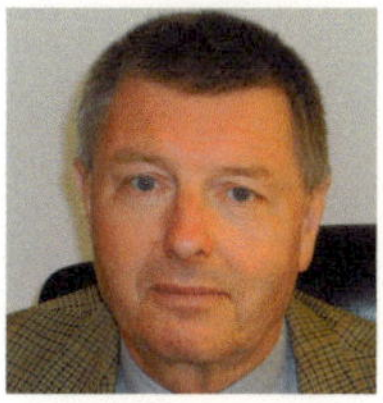

Dr. Reinhart T. Grundmann works currently as an independent medical expert. He is a professor of surgery at the University of Cologne and he has the qualification of general and vascular surgery. He is the former medical director of the B.Braun company and one of the leading providers of healthcare in the whole world. In the last eight years he has been working as the medical director of the Clinics Altotting-Burghausen, Germany. Dr. Grundmann was from 1992 until 2008 the managing director of the Zentralblatt fur Chirurgie and he is currently a member of the Editorial Board of World Journal of Gastrointestinal Surgery. He edited from 2001 to 2005 the Jahrbuch der Chirurgie- the book which provides an information on the latest developments in surgery. Dr. Grundmann already published more than 260 scientific publications, including books and the book chapters. His recent research interests lie in the field of efficiency and efectiveness in surgery. In this frame, he published a workflows on liver surgery, gastric cancer, obesity surgery and surgery for abdominal and carotide artery stenosis treatment.

Contents

Preface

This book considers mainly etiology, pathogenesis, and pathophysiology of aortic aneurysms (AA) and aneurysm rupture and addresses anyone engaged in treatment and prevention of AA. Multiple factors are implicated in AA pathogenesis, and are outlined here in detail by a team of specialist researchers. Initial pathological events in AA involve recruitment and infiltration of leukocytes into the aortic adventitia and media, which are associated with the production of inflammatory cytokines, chemokine, and reactive oxygen species. AA development is characterized by elastin fragmentation. As the aorta dilates due to loss of elastin and attenuation of the media, the arterial wall thickens as a result of remodeling. Collagen synthesis increases during the early stages of aneurysm formation, suggesting a repair process, but resulting in a less distensible vessel. Proteases identified in excess in AA and other aortic diseases include matrix metalloproteinases (MMPs), cathepsins, chymase and others. The elucidation of these issues will identify new targets for prophylactic and therapeutic intervention.

Prof. Dr. Reinhart T. Grundmann
Medical Expert
Burghausen
Germany

1

Etiology and Pathogenesis of Aortic Aneurysms

Carl W. Kotze and Islam G. Ahmed
University College London
United Kingdom

1. Introduction

The introduction of aneurysm screening programmes in North America and Europe has led to a significant increase in the number of new diagnoses. The pathobiology of aortic aneurysm (AA) is both complex and multifactorial, and is associated with several significant developmental risk factors. Understanding current concepts in the etiology and pathogenesis of AA is therefore imperative in fueling future research studies and in aiding the development of treatment guidelines.

In 2001, the Vascular Biology Research Program of the National Heart, Lung and Blood institute (Wassef et al, 2001) summarised abdominal aortic aneurysm (AAA) pathogenic mechanism into four broad areas: proteolytic degradation of the aortic wall connective tissue, inflammation and immune response, molecular genetics and biomechanical wall stress. More recently Nordon and colleagues investigated three possible models of AAA pathogenesis not mutually exclusive: AAAs secondary to a local disease process confined to the abdominal aorta resulting from atherosclerosis; a systemic dilating diathesis primarily governed by genotype; and diseased vascular tree as a consequence of a chronic inflammatory process. They concluded that the evidence suggest AAA disease being a systemic disease of the vasculature, with a predetermined genetic susceptibility leading to a phenotype governed by environmental factors. AAAs are therefore referred to by some researchers as a degenerative disease (Nordon et al, 2011).

AAAs are associated with atherosclerosis, transmural degenerative processes, neovascularization, degeneration of vascular smooth muscle cells, and a chronic inflammation, mainly located in the outer aortic wall. Literature describes the relevant mechanisms of the formation and progression of idiopathic ascending aortic aneurysm as destructive remodeling of the aortic wall, inflammation and angiogenesis, biomechanical wall stress, and molecular genetics. Aneurysm occurrence and expansion could be further influenced by the variability of local hemodynamic factors and factors intrinsic to the arterial segment along the aorta (Kirsch et al, 2006). Observational evidence now suggests that the intraluminal thrombus (ILT), together with adventitial angiogenic and immune responses, play important roles in the evolution of atherothrombosis from the initial stages through to clinical complications, which include the formation of aneurysms (Michel et al, 2010). The role of ILT in AA pathogenesis merits further discussion and will be explored in subsequent chapters.

Uncertainty exists as to the impact of reported AA risk factors since the incidence of AAA is increasing despite a general reduction in tobacco use and an ever-increasing incidence of diabetes, which has been shown to have a protective influence. A number of other factors have also been commonly associated with aneurysm formation. They include family history, advanced age, male sex, hypertension, aortic dissection and arteriosclerosis. The significance of AA risk factors will be further explored in subsequent chapters.

2. Structural considerations in AA

Multiple factors rather than a single process are implicated in AA pathogenesis. These result in the destructive changes in the connective tissue of the media and adventitia of the aortic wall and ultimately lead to aneurysm formation and eventual rupture. The media is composed of multiple elastic laminae alternating with circularly oriented vascular smooth muscle cells (VSMCs) and surrounded by a copious ground substance. The adventitia lacks lamellar architecture but is composed of loose connective tissue with fibroblasts and associated collagen fibers and vasa vasorum. Integrity of the aortic wall is dependent on balanced remodelling of the extracellular matrix (ECM), predominantly of elastin, collagen and VSMCs. (Dobrin & Mrkvicka, 1994; Tilson, 1988).

2.1 Elastin

The chief component of the media is elastin, a lamellar ECM protein consisting of soluble tropoelastin monomers. Elastin production by the VSMCs ceases when a patient reaches maturity, therefore these soluble tropoelastin monomers, which are cross-linked by lysine residues, have a half life of 40 to 70 yrs (Rucker & Tinker, 1977). This could explain the elderly predisposition to AA formation. Normally, more than 99% of total elastin in arteries is found in an insoluble cross-linked form that can be stretched as much as 70% of its initial length (Stromberg & Wiederhielm, 1969). Elastin is responsible for the load bearing property that behaves uniformly in both the circumferential and longitudinal directions at different locations across the wall thickness (Dobrin, 1999), thereby absorbing oscillating arterial shock waves, providing recoil and maintaining arterial structure.

2.2 Collagen

Collagen is the primary structural component of the arterial adventitia and has been identified in smaller quantities in the media. It is a stable triple helix composed of three polypeptide chains with repeating tripeptide sequences (Prockop, 1990) and is responsible for tensile strength and resistance of the arterial wall. In contrast to elastin, collagen is synthesized on a continual basis throughout life, thereby collagen content represents the net effect of synthesis and degradation. Type 1 fibrillar collagen accounts for aortic wall load bearing capability (over 20 times greater than that of elastin), while Type 3 collagen provides some extensile stretch (Menashi et al, 1987). Arterial distension in response to increasing intraluminal pressures are limited through the recruitment of inextensible collagen fibers (Dobrin, 1978). Structural damage occurs when collagen is extended beyond 2–4% from its uncoiled form (Dobrin, 1988).

2.3 Vascular Smooth Muscle Cells (VSMCs)

VSMCs as part of the ECM form an important structural element and perform a mediator role in AA disease by producing TGF-beta1, ECM and inhibitors of proteolysis (O'Callaghan

& Williams, 2000). Transition of VSMCs from a contractile to a synthetic phenotype is characterized by a change in cell morphology, resulting in the production of substances such as components of the ECM, growth factors, and proteases, which are important in remodeling the vascular wall (Lesauskaite et al, 2003). This was verified by an experimental study that reported cultured VSMCs from AAAs exhibited greater elastolytic activity than VSMCs from Aortic Occlusive Disease (AOD) (Patel et al, 1996). VSMC density depends on patient age, patient gender and the location of quantification in non-atherosclerotic aneurysms. Conversely, loss of VSMCs is a characteristic of atherosclerotic aortic aneurysms (Sakalihasan et al, 2005; Kirsch et al, 2006). In particular VSMC apoptosis has been associated with fibrous cap thinning, enlargement of the necrotic core, plaque calcification, medial expansion and degeneration, elastin breaks, and failure of outward remodeling. In addition, chronic VSMC apoptosis may mimic multiple features of medial degeneration seen in a variety of human pathologies (Clarke et al, 2008).

2.4 Experimental and clinical studies

Histological examination of aneurysms reveals a thinning of the media, disruption of the medial connective tissue structure, and the loss of elastin (Campa et al, 1987) culminating in the effacement of the lamellar architecture (White et al, 1993). The role of the aortic media in contributing to wall stability is emphasized through studies demonstrating AA formation following media destruction with surgical resection, freezing, or the injection of acetrizoate or other noxious agents (Economou et al, 1960). Other studies confirmed that both elastin and collagen content is decreased in AA walls with increased collagen cross-links (Carmo et al, 2002) and an increased collagen to elastin ratio. (Cohen et al, 1988) Loss of elastin appears to be accompanied by an increase in the collagen content of the arterial wall, resulting in an overall decrease in the elastin to collagen ratio (Halloran & Baxter, 1995). This reflects in experimental studies that suggest that aortic elastase is significantly higher in patients with AAAs, multiple aneurysms, and ruptured AAAs compared with AOD. Also elastase and its major serum inhibitor, alpha 1-antitrypsin, are significantly altered in the aortic wall in different types of infrarenal aortic disease (Cohen et al, 1988).

AA development is characterised by intial elastin fragmentation responsible for aneurysmal elongation and tortuosity. There is consensus that as the aorta dilates due to loss of elastin and attenuation of the media, the arterial wall thickens as a result of remodeling. Collagen synthesis increases during the early stages of aneurysm formation, suggesting a repair process (Shimizu et al, 2006). As the load bearing increases, more uncoiled collagen is recruited to load bear circumferentially (Goodall et al, 2002) resulting in a less distensible vessel. Collagen, because of its structural properties, must fail for significant dilatation and rupture to occur. This is confirmed as patients who are post aortic endarterectomy rarely incur AA disease. Dobrin et al. concluded that both elastin and collagen are possibly critical in AA dilatation with collagen failure resulting in gross expansion and rupture (Dobrin et al, 1994). This work confirmed experimental studies demonstrating that treatment with elastase leads to arterial dilatation and stiffening at physiologic pressures, whereas treatment with collagenase leads to arterial rupture without dilatation (Cohen et al, 1988). Cohen suggested that elastin degradation is a key step in the development of aneurysms, but that collagen degradation is ultimately required for aneurysm rupture. The integral role of VSMCs in AA disease is confirmed by an animal study that observed AAA prevention and regression after infusion with VSMCs (Allaire et al, 2002).

2.5 Structural considerations in TAA

Elastin lamellar units are found less frequently in AAA as compared to TAA, with an even more marked difference infrarenally. This relative paucity of elastin and collagen is thought to play a role, amongst other factors, in the predisposition for aneurysm development in the infrarenal aorta. The microscopic findings in TAAs are predominantly described as cystic medial degeneration, reflecting a non-inflammatory loss of medial VSMCs, fragmentation of elastic lamellae, and mucoid degeneration. In contrast, the histopathologic features of AAAs are characterized by severe intimal atherosclerosis, chronic transmural inflammation, neovascularization, and destructive remodeling of the elastic media (Diehm et al, 2007). Furthermore, ascending TAAs are associated with an underlying bicuspid aortic valve (BAV) with an estimated 75 % of patients who underwent BAV replacement demonstrating cystic medial necrosis on biopsy, compared to 14 % in patients who had tricuspid valve replacement. Inadequate levels of firillin-1 may be responsible for this weakness in aortic wall leading to BAV (Huntington et al, 1997).

	Ascending aorta	Abdominal aorta	Consequences
Elastin lamellae	-	number decreased/diameter	less provisional ECM
elastin/collagen	-	decreased	modified biomechanical properties
Embryonic origin of VSMCs	Neur-ectoderm	mesoderm	differences in responses to TGF-beta
Shear stress	-	decreased	control of inflammation
Thrombus in aneurysms	no	yes	neutrophils adsoption and protease release
VSMCs in aneurysms	unknown	decreased	homeostasis against inflammation, proteolysis

Table 1. Structural differences between TAA and AAA (Courtesy of Allaire, et al, 2009).

3. Molecular genetics in AA

Aortic aneurysms are a complex multi-factorial disease with genetic and environmental risk factors. Genetic factors have been shown to play a role in the etiology of TAA and AAA even though they are not associated aortic syndromes (Kuivaniemi et al, 2008). The genetic basis of aortic aneurysms was reviewed in 1991 (Kuivaniemi et al, 1991). The major determining factor in the appearance of aortic aneurysms may be an inborn defect of collagen type III or of another component of the connective tissue matrix. At least 20% of aneurysms result from inherited disorders (Verloes et al, 1995). Medial necrosis of the proximal aorta in aneurysms or dissections is associated with a number of conditions, including inherited connective tissue disorders such as Marfan syndrome and Ehlers–Danlos syndrome type IV. It can also present along with bicuspid aortic valve, coarctation of the aorta, adult polycystic kidney disease and Turner syndrome (Caglayan & Dundar, 2009).

3.1 AAA

3.1.1 Genetic considerations in AAA

Screening studies suggest that having a first-degree relative with a AAA is associated with an odds ratio of 1.9 to 2.4 of developing a similar problem. AAAs develop in 20% of brothers of patients with the condition (Rizzo et al, 1989). These and other findings including the presence of multiple aneurysms and systemic abnormalities in aneurysm patients e.g., increased connective tissue laxity; all emphasize a role for genetic factors in AAAs.

A small number of studies have concentrated on multiplex AAA families (with at least 2 affected members) (Platsoucas et al, 2006; Oleszak et al, 2004). Genome-wide scans of these patients have suggested a role for genes located on chromosome 19q13 and 4q31.47. Candidate genes in these regions include interleukin (IL)-15, endothelin receptor A, programmed cell death 5, and LDL receptor-related protein 3.47 (Kuivaniemi et al, 2008).

3.2 TAA

Since more than 40% of patients with TAA are asymptomatic at the time of diagnosis, such aneurysms are typically discovered accidentally through routine examination or when complications arise. Once one aneurysm has been discovered, the patient is at increased risk for developing another aneurysm (Lawrie et al, 1993; Crawford et al, 1989). Therefore, lifelong follow-up is required in these patients. If any mutation is found in the patients affected, the mutation should then be investigated in their relatives, and hence genetic counseling should be given. Because of this increased risk, according to target diseases, chromosomal and gene analysis are essential in selected cases with aneurysms or dissections, especially in inherited forms (Caglayan & Dundar, 2009).

3.2.1 Genetic considerations in TAA

Although AAA's have been well characterized in terms of familial clustering, risk factors, growth rates, and possible modes of inheritance, less is known about thoracic aortic aneurysm (TAA). Rapid advances are being made in the understanding of TAA disease at the molecular genetic level. In pedigrees with several generations of multiply affected family members, chromosomal loci have been identified. These relate to the TAA phenotype by using the methods of linkage analysis and gene sequencing. Thus far, these loci have been mapped to the 5q13-14, 11q 23.2-24, and 3p24-25 chromosome sites (Vaughan et al, 2001; Hasham et al, 2002; Kakko et al, 2003). Most recently, important work has localized the mutation on the 3p24-25 chromosome to the transforming growth factor-receptor type II (Pannu et al, 2005). Albornoz and his colleagues evaluated 88 familial pedigrees with TAA and found that 70 (79.5%) had an inheritance pattern that was most consistent with a dominant mode of inheritance: 30 were autosomal dominant, 24 were autosomal dominant versus X-linked dominant, 15 were autosomal dominant with decreased penetrance, and there was one pair of monozygotic probands with a likely autosomal dominant spontaneous mutation. The other 18 pedigrees (20.5%) were most consistent with a recessive inheritance pattern, eight being autosomal recessive versus X-linked recessive, five autosomal recessive, and five autosomal recessive versus autosomal dominant with decreased penetrance. (Albornoz et al, 2006).

Affected Aortic Segment	Familial disorder	Mode of inheritance	Gene linked
Ascending thoracic / abdominal	Ehlers-Danlos syndrome type IV	Autosomal dominant	COLA3A1
Ascending	Marfan Syndrome	Autosomal dominant	FBN1 TGFβR2
	Turner Syndrome	Chrosomal	
	Osteogenesis imperfecta	Autosomal dominant	COLA1A1
Thoracic	Autosomal dominant adult polycystic kidney disease	Autosomal dominant	PKD1,PKD2
Abdominal	Homocystinuria	Autosomal recessive	CBS
	Pseudoxanthoma elasticum	Autosomal recessive	ABCC6

Table 2. Genetic diseases and Aortic Aneurysms

3.3 General behaviour of familial aneurysms

3.3.1 Aneurysm expansion

TAA is a lethal disease and the size of the aneurysm has a profound impact on aortic dissection and death (Coady et al, 1999). The growth rate of TAA is highly variable ranging from 0.03 to 0.22 cm per year. Genetic factors may play an important role in aortic growth rates. The data suggests that genetic etiology permits more rapid aortic dilatation, thus increasing the risk for aortic dissection. Physicians must know how to distinguish between syndromic and non-syndromic forms of aortic aneurysm and dissection. As a result family history is a most important factor in evaluating the patients who have aortic aneurysms or dissection (Caglayan & Dundar, 2009).

Aneurysms affecting the thoracic aorta in patients with Marfan syndrome behave more aggressively than TAA in patients without Marfan syndrome. However, the natural history of TAA in patients who do not have Marfan syndrome but who demonstrate a family history that is positive for aortic aneurysms has not been not well-described (Coady et al, 1997). It has also been reported that the presence of an aortic dissection significantly increases the aneurysm growth rate (Coady et al, 1997). Coady and colleagues clearly demonstrated that patients with familial nonsyndromic aneurysms and superimposed aortic dissections display a faster rate of aneurysmal growth (0.33 cm/y,) when compared with the overall growth rate of aortic dissections alone. The reasons for faster growth rates in patients exhibiting familial patterns and with concomitant aortic dissections are not clear, but may reflect a compounded environmental insult on a genetically weakened aortic wall (Coady et al, 1999).

3.3.2 Dissection

In most adults, the risk of aortic dissection or rupture becomes significant when the maximal aortic dimension reaches about 5.5 cm. However, in individuals with TGFBR2 mutations, dissection of the aorta may occur before the aorta extends to 5.0 cm (Loeys et al, 2005). Even patients with Loeys-Dietz syndrome (LDS) syndrome, both transforming growth factor, beta receptor 1 (TGFBR1) and two mutations have been described and dissections may occur under 5.0 cm (Caglayan & Dundar, 2009).

In the near future, new genetic studies such as single nucleotide polymorphisms (SNP) and RNA expression studies may help underlie genetic based therapies and develop more useful, simple and cheap diagnostic genetic tests for susceptible patients.

4. Haemodynamic factors and biomechanical wall stress considerations in AA

The pathobiology of AA is thought to be a multifactorial process that includes biological, biomechanical, and biochemical processes. Contrary to current understanding of biological and biochemical factors, the role of biomechanical factors in AA pathobiology is poorly understood. It is generally recognized that AAAs can continuously expand, dissect and even potentially rupture when the stress acting on the wall exceeds the strength of the wall. Wall stress simulation based on a patient-specific AAA model appears to give a more accurate rupture risk assessment than AAA diameter alone (Li et al, 2010).

4.1 Haemodynamic forces

The artery wall is subject to three distinct fluid-induced forces: (1) pressure created by hydrostatic forces, (2) circumferential stretch exerting longitudinal forces, and (3) shear stress created by the movement of blood. The net force includes a component perpendicular to the wall, the pressure; and a component along the wall, the shear stress. Disturbed flow conditions, such as turbulence, contribute to aneurysm growth by causing injury to the endothelium and accelerating degeneration of the arterial wall. Areas of flow oscillation and extremes in shear stress (high or low) correlate with development of atherosclerosis in the aorta (Ku et al, 1985). Although clinical studies show that flow within AAAs can be smooth and laminar or irregular and turbulent, little information is available on effects of wall shear stress in aneurysms (Miller, 2002).

Intra-aneurysmal flow is affected by the geometry of the aneurysm sac and surrounding vasculature; including the existence, size, and symmetry of branches arising near the aneurysm; and the position of the aneurysm sac relative to the parent vessel (e.g. sidewall, terminal, or bifurcation). Effort has been made to correlate rupture with these various geometric features. (Zeng et al, 2011)

4.2 Effect on aneurysm expansion

Vascular endothelial cells are constantly exposed to fluid shear stress, the frictional force generated by blood flow over the vascular endothelium. The importance of shear stress in vascular biology and pathophysiology has been highlighted by the focal development patterns of atherosclerosis in hemodynamically defined regions. For example, the regions of branched and curved arteries exposed to disturbed flow conditions, including oscillatory and low mean shear stresses (OS), correspond to atheroprone areas. In contrast, straight arteries exposed to pulsatile high levels of laminar shear stress (LS) are relatively well protected from atherosclerotic plaque development (Zarins et al, 1983). Changes in blood flow have been shown to be a critical factor inducing arterial remodeling (Manu & Plattet, 2006).

The increase in shear stress is also associated with a reduction in reactive oxidative stress (ROS). The flow-mediated increase in shear stress does not decrease oxidative stress in AAAs by reducing the inflammatory cell infiltrate, but through the expression of hemeoxygenase (HO-1) in macrophages. Activation of HO-1 expression is an adaptive cellular response to survive exposure to environmental stresses (Immenschuh & Ramadori, 2000). HO-1 has anti-

inflammatory effects and may play a beneficial role in reducing oxidative reactions through the production of the antioxidants biliverdin and bilirubin (Miller, 2002).
Because of limitations in studying hemodynamics in vivo, in vitro models of AAAs have often been used to analyze pressure and flow patterns. However, these biomechanical designs often use an axisymmetric model, whereas AAAs, particularly in advanced stages, are asymmetric, resulting in growth away from the lumen's centerline. Interpretation of mechanical models can also be limited if they neglect effects of branch arteries, or by their use of steady flow, rigid walls; and homogenous and incompressible fluid. Understanding the biology of AAA development and expansion requires experiments in animal models. Unfortunately, in vivo studies are complicated by controversy regarding appropriate animal models of human AAAs (Miller, 2002).

4.3 Effect on aneurysm rupture

Rupture of the aneurysm can be seen as a structural failure when the induced mechanical stresses acting on the weakened AAA wall exceed its local mechanical failure strength. The external forces include blood pressure and wall shear stress. Stress in the AAA wall is due to the influence of other concomitant factors, including the shape of the aneurysm, the characteristics of the wall material, the shape and characteristics of the intraluminal thrombus (ILT) when present, the eccentricity of the AAA, and the interaction between the fluid and solid domains (Li et al, 2010).

4.4 Haemodynamic factors and biomechanical wall stress considerations in TAA

The influence of biomechanical factors in TAA is scarcely reported, therefore the role that haemodymic factors play in TAA pathobiology remains unknown. Nevertheless, weakening of the aortic wall is compounded by increased shear stress, especially in the ascending aorta (Ramanath et al, 2009). An experimental study of a cylindrical model of TAA demonstrates that mean circumferential stress depends on the aortic diameter and systolic blood pressure but not on age or clinical diagnosis supporting the clinical importance of blood pressure control and serial evaluation of aortic diameter in these patients (Okamoto et al, 2003). Considering the functional complexity and structural differences of TAA compared to AAA, several hemodynamic factors might contribute to the development of TAA. However the predilection of aneurysm formation infrarenally suggests other factors may overrule haemodynamic factors in AA pathogenesis.

4.5 Current limitations

Although rupture is determined by the comparison of wall stress and wall strength, accurate wall strength measurement in vivo is currently not possible. Therefore, computed wall stresses at one time point may not necessarily provide an estimation of the risk of rupture without knowing the strength value at that time point. However, by following up patients and performing wall stress analysis based on follow-up images, the change in wall stresses may be more useful in identifying aneurysm stability (Li et al, 2010).

5. Enzymatic activity in AA

Proteolytic degeneration is known to cause AA formation and lead to disease progression. Proteases identified in excess in AA and other aortic diseases includes matrix metalloproteinases (MMPs), cathepsins, chymase and tryptase, neutrophil-derived serine elastase and the enzymes of the plasmid pathway, tissue plasminogen activator (tPA), Urokinase-type Plasminogen Activator (uPA) and plasmin (Choke et al, 2005). These proteolytic enzymes are involved in regulating and remodeling the ECM.

5.1 Experimental and clinical studies

Pioneering work in animal models has demonstrated the role of proteolysis in AA. These experimental studies showed elongation and dilatation following treatment with elastase, and rupture post collagenase infusion. More recently, an in vivo study of aortic wall treated with doxycycline loaded, controlled-release, biodegradable fiber led to preservation of elastin content, decreased MMPs (most notably MMP-2 and MMP-9) and increased tissue inhibitor of metalloproteases (TIMP-1) (Yamawaki-Ogata et al, 2010). A number of MMPs, including elastases, collagenases, gelatinases and stromelysin, are found in increased concentrations in the media of the AAA and are normally inhibited by TIMP.

MMPs and other proteinases derived from macrophages and VSMCs are secreted into the extracellular matrix in response to stimulation by the products of elastin degradation (Ailawadi et al, 2003). Inflammatory infiltrates and invading neovessels are relevant sources of MMPs in the AAA wall and may substantially contribute to aneurysm wall instability (Reeps et al, 2009). In AA disease evidence suggests that the balance of vessel wall remodeling between MMPs, TIMPS, and other protease inhibitors favors elastin and collagen degradation with the net pathological effect of ECM destruction.

5.1.1 MMP-9 (92-kd gelatinase)

MMP-9 predominantly secreted by macrophages, monocytes and VSMCs is the most comprehensively studied of the metalloproteases. MMP-9 concentrations are higher in patients with AAA compared to subjects without AAA or AOD. Interestingly, Takagi observed that increased MMP-9 serum levels return to normal after aneurysm repair (Hisato Takagi et al, 2009). Furthermore, an experimental study showed that targeted gene disruption of MMP-9 prevented aneurysmal degeneration in murine models (Pyo et al, 2000). Recently, a correlation was found between AAA rupture and elevated plasma levels of MMP-9 and MMP-1 (Wilson et al, 2008).

5.1.2 MMP-2 (72-kd gelatinase)

Evidence suggests MMP-2 may be the most integral protease in ECM degeneration. MMP-2 sourced by adventitial VSMCs and fibroblasts is uniquely activated by membrane type (MT)-MMPs. MMP-2 has the ability to degrade both elastin and collagen, and possibly plays a role in early AA development. MMP-2 complements and facilitates the degenerative activity of MMP-9 in transgenic murine models, however some studies suggest that MMP-2 has greater elastolytic activity compared to MMP-9. MMP-2 levels are increased in subjects with AA compared to those with AOD or without AA disease. It is found predominantly in its active form (62-kd), which is closely associated with its substrates, which provide additional support of its role in ECM degradation. Convincing evidence from a rat aneurysm model demonstrated that the inhibition of AA formation following TIMP-1 over-expression, resulted in an activation blockade of both MMP-2 and MMP–9. Furthermore, Wilton concluded patients with larger aortic diameters have increased MMP-2/TIMP-1 ratios (Wilton et al, 2007).

5.1.3 MMP- 3

Matrix metalloproteinase-3 (MMP-3) degrades the ECM and may lead to the development of dilatative pathology of the ascending thoracic aorta (Lesauskaite et al, 2008). MMP-3 gene inactivation in mice demonstrated MMP-3 possibly causes degradation of matrix components, and promotes aneurysm formation by degradation of the elastica lamina (Silence et al, 2001).

5.1.4 MMP-12 (54-kd macrophage metalloelastase)

MMP-12 is involved in AA pathogenesis and shows a high affinity for elastin. In its active form the 22-kd enzyme degrades elastin (Longo et al, 2005). AA development in apolipoprotein E-knockout mice reported MMP-12 predominance in elastolytic activity. Deficiency of MMP-12 in the mice conferred protection against medial destruction and ectasia (Luttun et al, 2004).

5.1.5 Collagenases

Increasing collagenolytic activity has been identified in AAs, however collagen proteolysis is mostly associated with the terminal event of AA rupture. This is confirmed by greater levels of activity measured in specimens of ruptured aneurysms. (Busuttil et al, 1980).

5.1.6 MMP-1 (Collagenase-1)

MMP-1 localises within the mesenchymal cells (VSMCs, fibroblasts and endothelial cells) and is up-regulated by inflammatory mediators, however macrophage involvement has been described. Increased pro MMP-1, MMP-1 protein and mRNA levels have been reported in AAA compared to healthy aorta (Irizarry et al, 1993).

5.1.7 MMP-8 (Collagenase-2) (Matrilysin)

Studies report inconsistent expression of MMP-8 in AOD and AAA tissue, however, MMP-8 is stored as pre-formed protein in granules. Therefore MMP-8 mRNA may not accurately reflect protein concentration. Prominent expression of MMP-8 has been described in acute aortic dissection (Li et al, 2010).

5.1.8 MMP-13 (Collagenase-3)

MMP-13 is localised to VSMCs in close spatial proximity to collagen. Increased expression of MMP-13 in AAA compared to AOD tissue has been documented (Mao et al, 1999).

5.1.9 Inhibition of MMPs

Primary control of the activity of MMPs is achieved through tissue inhibitor of metalloproteinase (TIMP), by the formation of non-covalent complexes (Choke et al, 2005). TIMP-2, a broad-spectrum MMP inhibitor, and PAI-1, an inhibitor of tPA and uPA, are less expressed in AAA walls than in AOD, suggesting that ECM destruction is caused by a decrease in inhibitors and an increase in proteases (Allaire et al, 2009). Alpha-1-antitrypsin and Alpha-2-macroglobulin may suppress elastolysis, which is responsible for 90% of the inhibition of circulating MMPs, (Cohen et al, 1990). Treatment with atorvastatin decreases MMP expression and activity and leads to a reduction of TGF-beta signaling in the central region of human AAAs (Schweitzer et al, 2010). Ezetimibe combination therapy reduces aortic wall proteolysis and inflammation, key processes that drive AAA expansion (Dawson et al, 2011).

5.2 Proteolytic consideration in TAA

The hypothetical model of AAA cellular pathogenesis cannot completely explain the formation of dilatative pathology of the ascending thoracic aorta. The cellular expression of MMP-9 and their tissue inhibitors TIMP-1, TIMP-2, and TIMP-3 differ in the dilatative pathology of abdominal and thoracic aortas (Lesauskaite et al, 2006).

Overall a diminished expression of MMPs and tissue inhibitors relative to aged control AAAs in TAA, is documented. This may represent a loss of VSMCs in non-atherosclerotic TAA. Also, MT1-MMP plays a dynamic multifunctional role is TAA development (Jones et al, 2010). In Marfans syndrome MMP-2 and MMP-9 are found to be upregulated in TAA (Chung et al, 2007). Furthermore, animal studies show elevated MMP-9, MMP-2 and disintegrin and metalloproteinase domain-containing proteins 10 and 17 (ADAM-10 and -17) expressed in calcium chloride induced TAAs. Murine studies depleted of MMP-9 gene have demonstrated attenuated TAA formation (Ikonomidis et al, 2005).

6. Inflammatory changes in AA

AA is best described as a chronic inflammatory condition with an associated proteolytic imbalance. The most important pathological feature of human AA is probably the infiltration of inflammatory cells. The chronic infiltration consists mainly of macrophages, lymphocytes and plasma cells. It is suggested that these inflammatory cells and others play a regulatory role through release of a cascade of cytokines. This process results in the expression of cell adhesion molecules, increased protease expression, and the release of reactive oxygen species causing degradation of the ECM through the activation of MMPs and TIMP (Shah, 1997).

The recruitment of macrophages by chemotactic agents is possibly triggered by exposed elastin degradation products. Lymphocyte activation may be mediated by micro-organisms as well as by auto-antigens from structural degradation. TNF-alpha and INF-gamma appear to be the most consistently upregulated cytokines in patients with large AAAs. (Golledge et al, 2009). These inflammatory cytokines play multiple roles in regulating mesenchymal cell matrix metabolism, endothelial cell growth and proliferation, lymphocyte activation, antigen presenting cell (APC) function, major histocompatibility (MHC) class II molecule expression, vascular adhesion molecule expression, and even matrix degrading protease expression of surrounding cells (Wills et al, 1996).

Although AA and AOD are characterised by underlying inflammation, immunohistological studies have concluded that T- and B-cell predominance is localised to the outer media and adventitia in AA; compared to largely T–cell involvement localised to the intima and inner media in AOD. Furthermore, an autoimmune component to AA disease has been suggested after localisation of B lymphocytes in the media and considerable deposits of immunoglobulins (IgG) and complement in the wall of AA. (Lindholt & Shi, 2006).

6.1 Experimental and clinical studies

Key features of human AA include intense inflammation, increased expression of MMP-2 and MMP-9, and local ECM destruction. It became evident that inflammation plays an integral role in aneurysm pathogenesis following novel experimental animal models that demonstrated key features of human aneurysm following transmural chemical injury induced by calcium chloride treatment of vessel adventitia. Interestingly, aneurysm formation only developed after the inflammatory response was present, suggesting that inflammation occurring in response to chemical and mechanical injury is responsible for aneurysm development, rather than direct elastolysis. The calcium chloride murine model further indicates that CD4+ lymphocytes may be central in orchestrating production of MMP-2 and MMP-9 through interferon gamma (Xiong et al, 2004; Gertz et al, 1988). Anidjar and Dobrin recognized that exposure of the aorta caused destruction of elastic lamellae with up to a 4-fold increase in AA diameter at 6 days following elastase treatment. This increase was also associated with media infiltration of a large number of activated macrophages and T-cells (Anidjar et al, 1994). Characteristics of the elastase infusion model demonstrated that inflammatory cell infiltrate is accompanied by an increase in MMP-2 and MMP-9. Interestingly, the infiltration of macrophages and T-lymphocytes is not the prominent feature in the ruptured edges of AAAs and is even less prominent in non-ruptured areas or walls of the same AAAs. Rather, ruptured areas present significantly increased amounts of immature micro-vessels, with an excess of total and activated MMPs (Choke et al, 2006). Furthermore, prostaglandins (PG) and leukotrienes may also contribute to AAA in that the deficiency of 5-lipoxygenase attenuates aneurysm formation of atherosclerotic apolipoprotein E-deficient mice, suggesting a role for the 5-LO pathway in AAA formation (Shimizu et al, 2006).

6.2 Inflammatory cells involved in AA

6.2.1 Lymphocytes

It is suggested that Th1 and Th2-restricted T lymphocyte are the most commonly found infiltrates in AAA walls and are activated by antigen presenting cells such as macrophages, VSMCs, and endothelial cells. These inflammatory cells are integral for the regulation of the immune response in AAA. However, the specific regulatory traits of components of the inflammatory cascades and of proteases that cause aneurysmal growth remain largely unresolved. This reflects in earlier mouse studies which designated AAA disease as a T-helper (Th)-2-type inflammatory disease and identified T-helper(Th)-2-restricted CD3C T as the dominant influx. Later human studies suggested differently with AAA disease labeled as Th1-dominated or as a general pro-inflammatory condition (Abdul-Hussein et al, 2010). Local production of Th1 cytokines (Interferon-gamma (IFN-gamma), Interleukin-2 (IL-2), IL-12, IL-15 and IL-18 possibly enhances macrophage expression of MMPs, whereas Th2 cytokines (IL-4, 5, 8, and 10, Tumor necrosis factor-alpha (TNF-alpha), INF-gamma and CD40 ligand) appear to suppress macrophage MMP production and limit disease progression (Lindholt & Shi, 2006). In addition T-helper (Th)-2 cells secrete an FAS-ligand and FAP-1 resulting in apoptosis of VSMCs and Th1 cells (Shonbeck et al, 2002). Cytokines TNF-alpha and IL-8 cause inflammatory cell recruitment that is responsible for stimulating neoangiogenesis. INF-gamma stimulates cathepsin production for further Th2 activation, B-cell differentiation and Ig secretion.

In most cases, the default pathway will be a Th1-dominant for stenotic arterial lesions; however, when the local environment is skewed toward Th2 predominance, aneurysms will develop (Shimizu et al, 2006). More recently a study comparing inflammatory and proteolytic processes in AAA and popliteal artery aneurysm, characterized degenerative aneurysmal disease as a general inflammatory condition that is dominated by profound activation of the nuclear factor-kappa-B and activator protein-1 pathways. There is also hyperexpression of IL-6 and IL-8, and neutrophil involvement (Adul-Hussein et al, 2010).

6.2.2 Macrophages

Inflammation is characterised by macrophage migration from the onset of AA formation. Elastin degradation products are possibly responsible for the recruitment of macrophages by chemotactic agents. Heamodynamic forces may regulate macrophage adhesion, transmural migration and survival (Sho et al, 2004). A recent animal study confirmed that MT1-MMP acts directly to regulate macrophage secretion (Xiong et al, 2009). This antigen presenting cell is suggested to be a central role player in the immune response and subsequent ECM destruction. It is mostly localised in the adventitia of the AA wall. Through the secretion of cytokines (IL-1b, IL-6, IL-8, and TNF-alpha) and proteases (in particular MMP-9) these macrophages recruit inflammatory cells and stimulate cytokine production, protease production, B-cell differentiation, Ig secretion, cytotoxic T-cell differentiation and neovascularization. (Lindholt & Shi, 2006). In addition to producing cytokines and proteases, these cells also produce TIMP, confirming the governing role of macrophages in AA immune response. Animal studies confirmed the paramount role of macrophages in AA inflammatory response by demonstrating human-like aortic aneurysmal degradation without further manipulation following the application of macrophages and plasmin to the aorta (Werb et al, 2001).

6.2.3 Endothelial cells

Endothelial cells have been localised in AA and are found in approximation to neovascularisation. A prominent role for endothelial cells in the inflammatory response has been suggested following histological study reports of a positive association between the degree of inflammation and the degree of neovascularisation. It is suggested that these inflammatory cells play a role in ECM remodeling through the secretion of IL-1b and IL-8, which stimulate intercellular adhesion molecule-1 (ICAM-1) presentation, thus causing recruitment of additional inflammatory cells, attraction of lymphocytes, stimulation of endothelial proliferation, stimulation of B-cell differentiation and Ig secretion. In addition, like macrophages, the proliferating endothelium also produces various MMPs and TIMP (Lindholdt & Shi, 2006). To this end an experimental study has demonstrated that doxycycline not only inhibits MMP-8 and MMP-9 activity, but also the synthesis of MMPs in human endothelial cells (Hanemaaijer et al, 1998).

6.2.4 Fibroblasts

Although fibroblasts are commonly identified in the adventitia of AAA and have a recognized function in atherosclerosis, the role of the fibroblast in aneurysm pathogenesis is uncertain. Fibroblasts secrete cytokine IL-6 which is suggested to cause a stimulatory cascade of B-cell and cytotoxic T-cell differentiation and MMP stimulation (Thompson & Parks, 1996).

6.3 Infection and AA

An infectious cause of aneurysm formation has also been suggested. Between 30% and 50% of AAAs are associated with *Chlamydia* and *Herpes* virus infections. *Chlamydia* has been shown to induce AAA in rabbits and antichlamydial antibodies are commonly detected in AAA patients, however a causal relationship remains to be established. Studies have suggested that these infections play a role in elastolysis, possibly creating and augmenting an autoimmune response through particle mimicking. Lindholt et al. found that serum antibodies against C. Pneumonia have been associated with AAA expansion and cross-reaction with AAA structural proteins. Thus, immune responses mediated by microorganisms and autoantigens may play a pivotal role in AAA pathogenesis (Lindholt et al, 1999).

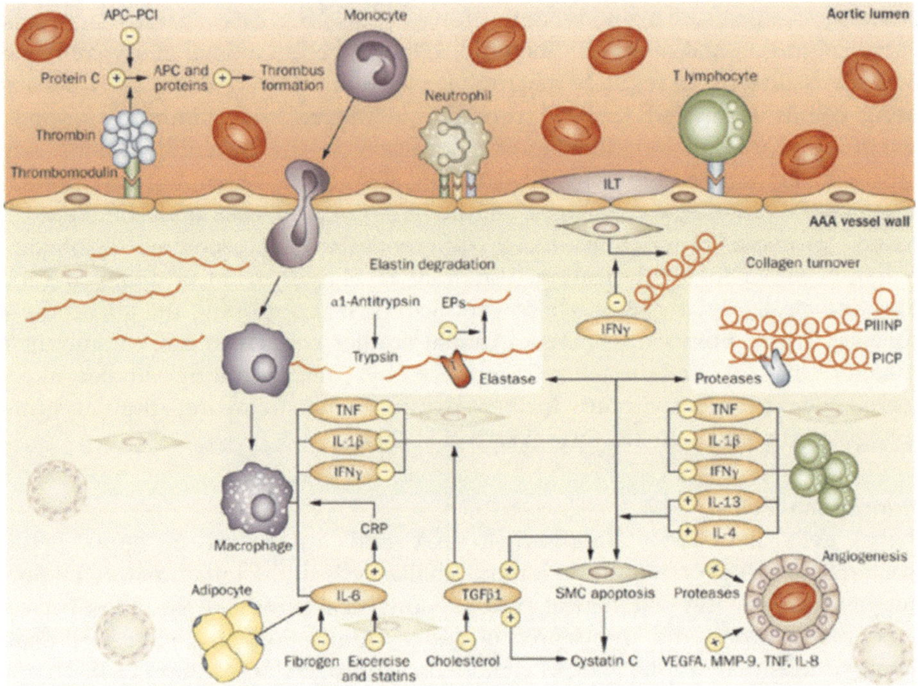

Fig. 1. Schematic diagram of the mechanisms implicated in abdominal aortic aneurysm, which primarily involve two main processes: inflammation and extracellular matrix turnover (Courtesy of Hellenthal et al, 2009).

6.4 Reactive oxygen species and AA

Reactive oxygen species such as superoxide (O2-) have also been shown to be raised in human AAAs. Elastase infusion in animal models has been shown to increase nitric oxide synthase expression and decrease the expression of the antioxidant, superoxide dismutase. O2- levels in human aneurysmal tissue are 2.5-fold higher than in adjacent nonaneurysmal aortic tissue and 10-fold higher than in control aorta (Miller et al, 2002).

6.5 Inflammation considerations in TAA

Developmental variation between TAA and AAA leads to differences in cellular responses to similar biological responses (El-Hamansy & Yacoub, 2009). Similar to AAA, histological studies demonstrate inflammatory cells in the adventitia and media of the aortic wall. In particular TAA infiltrate consistently shows CD3+, CD45+, CD68+ cells in the adventitia along with a prominent vasovasorum (possibly suggesting its role as conduit) and local endothelial activation (El-Hamansy & Yacoub 2009). Immunohistochemical staining showed that T- lymphocytes followed by macrophages were the predominant inflammatory cell in sporadic TAA (Guo et al, 2000). A Th1-type immune response is predominant in TAA as mRNA levels of INF-y are significantly increased compared to controls. Specific inflammatory pathways implicated in TAA formation remain unknown. However, transforming growth factor Beta (TGF-B), a cytokine, is recognized to be central in TAA pathogenesis causing ECM degeneration through the production of plasminogen activators and the release of MMP-2 and MMP-9. Reduced or mutated forms of fibrillin 1 release active

TGF-B, which in turn activates mitogen kinase activated pathways in VSMCs. Emilin 1, however, inhibits TGF-B signaling (El-Hamamsy & Yacoub 2009). 'Mycotic' aneurysms are found in less than 1% of patients with TAA. Salmonella, Staphylococcus and Mycobacterium species are mostly identified in blood cultures and tissue samples of subjects with AA disease (Koeppel et al, 2000). The role of oxidative stress is well described in AAA, however this remains to be established in TAA disease.

7. Implications for AA management

Current treatment of AA targets risk factors and the reduction of inflammation and proteolysis in AA walls. To this extent AA repair (open or endovascular) is currently practiced when aneurysms reach the recommended size for intervention or become symptomatic. The role of in vivo imaging techniques in vascular inflammation, such as Hybrid Positron Emmission Tomography / CT, that reflects the macrophage metabolic activity, may help to clarify the role of inflammation in AA pathogenesis and aid in the evaluation of treatment response. Currently, the potential role of pharmacotherapy in attenuation of AA growth is under investigation. Evidence suggests that smoking cessation may slow aneurysm growth and reduce the risk of rupture; therefore all AA patients should be counseled on the risks of smoking.

Antihypertensive medication has been investigated in the past, as hypertension is regarded as a potential significant risk factor for AA disease. A meta-analysis did suggest a significantly attenuated growth rate by β-blockers, however randomised control trials reported no benefit in the β-blocker (propanolol) group (Guessous et al, 2008) and a greater stroke and all-cause mortality with a short peri-operative course of β-blockers. Angiotensin converting enzyme (ACE) inhibitors have been demonstrated to cause AA attenuation in animal models, however no clinical trial has been conducted to confirm this. The exact mechanism by which ACE inhibitors restrict aneurysm growth is unknown; however its ability to bind zinc, an important cofactor for MMP activity, has been suggested. Nevertheless, a population based study suggested that patients taking ACE inhibitors were less likely to present with rupture (Hackman et al, 2006). TGF-β antagonists such as TGF-β–neutralizing antibody or the angiotensin II type 1 receptor (AT1) blocker, losartan, have demonstrated prevention of AA in a mouse model of Marfan Syndrome (Habashi et al, 2006) but no significant proven effect in human AAA. Distinguishing TAA from AAAs might explain the differential findings regarding the beneficial effects of angiotensin II type 1 receptor (AT1) blocker on various aortic aneurysmal pathologies. 3-Hydroxy-3-methylglutaryl coenzyme A reductase inhibitors (statins) restrict aneurysm growth through reduction of IL6 and MMPs (in particular MMP-9) in experimental models. However, a recent meta-analysis concluded that reduction in AAA expansion rate due to statins is not significant (Twine & Williams, 2010). Tetracyclines such as doxicycline, inhibit MMPs in animal models and have been shown to significantly reduce the growth of AAA. This has been confirmed clinically by a small scale, randomised, placebo controlled pilot study (Mosorin et al, 2001). Furthermore a macrolide antibiotic (Roxithromycin) used in a small randomised clinical trial reported a 44% reduction in AAA growth over 12 months, with the effect gradually tailing off up to 5 years (Vammen et al, 2001). Non-steroidal anti-inflammatory drug, Indomethacin prevents elastase induced AAA in animal models through CoX 2 inhibition, leading to reduction of MMP-9 and PGE2 (Miralles et al, 1999). More recently, the antioxidant properties of Vitamin E have been investigated in AAA models. It has been shown to block the induction of AAA in Angiotensin II-infused Apo-E knockout mice via reduction of macrophage infiltration and reduction of a chemotactic cytokine, suggesting that inhibition of oxidative stress in aneurysm tissue may play a significant role in AA pathobiology and be a possible treatment target (Gavrilla et al, 2005).

8. Conclusion

Interaction of multiple factors rather than a single process is responsible for the failure of the integrity of the aortic wall, which result in AA formation and progression. Despite several similarities in etiology and pathogenic mechanisms, it appears that TAA differs in many ways from AAA. Current areas of interest include proteolytic degradation of the arterial wall, inflammation and the immune response, biomechanical wall stress, and molecular genetics. Knowledge of the pathobiology of AA has lead to more targeted imaging methods and treatment trial design to investigate various pathobiological mechanisms of AA progression. Although some agents show promise, large controlled trials are needed to demonstrate clinically significant benefits. Future research should take into consideration knowledge gained of the differences between TAA and AAA pathobiology when designing clinical trials, in order to unravel the specificities of these different events in AA. As it stands surgical treatment of AA disease continues to be the most effective means of addressing the majority of factors involved in AA formation and progression.

9. References

Abdul-Hussien, H.; Hanemaaijer, R.; Kleemann, R.; Verhaaren, B.; Hajo van Bockel, J.; Lindeman, J. (2010). The pathophysiology of abdominal aortic aneurysm growth: Corresponding and discordant inflammatory and proteolytic processes in abdominal aortic and popliteal artery aneurysms. *Journal of Vascular Surgery*, Vol.51, No.6, (June 2010), pp. 1479-87, ISSN 1097-6809

Ailawadi, G.; Eliason, J.; Upchurch, G. (2003). Current concepts in the pathogenesis of abdominal aortic aneurysm. *Journal of Vascular Surgery*, Vol.38, No.3, (September 2003), pp. 584-8, ISSN 1097-6809

Albornoz, G.; Coady, MA.; Roberts, M.; Davies, R.; Tranquilli, M.; Rizzo, J.; Elefteriades, J. (2006). Familial thoracic aortic aneurysms and dissections: incidence, modes of inheritance, and phenotypic patterns. *Annals of Thoracic Surgery*, Vol.82, No.4, (October 2006), pp. 1400 –1405, doi:10.1016/j.athoracsur.2006.04.098

Alexander J. (2004). The pathobiology of aortic aneurysms. *Journal of Surgical Research*, Vol. 117, No. 1, (March 2004), pp. 163-175. doi:10.1016/j.jss.2003.11.011.

Allaire, E.; Muscatelli-Groux, B.; Mandet, C.; Guinault, A.; Bruneval, P.; Desgranges, P.; Clowes, A.; Méllière, D.; Becquemin, J. (2002). Paracrine effect of vascular smooth muscle cells in the prevention of aortic aneurysm formation. *Journal of Vascular Surgery*, Vol.36, No.5 (November 2002), pp. 1018-26, doi:10.1067/mva.2002.12734

Allaire, E.; Schneider, F.; Saucy, F.; Dai, J.; Cochennec, F.; Michineau, S.; Zidi, M.; Becquemin, J.; Kirsch, M.; Gervais, M. (2009). New insight in aetiopathogenesis of aortic diseases. *European Journal of Vascular and Endovascular Surgery*, Vol.37, No.5 (May 2009), pp. 531-7, doi:10.1016/j.ejvs.2009.02.002

Anidjar, S.; Dobrin, P.; Chejfec, G.; Michel, J. (1994). Experimental study of determinants of aneurismal expansion of the abdominal aorta. *Annals of Vascular Surgery,* Vol.8, No.2, (March 1994), pp. 127-36, ISSN 0195-6108

Busuttil, R.; Abou-Zamzam, A.; Machleder, H. (1980). Collagenase activity of the human aorta. A comparison of patients with and without abdominal aortic aneurysms. *Archives of Surgery,* Vol.115, No.11, (November 1980), pp. 1373-8, ISSN 0004-0010

Caglayan, A.; Dundar, M. (2009). Inherited diseases and syndromes leading to aortic aneurysms and dissections. *European Journal of Cardiothoracic Surgery,* Vol.35, No.6, (June 2009), pp. 931-940 ISSN 0305-1048

Campa, J.; Greenhalgh, R.; Powell, J. (1987). Elastin degradation in abdominal aortic aneurysms. *Atherosclerosis,* Vol.65, No.1-2, (May 1987), pp.13-21, ISSN: 0021- 9150

Carmo, M.; Colombo, L.; Bruno, A.; Corsi, F.; Roncoroni, L.; Cuttin, M.; Radice, F.; Mussini, E.; Settembrini, P. (2002). Alteration of elastin, collagen and their cross-links in abdominal aortic aneurysms. *European Journal of Vascular and Endovascular Surgery,* Vol.23, No.6, (June 2002), pp. 543-549

Choke, E.; Cockerill, G.; Wilson, W.; Sayed, S.; Dawson, J.; Loftus, I.; Thompson, M. (2005). A review of biological factors implicated in abdominal aortic aneurysm rupture. *European Journal of Vascular and Endovascular Surgery,* Vol.30, No.3, (September 2005) pp. 227-44, ISSN 1078-5884

Choke, E.; Cockerill, G.; Dawson, J.; Wilson, R.; Jones, A.; Loftus, I.; Thompson, M. (2006). Increased angiogenesis at the site of abdominal aortic aneurysm rupture. *Annals of New York Academic Science,* Vol.1085, (November 2006), pp. 315-9, DOI 10.1196/annals.1383.007

Chung, A.; Au Yeung, K.; Sandor, G.; Judge, D.; Dietz, H.; van Breemen, C. (2007). Loss of elastic fiber integrity and reduction of vascular smooth muscle contraction resulting from the upregulated activities of matrix metalloproteinase-2 and -9 in the thoracic aortic aneurysm in Marfan syndrome. *Circulation Research.* Vol.101, No.5, (August 2007), pp. 512-22, ISSN 1524-4571

Clarke, M.; Littlewood, T.; Figg, N.; Maguire, J.; Davenport, A.; Goddard, M.; Bennett, M. (2008). Chronic apoptosis of vascular smooth muscle cells accelerates atherosclerosis and promotes calcification and medial degeneration. *Circulation Research.* Vol.102, No.12, (June 2008), pp. 1529-38, ISSN: 1524-4571

Coady, M.; Rizzo, J.; Hammond, G. (1997). What is the appropriate size criterion for resection of thoracic aortic aneurysms? *Journal of Thoracic and Cardiovascular Surgery,* Vol.113, No.3, (March 1997), pp. 476-91, ISSN 0022-5223

Cohen, J.; Mandell, C.; Chang, J.; Wise, L. (1988). Elastin metabolism of the infrarenal aorta. *Journal of Vascular Surgery,* Vol. 7, No. 2, (February 1988), pp. 210-214

Cohen, J.; Sarfati, I.; Ratner, L.; Tilson, D. (1990). Alpha 1-antitrypsin phenotypes in patients With abdominal aortic aneurysms. *Journal of Surgical Research,* Vol. 49, No. 4, (October 1990), pp. 319-21, ISSN 0022-4804

Crawford, E.; Svensson, L.; Coselli, J.; Safi, H.; Hess, K. (1989). Surgical treatment of aneurysm and/or dissection of the ascending aorta, transverse aortic arch, and ascending aorta and transverse aortic arch. Factors influencing survival in 717 patients . *Journal of Thoracic and Cardiovascular Surgery,* Vol.98, No.5 pt 1, (November 1989), pp.659-73, ISSN 0022-5223

Dawson, J.; Choke, E.; Loftus, I.; Cockerill, G.; Thompson, M. (2011). A randomised placebo-controlled double-blind trial to evaluate lipid-lowering pharmacotherapy on proteolysis and inflammation in abdominal aortic aneurysms. *European Journal of Vascular and Endovascular Surgery*, Vol.41, No.1, (January 2011), pp. 28-35, doi:10.1016/j.ejvs.2010.08.023

Diehm, N.; Dick, F.; Schaffner, T.; Schmidli, J.; Kalka, C.; Di Santo, S.; Voelzmann, J.; Baumgartner, I. (2007). Novel Insight Into the Pathobiology of Abdominal Aortic Aneurysm and Potential Future Treatment Concepts. *Progress in Cardiovascular Diseases*, Vol.50, No.3, (November 2007), pp. 209-217,doi:10.1016/j.pcad.2007.05.001

Dobrin, P. (1978). Physiological Properties of Arteries. *Physiological Reviews*, Vol.58, No.2, (April 1978), pp. 397-460

Dobrin, P. (1988). Mechanics of normal and diseased blood vessels. *Annals of Vascular Surgery*, Vol.2, No.3, (July 1988), pp. 283-94.

Dobrin, P.; Mrkvicka R. (1994). Failure of elastin or collagen as possible critical connective Tissue alterations underlying aneurysmal dilatation. *Cardiovascular Surgery*, Vol.2, No.4, (August 1994), pp.484–488

Dobrin, P. (1999). Distribution of lamellar deformations: implications for properties of the arterial media. *Hypertension*, Vol.33, No.3, (March 1999), pp. 806-810

Economou, S.; Taylor, C.; Beattie, E.; Davis, C. Persistent experimental aortic aneurysms in dogs. *Surgery*, Vol.47, (January 1960), pp. 21-8

El-Hamamsy, I.; Yacoub, M. (2009). Cellular and molecular mechanisms of thoracic aortic aneurysms. *Nature Review Cardiology*, Vol.6, No.12, (December 2009), pp. 771-86, ISSN 1759-5002

Gavrila, D.; Li, W.; McCormick, M.; Thomas, M.; Daugherty, A.; Cassis, L.; Miller, F.; Oberley, L.; Dellsperger, K.; Weintraub, N. (2005). Vitamin E inhibits abdominal aortic aneurysm formation in angiotensin II-infused apolipoprotein E-deficient mice. *Arteriosclerosis Thrombosis Vascular Biology*, Vol.25, No.8, (August 2005), pp. 1671-7, ISSN 1524-4636

Gertz, S.; Kurgan, A.; Eisenberg, D. (1988). Aneurysm of the rabbit common carotid artery induced by periarterial application of calcium chloride in vivo. *Journal of Clinical Investigation*, Vol.81, No.3, (March 1988), pp. 649-56, doi: 10.1172/JCI113368

Golledge, A.; Walker, P.; Norman, P.; Golledge, J. (2009). A systematic review of studies examining inflammation associated cytokines in human abdominal aortic aneurysm samples. *Disease Markers*, Vol.26, No.4, (September 2009), pp. 181-8. Review. ISSN 0278-0240.

Goodall, S.; Porter, K.; Bell, P.; Thompson, M. (2002) Enhanced invasive properties exhibited by smooth muscle cells are associated with elevated production of MMP-2 in patients with aortic aneurysms. *European Journal of Vascular and Endovascular Surgery*, Vol.24, No.1, (July 2002), pp. 72-80

Guessous, I.; Periard, D.; Lorenzetti, D.; Cornuz, J.; Ghali, W. The efficacy of pharmacotherapy for decreasing the expansion rate of abdominal aortic aneurysms: a systematic review and meta-analysis. *PLoS One*, Vol.26, No.3, (March 2008), e1895.

Guo, D.; Papke, C.; He, R.; Milewicz, D. (2006). Pathogenesis of thoracic and abdominal aortic aneurysms. *Annals of the New York Academy of Science*, Vol.1085, (November 2006), pp. 339-52. Review

Habashi, J.; Judge, D.; Holm, T.; Cohn, R.; Loeys, B.; Cooper, T.; Myers, L.; Klein, E.; Liu, G.; Calvi, C.; Podowski, M.; Neptune, E.; Halushka, M.; Bedja, D.; Gabrielson, K.; Rifkin, D.; Carta, L.; Ramirez, F.; Huso, D.; Dietz, H. (2005). Losartan, an AT1 antagonist, prevents aortic aneurysm in a mouse model of Marfan syndrome. *Science,* Vol.7, No.312, (April 2006), pp.117-21, ISSN 0036-8075

Hackman, D.; Thiruchelvam, D.; Redelmeier, D. (2006). Angiotensin-converting enzyme inhibitors and aortic rupture: a population-based case-control study. *Lancet,* Vol.368, No.9536, (August 2006), pp. 659–65

Halloran, B.; Baxter, B. (1995) Pathogenesis of aneurysms. *Seminars in Vascular Surgery,* Vol.8, No.2, (June 1995), pp. 85–92

Hanemaaijer, R.; Visser, H.; Koolwijk, P.; Sorsa, T.; Salo, T.; Golub, L.; van Hinsbergh, V. Inhibition of MMP synthesis by doxycycline and chemically modified tetracyclines (CMTs) in human endothelial cells. *Advances in Dental Research,* Vol.12, No.2, (November 1998), pp. 114-8, doi 10.1177/08959374980120010301.

Hasham, S.; Guo, D.; Milewicz, D. (2002). Genetic basis of thoracic aortic aneurysms and dissections. *Current Opinion in Cardiology,* Vol.17, No. 6, (November 2002), pp.677–683, ISSN 0268-4705

Hellenthal, F.; Buurman, W.; Wodzig, W.; Schurink, G. (2009). Biomarkers of abdominal Aortic aneurysm progression. Part 2: inflammation. *Nature Review Cardiology,* Vol.6, No.8, (August 2009), pp. 543-52, doi:10.1038/nrcardio.2009.102

Huntington, K.; Hunter, A.; Chan, K. (1997). A prospective study to assess the frequency of Familial clustering of congenital bicuspid aortic valve. *Journal of The American College of Cardiology,* Vol.30, No.7, (December 1997), pp. 1809-12

Ikonomidis, J.; Barbour, J.; Amani, Z.; Stroud, R.; Herron, A.; McClister, D.; Camens, S.; Lindsey, M.; Mukherjee, R.; Spinale, F. (2005). Effects of deletion of the matrix metalloproteinase 9 gene on development of murine thoracic aortic aneurysms. *Circulation,* Vol.112, No.9, (August 2005), pp. I242-8, doi: 10.1161/CIRCULATIONAHA.104.526152.

Immenschuh, S.; Ramadori, G. (2000). Gene regulation of heme oxygenase-1 as a therapeutic target. *Biochemical Pharmacology,* Vol.60, No.8, (October 2000), pp.1121–1128, doi:10.1016/S0006-2952(00)00443-3

Inzoli, F.; Boschetti, F.; Zappa, M.; Longo, T.; Fumero, R. (1993). Biomechanical factors in abdominal aortic aneurysm rupture. *European Journal of Vascular Surgery,* Vol.7, No.6, (November 1993), pp.667–674, ISSN 0950-821X

Irizarry, E.; Newman, K.; Gandhi, R.; Nackman, G.; Halpern, V.; Wishner, S.; Scholes, J.; Tilson, M. (1993). Demonstration of interstitial collagenase in abdominal aortic aneurysm disease. *Journal of Surgical Research,* Vol.54, No.6, (June 1993), pp. 571-4, doi 10.1006/jsre.1993.1087

Jones, J.; Zavadzkas, J.; Chang, E.; Sheats, N.; Koval, C.; Stroud, R.; Spinale, F.; Ikonomidis, J. (2010). Cellular phenotype transformation occurs during thoracic aortic aneurysm development. *Journal of Thoracic Cardiovascular Surgery,* Vol.140, No.3, (September 2010), pp. 653-9, doi 10.1016/j.jtcvs.2009.12.033

Kakko, S.; Raisanen, T.; Tamminen, M. (2003). Candidate locus analysis of familial ascending aortic aneurysms and dissections confirms the linkage to the chromosome 5q13-14 in Finnish families. *Journal of Thoracic and Cardiovascular Surgery,* Vol.126, No. 1, (July 2003), pp. 106-13, doi 10.1016/S0022-5223(03)00037-0

Kirsch, M.; Radu, C.; Allaire, E.; Loisance, D. (2006) Pathobiology of Idiopathic Ascending Aortic Aneurysms. *Asian Cardiovascular Thoracic Annals,* vol.14 no.3, (June 2006), pp. 254-260

Koeppel, T.; Gahlen, J.; Diehl, S.; Prosst, R.; Dueber, C. (2004). Mycotic aneurysm of the abdominal aorta with retroperitoneal abscess: successful endovascular repair. *Journal of Vascular Surgery*, Vol.40, No.1, (July 2004), pp. 164-6, doi:10.1016/j.jvs.2004.02.046.

Ku, D.; Giddens, D.; Zarins, C.; Glagov, S. (1985). Pulsatile flow and atherosclerosis in the human carotid bifurcation: positive correlation between plaque location and low oscillating shear stress. *Arteriosclerosis,* Vol.5, No.3, (June 1985), pp. 293–302, ISSN: 1079-5642

Kuivaniemi, H.; Tromp, G.; Prockop, D. (1991). Genetic causes of aortic aneurysms. Unlearning at least part of what the textbooks say. *Journal of Clinical Investigation,* Vol.88, No.5, (November 1991), pp. 1441-1444, ISSN 0268-4705

Kuivaniemi, H.; Platsoucas, C.; Tilson; M. (2008). Aortic Aneurysms: An Immune Disease with a Strong Genetic Component. *Circulation*, Vol.117, No.2, (Jan 2008), pp. 242-252, ISSN 1524-4539

Lawrie, G.; Earle, N.; DeBakey, M.(1993). Long-term fate of the aortic root and aortic valve after ascending aneurysm surgery. *Annals of Surgery,* Vol.217, No.6 , (June 1993), pp.711-20. ISSN 0003-4932

Lesauskaite, V.; Ivanoviene, I.; Valanciute, A. (2003). Programmed cellular death and atherogenesis: from molecular mechanisms to clinical aspects. *Medicina*, Vol.39, No.6, (January 2003), pp. 529-34

Lesauskaite, V.; Epistolato, M.; Castagnini, M.; Urbonavicius, S.; Tanganelli P. (2006). Expression of matrix metalloproteinases, their tissue inhibitors, and osteopontin in the wall of thoracic and abdominal aortas with dilatative pathology. *Human Pathololy*, Vol.37, No.8, (August 2006), pp. 1076-84, doi:10.1016/j.humpath.2006.03.017

Lesauskaite, V.; Sinkūnaite, G.; Benetis, R.; Grabauskas, V.; Vaskelyte, J.; Smalinskiene, A.; Simonyte, S.; Jariene, G.; Tatarūnas, V.; Klumbiene, J.; Petkeviciene, J.; Kinduris, S.; Giedraitis, S.; Sakalauskas, J.; Bolys, R.; Sirvinskas, E.; Lenkutis, T.; Pangonyte, D. (2008). Matrix metalloproteinase-3 gene polymorphism and dilatative pathology of ascending thoracic aorta. *Medicina* (Kaunas), Vol.44, No.5, (February 2008), pp. 386-91

Li, Z.; Sadat, U.; U-King-Im, J.; Tang, T.; Bowden, D.; Hayes, P, Gillard, J. (2010). Association between aneurysm shoulder stress and abdominal aortic aneurysm expansion: A Longitudinal Follow-Up Study. *Circulation,* Vol.122, No.18, (November 2010), pp. 1815-1822, doi 10.1161/CIRCULATIONAHA.110.93981

Li, Y.; Shao, A.; Jiang, H.; Dong, G.; Xu, B.; Yi, J.; Jing, H. (2010). The prominent expression of plasma matrix metalloproteinase-8 in acute thoracic aortic dissection. *Journal of Surgical Research,* Vol.163, No.2, (October 2010), e99-104, Epub 2010, doi 10.1016/j.jss.2010.05.030

Lindholt, J.; Fasting, H.; Henneberg, E.; Ostergaard, L. (1999). A review of Chlamydia pneumoniae and atherosclerosis. *European Journal of Vascular and Endovascular Surgery*, Vol.17, No.4, (April 1999), pp. 283-9, Review, doi 10.1053/ejvs.1998.0757

Lindholt, J.; Shi, G. Chronic inflammation, immune response, and infection in abdominal aortic aneurysms. *European Journal of Vascular and Endovascular Surgery*, Vol.31, No.5, (May 2006), pp. 453-63, Review, doi 10.1016/j.ejvs.2005.10.030

Loeys, B.; Chen, J.; Neptune, E.; Judge, D.; Podowski, M.; Holm, T.; Meyers, J.; Leitch, C.; Katsanis, N.; Sharifi, N.; Xu, F.; Myers, L.; Spevak, P.; Cameron, D.; De Backer, J.; Hellemans, J.; Chen, Y.; Davis, E.; Webb, C.; Kress, W.; Coucke, P.; Rifkin, D.; De Paepe A.; Dietz H. (2005). A syndrome of altered cardiovascular, craniofacial, neurocognitive and skeletal development caused by mutations in TGFBR1 or TGFBR2. *Nature Genetics*,Vol.37, No.3, (March 2005), pp. 275—81, doi:10.1038/ng1511

Longo, G.; Buda, S.; Fiotta, N.; Xiong, W.; Griener, T.; Shapiro, S.; Baxter, B. (2005). MMP-12 has a role in abdominal aortic aneurysms in mice. *Surgery*, Vol.137, No.4, (April 2005), pp. 457-62.

Luttun ,A.; Lutgens, E.; Manderveld, A.; Maris, K.; Collen, D.; Carmeliet, P.; Moons, L. (2004). Loss of matrix metalloproteinase-9 or matrix metalloproteinase-12 protects apolipoprotein E-deficient mice against atherosclerotic media destruction but differentially affects plaque growth. *Circulation*, Vol.109, No.11, (March 2004), pp. 1408-14, ISSN 1524-4539

Mao, D.; Lee, J.; VanVickle, S.; Thompson, R. (1999). Expression of collagenase-3 (MMP-13) in human abdominal aortic aneurysms and vascular smooth muscle cells in culture. *Biochemistry Biophysics Research Communications*, Vol.261, No.3, (August 1999), pp. 904-10., doi10.1006/bbrc.1999.1142

Menashi, S.; Campa, J.; Greenhalgh, R.; Powell, J. (1987). Collagen in abdominal aortic aneurysm: Typing, content, and degradation. *Journal of Vascular Surgery*, Vol.6, No.6, (December 1987), pp. 578-582

Michel, J.; Ventura, J.; Egido, J.; Sakalihasan, N.; Treska, V.; Lindholt, J.; Allaire, E.; Thorsteinsdottir, U.; Cockerill, G.; Swedenborg, J. For the FAD EU consortium. (2011) Novel aspects of the pathogenesis of Aneurysms of the Abdominal Aorta in humans. *Cardiovascular Research*, Vol. 90 No.1, (April 2011), pp. 18-27 ISSN 0008-636

Miller, F.; Sharp, W.; Fang, X.; Oberley, L.; Oberley, T.; Weintraub, N. (2002). Oxidative stress in human abdominal aortic aneurysms: a potential mediator of aneurysmal remodeling. *Arteriosclerosis Thrombosis Vascular Bioloiy*, Vol.22, No.1, (April 2002), pp. 560–565, ISSN 1524-4636

Miller, F. (2002). Aortic Aneurysms: It's All About the Stress. *Arteriosclerosis, Thrombosis and Vascular Biology*, Vol.22, No.12, (December 2002), pp. 1948-1949, DOI 10.1161/01.ATV.0000047947.37203.82

Miralles, M.; Wester, W.; Sicard, G.; Thompson, R.; Reilly, J. (1999) Indomethacin inhibits expansion of experimental aortic aneurysms via inhibition of the cox2 isoform of cyclooxygenase. *Journal of Vascular Surgery*, Vol.29, No.5, (May1999), pp.884-92

Mosorin, M.; Juvonen, J.; Biancari, F.; Satta, J.; Surcel, H.; Leinonen, M.; Saikku, P.; Juvonen, T. (2001). Use of doxycycline to decrease the growth rate of abdominal aortic aneurysms: a randomized, double-blind, placebo-controlled pilot study. *Journal of Vascular Surgery*, Vol.34, No,4, (October 2001), pp 606-10

Nordon, I.; Hinchliffe, R.; Loftus, I.; Thompson, M. (2011). Pathophysiology and epidemiology of abdominal aortic aneurysms. *Nature Reviews Cardiology*, Vol.8, No.2, (February 2011), pp. 92-102, ISSN 1759-5002

O'Callaghan, C.; Williams, B. (2000) Mechanical strain-induced extracellular matrix production by human vascular smooth muscle cells: role of TGF-ß1. *Hypertension*, Vol.36, No.3, (September 2000), pp. 319–324, ISSN 1524-4563

Okamoto, R.; Xu, H.; Kouchoukos, N.; Moon, M.; Sundt, T. (2003). The influence of Mechanical properties on wall stress and distensibility of the dilated ascending aorta. *Journal of Thoracic Cardiovascular Surgery*, Vol.126, No.3, (September 2003), pp. 842-50, ISSN 0022-5223

Oleszak, E.; Chang J.; Friedman, H.; Katsetos, C.; Platsoucas, C. (2004). Theiler's virus infection: a model for multiple sclerosis. *Clinical Microbiology Reviews*, Vol.17, No.1, (January 2004), pp.174 –207, ISSN 0079-645X

Pannu, H.; Fadulu, V.; Chang, J. (2005). Mutations in transforming growth factor-_ receptor type ii cause familial thoracic aortic aneurysms and dissections. *Circulation*, Vol.112, No.4, (July 2005), pp. 513–20, ISSN 0009-7322

Patel, M.; Melrose, J.; Ghosh, P.; Appleberg, M. (1996). Increased synthesis of matrix Metalloproteinases by aortic smooth muscle cells is implicated in the etiopathogenesis of abdominal aortic aneurysms. *Journal of Vascular Surgery*, Vol.24, No.1, (July 1996), pp. 82-92

Platsoucas, C.; Lu, S.; Nwaneshiudu, I.; Solomides, C.; Agelan, A.; Ntaoula, N.; Purev, E.; Li, L.; Kratsios, P.; Mylonas, E.; Jung, W.; Evans, K.; Roberts, S.; Lu, Y.; Layvi, R.; Lin, W.; Zhang, X.; Gaughan, J.; Monos, D.; Oleszak, E.; White, J. (2006). Abdominal aortic aneurysm is a specific antigen-driven T cell disease. *Annals of the New York Academy of Sciences*, Vol.1085, (November 2006), pp. 224 –235, ISSN 0077-8923

Prockop, D. (1990). Mutations that alter the primary structure of type I collagen. The perils of a system for generating large structures by the principle of nucleated growth. *The Journal of Biological Chemistry*, Vol.265, No.26, (September 1990), pp. 15349 -15352. ISSN: 0021-9258

Pyo, R.; Lee, J.; Shipley, J.; Curci, J.; Mao, D.; Ziporin, S.; Ennis, T.; Shapiro, S.; Senior, R.; Thompson R. (2000). Targeted gene disruption of matrix metalloproteinase-9 (gelatinase B) suppresses development of experimental abdominal aortic aneurysms. *Journal of Clinical Investigation*, Vol.105, No.11, (June 2000), pp. 1641-9, doi 10.1172/JC18931

Ramanath, V.; Oh, J.; Sundt, T.; Eagle, K. (2009). Acute aortic syndromes and thoracic aortic aneurysm. *Mayo Clinical Proceedings*, Vol.84, No.5, (May 2009), pp. 465-81, ISSN 0025-6196

Ramanath, V.; Oh, J.; Sundt, T.; Eagle, K. (2009). Acute aortic syndromes and thoracic aortic aneurysm. *Mayo Clinical Proceedings*, Vol.84, No.5, (May 2009), pp. 465-81, ISSN 0025-6196

Reeps, C.; Gee, M.; Maier, A.; Pelisek, J.; Gurdan, M.; Wall, W.; Mariss, J.; Eckstein, H.; Essler, M. (2009). Glucose metabolism in the vessel wall correlates with mechanical instability and inflammatory changes in a patient with a growing aneurysm of the abdominal aorta. *Circulation: Cardiovascular Imaging*, Vol. 2, No. 6, (November 2009) pp. 507-9. doi 10.1161/CIRCIMAGING.109.858712

Rizzo, R.; McCarthy, W.; Dixit, S.; Lilly, M.; Shively, V.; Flinn, W.; Yao, J. (1989). Collagen types and matrix protein content in human abdominal aortic aneurysms. *Journal of Vascular Surgery*, Vol.10, No.4, (October 1989), pp.365–373, ISSN 1018–1172

Rucker, R.; Tinker, D. (1977) Structure and metabolism of arterial elastin. *International Review of Experimental Pathology*, Vol.17, (January 1977), pp. 1-47.

Sakalihasan, N.; Limet, R.; Defawe, O. (2005). Abdominal aortic aneurysm. *The Lancet*, Vol.365, No.9470, (January 2005), pp. 1577-1589, doi:10.1016/S0140-6736(05)66459-8

Schönbeck, U.; Sukhova, G.; Gerdes, N.; Libby, P. T(H)2 predominant immune responses prevail in human abdominal aortic aneurysm. *American Journal of Pathology*, Vol.161, No.2, (August 2002), pp. 499-506, ISSN 0002-9440

Schweitzer, M.; Mitmaker, B.; Obrand, D.; Sheiner, N.; Abraham, C.; Dostanic, S.; Meilleur, M.; Sugahara, T.; Chalifour, L.; (2010). Atorvastatin modulates matrix metalloproteinase expression, activity, and signaling in abdominal aortic aneurysms. *Vascular and Endovascular Surgery*, Vol.44, No.2, (February 2010), pp116-22, doi:10.1177/1538574409348352

Shimizu, K.; Shichiri, M.; Libby, P.; Lee, R.; Mitchell, R. (2004). Th2-predominant inflammation and blockade of IFN-gamma signaling induce aneurysms in allografted aortas. *Journal of Clinical Investigation*, Vol.114, No.2, (July 2004), pp.300-8, doi 10.1172/JC1200419855

Shimizu, K.; Mitchell, R.; Libby, P. (2006). Inflammation and cellular immune responses in Abdominal aortic aneurysms. *Arteriosclerosis Thrombosis and Vascular Biology*, Vol.26, No.5, (May 2006), pp. 987-94. ISSN: 1524-4636

Shah, P. (1997). Inflammation, metalloproteinases, and increased proteolysis: an emerging pathophysiological paradigm in aortic aneurysm. *Circulation*,Vol.96, No.7, (October 1997), pp. 2115-7.

Sho, E.; Sho, M.; Hoshina. K.; Kimura, H.; Nakahashi, T.; Dalman, R. (2004). Hemodynamic Forces regulate mural macrophage infiltration in experimental aortic aneurysms. *Experimental Molecular Pathology*. Vol.76, No.6, (April 2004), pp. 108-16, doi10.1016/j.yexmp.2003.11.003

Silence, J.; Lupu, F.; Collen, D.; Lijnen, H. (2001). Persistence of atherosclerotic plaque but reduced aneurysm formation in mice with stromelysin-1 (MMP-3) gene inactivation. *Arteriosclerosis Thrombosis Vascular Biololoy*, Vol.21, No.9, (September 2001), pp. 1440-5, ISSN 1524-4636

Stromberg, D.; Wiederhielm, C. (1969). Viscoelastic description of a collagenous tissue in simple elongation. *Journal of Applied Physiology*, Vol.26, No.6, (June 1969), pp. 857-62

Takagi, H.; Manabe, H.; Kawai, N.; Goto, S.; Umemoto, T. (2009). Circulating matrix metalloproteinase-9 concentrations and abdominal aortic aneurysm presence: a meta-analysis. *Interacteractive Cardiovascular Thoracacic Surgery*, Vol.9, No.3, (September 2009), pp. 437-40, Review, doi 10.1510/icvts.2009.208835

Thompson, R.; Parks, W. (1996). Role of matrix metalloproteinases in abdominal aortic aneurysms. *Annals of the New York Academy of Sciences*, Vol.18, No.800, (November1996), pp. 157-74, Review, doi 10.1111/j.1749-6632.1996.tb33307.x

Twine, C.; Williams I. (2010) Systematic review and meta-analysis of the effects of statin therapy on abdominal aortic aneurysms. *British Journal of Surgery*, Vol.98, No.3, (March 2011), pp 346-53, doi 10.1002/bjs.7343

Vammen, S.; Lindholt, J.; Ostergaard, L.; Fasting, H.; Henneberg, E. (2001). Randomized double-blind controlled trial of roxithromycin for prevention of abdominal aortic aneurysm expansion. *British Journal of Surgery*, Vol.88, No.8, (August 2001), pp. 1066-72, ISSN 1365-2168

Vaughan, C.; Casey, M.; He, J. (2001). Identification of a chromosome 11q23.2-q24 locus for Familial aortic aneurysm disease, a genetically heterogeneous disorder. *Circulation*, Vol.103, No.20, (May 2001), pp. 2469 -2475, ISSN 0009-7322

Verloes, A.; Sakalihasan, N.; Koulischer, L.; Limet, R. (1995). Aneurysms of the abdominal aorta: familial and genetic aspects in three hundred thirteen pedigrees. *Journal of Vascular Surgery*, Vol.21, No.4, (April 1995), pp.646-655, ISSN 0741-5214

Wassef, M.; Baxter, T.; Chisholm, R.; Dalman, R.; Fillinger, M.; Heinecke, J.; Humphrey, J.; Kuivaniemi, H.; Parks, W.; Pearce, W.; Platsoucas, C.; Sukhova, G.; Thompson, R.; Tilson, D.; & Zarins, C. (2001). Pathogenesis of abdominal aortic aneurysms: A multidisciplinary research program supported by the National Heart, Lung, and

Blood Institute. *Journal of Vascular Surgery,* Vol.34, No 4, (October 2001), pp. 730-8. doi:10.1067/mva.2001.116966

Werb, Z.; Bainton, D.; Jones, P. (1980). Degradation of connective tissue matrices by macrophages. III. Morphological and biochemical studies on extracellular, pericellular, and intracellular events in matrix proteolysis by macrophages in culture. *Journal of Experimental Medicine,* Vol.152, No.6, (December 1980), pp. 1537-53. ISSN: 1540-9538

White, J.; Haas, K.; Phillips, S.; Comerota, A. (1993). Adventitial elastolysis is a primary event in aneurysm formation. *Journal of Vascular Surgery,* Vol.17, No. 2, (February 1993), pp. 371-80. doi:10.1067/mva.1993.43023

Wills, A.; Thompson, M.; Crowther, M.; Sayers, R.; Bell, P. (1996). Pathogenesis of abdominal aortic aneurysms-cellular and biochemical mechanisms. *European Journal of Vascular and Endovascular Surgery,* Vol.12, No.4, (November 1996), pp. 391-400, Review, ISSN 0741-5214

Wilson, W.; Anderton, M.; Choke, E.; Dawson, J.; Loftus, I.; Thompson, M. (2008). Elevated plasma MMP1 and MMP9 are associated with abdominal aortic aneurysm rupture. *European Journal of Vascular an Endovascular Surgery.* Vol.35, No.5, (May 2008), pp. 580-4, doi:10.1016/j.ejvs.2007.12.004

Wilton, E.; Bland, M.; Thompson, M.; Jahangiri, M. (2008). Matrix metalloproteinase expression in the ascending aorta and aortic valve. *Interactive Cardiovascular Thoracic Surgery,* Vol.7, No.1, (February 2008), pp. 37-4, doi:10.1510/icvts.2007.163311

Xiong, W.; Zhao, Y.; Prall, A.; Greiner, T.; Baxter, B. (2004). Key roles of CD4+ T cells and IFN-γ in the development of abdominal aortic aneurysms in a murine model. *Journal of Immunology,* Vol.172, No.4, (February 2004), pp. 2607–12. ISSN: 0022-1767

Xiong, W.; Knispel, R.; MacTaggart, J.; Greiner, T.; Weiss, S.; Baxter, B. (2009). Membrane-type 1 matrix metalloproteinase regulates macrophage-dependent elastolytic activity and aneurysm formation in vivo. *Journal of Biological Chemistry,* Vol. 284, No.3, (January 2009), pp. 1765-71, doi 10.1074/jbc.M806239200

Yamawaki-Ogata, A.; Hashizume, R.; Satake, M.; Kaneko, H.; Mizutani, S.; Moritan, T.; Ueda, Y.; Narita, Y. (2010). A doxycycline loaded, controlled-release, biodegradable fiber for the treatment of aortic aneurysms. *Biomaterials,* Vol.31, No.36, (December 2010), pp. 9554-64. ISSN:0142-9612

Zarins, C.; Giddens, D.; Bharadvaj, B.; Sottiurai, V.; Mabon, R.; Glagov, S. (1983). Carotid bifurcation atherosclerosis. Quantitative correlation of plaque localization with flow velocity profiles and wall shear stress. *Circulation Research.* Vol.53, No.4, (October 1983), pp. 502–514, ISSN 0009-7330

Zeng, Z.; Kallmes, D.; Durka, M.; Ding, Y.; Lewis, D.; Kadirvel, R.; Robertson, A. (2011). Hemodynamics and anatomy of elastase-induced rabbit aneurysm models: similarity to human cerebral aneurysms? *American Journal of Neuroradiology,* Vol.32, No.3, (March 2011), pp. 595-601, doi 10.3174/ajnr.A2324

2

Matrix Metalloproteinases in Aortic Aneurysm – Executors or Executioners?

Tomasz Grzela, Barbara Bikowska and Małgorzata Litwiniuk
The Medical University of Warsaw
Poland

1. Introduction

Despite numerous studies focusing on the aortic aneurysm pathogenesis, the mechanism of aneurysm formation, especially - initiation of this process, remains unclear. The research concerning both, structural and molecular studies, is based on two main data sources. The first source of information are patients with already formed aneurysm, and with well defined biochemical and morphological changes in aortic wall architecture. The other source of data are experimental studies based on laboratory animals with artificially induced aneurysms. This approach enables verification of various hypotheses concerning pathogenesis of aortic aneurysm. Regrettably, animal aneurysm models, although similar, are not exactly the same, as human pathology. Thus, since the link between both mentioned data sources is still lacking, the knowledge achieved to date, even being highly profound, is not sufficient to fully understand this disease. Besides well defined factors, predisposing to formation of aortic aneurysm (patient's age, cigarette smoking, arterial hypertension, atherosclerosis, as well as the Marfan's and the Ehlers-Danlos's syndrome-associated mutations), increasing popularity is currently being gained by the hypothesis concerning the pivotal role of proteolytic enzymes - matrix metalloproteinases (MMPs) in aortic wall destruction. The involvement of MMPs in extracellular matrix damage in aortic aneurysm is doubtless. However, it needs to be elucidated, what the sequence of events is and what the exact role of MMPs is in these events. MMPs could play a role of "executioners", that are produced and activated in the aortic wall as constituents of inflammatory reaction, in response to some yet poorly defined triggers. On the other hand, it is plausible, that aortic wall destruction, followed by inflammatory response to tissue degradation products, results from primary local overproduction and/or activation of proteases. It could be due to some mutations or polymorphisms of MMP genes, or some impairment in their controlling mechanisms. In that circumstance MMPs could rather be considered as "executors", with causative role in aortic aneurysm pathogenesis. Although the majority of studies suggest the first scenario as being more possible, there is some evidence, that could support the second alternative, too.

2. Chronic inflammation – where the chaos begins…

The histopathological assessment of aneurismal aortic wall specimens reveals widespread chronic inflammatory reaction. This reaction is associated with extensive destruction of elastic fibers in the tunica media layer, and infiltration of both, media and adventitia, by macrophages and lymphocytes, mainly the Th2 subset. Moreover, as has been found recently, outer media and adventitia of human aortic aneurysm samples contain numerous mast cells (Miyake & Morishita, 2009; Michel et al., 2011). In addition to the previously mentioned lymphocytes and macrophages, mast cells are currently recognized as a third considerable source of pro-inflammatory cytokines, including tumor necrosis factor (TNF), various chemokines, and interleukins. Furthermore, in cooperation with macrophages, mast cells produce and release large quantities of various proteases and, thus, they are also actively engaged in aortic wall destruction (Tsuruda et al., 2008). However, a trigger of inflammatory reaction still remains to be a missing component of this scenario.

2.1 Chronic proteolytic atherothrombosis – a new concept

Recently, it has been proposed, that the aneurysm pathogenesis could be explained, at least to some extent, by the model of chronic proteolytic atherothrombosis (Michel et al., 2011). This model is based on the observation that the development of aortic aneurysms is accompanied by the formation of chronic intraluminal thrombus inside the aneurysmal sac. It has been shown that the presence of intraluminal thrombus is associated with widespread degradation of elastic fibers, increased apoptosis and loss of vascular smooth muscle cells (VSMC) in tunica media, and with extensive inflammatory reaction in adventitia. It may suggest, that the thrombus rather, than the aortic wall, could be the primary source of various pro-inflammatory factors, including proteolytic enzymes (Michel et al., 2011). On the other hand, one can argue that formation of thrombus on the inner, luminal surface of the aortic wall could be secondary to already existing aortic wall inflammation, due to the damage of endothelium and tunica intima. Nevertheless, it is plausible, that independently of the sequence of events, the thrombus-aortic wall interface may be "the place, where the chaos begins"…

The pathophysiological role of intraluminal thrombus may be described by various activities of its components. The first activity could be a generation of free radicals and induction of oxidative stress reaction, mainly due to a degradation of red blood cells and release of the potent pro-oxidant mediator – iron-rich hemoglobin. The oxidative stress leads to the production of reactive oxygen and reactive nitrogen species, which are both components of a self-augmenting mechanism (Miyake & Morishita, 2009). Reactive oxygen and nitric oxide increase expression of pro-inflammatory cytokines, followed by further up-regulation of reactive oxygen species production, peroxidation of membrane phospholipids and generation of eicosanoids and pro-apoptotic ceramides. Finally, reactive oxygen species induce activation of nuclear factor kappa-B (NF-κB), that leads to additional increase in MMPs expression and initiates the apoptosis of VSMC in the aortic wall. In addition to erythrocytes, intraluminal thrombus consists of an approximately 12-fold higher number of neutrophils, as compared to circulating blood (Michel et al., 2011). These cells produce a large number of proteinases, including elastase, cathepsin, MMP-8 and -9. Moreover, strong proteolytic activity between the thrombus and the adjacent aneurysm wall is revealed by the plasmin. This activity, although originally aimed at the thrombus fibrin network, may also contribute to aortic wall destruction. It may occur mainly through degradation of fibronectin, thus resulting in mesenchymal cells detachment and apoptosis, as well as direct activation of pro-MMPs.

2.2 *Chlamydia pneumoniae* and MMPs in aortic aneurysm

According to "infection hypothesis", the chronic inflammatory reaction, which takes place in the aortic wall, may be initiated by some pathogens. However, studies focusing on the presumed importance of various *Chlamydia* species, *Helicobacter pylori, Borrelia burgdorferi, Cytomegalovirus, Herpes simplex virus,* and most recently, some comensal, or weak pathogenic bacteria from the oral cavity, including *Porphyromonas gingivalis* and *Streptococcus mutans,* have failed to reveal a direct relationship between the presence of pathogen and aneurysm formation. Nevertheless, there is still no consensus in the debate concerning the significance of intracellular bacteria *Chlamydia (Chlamydophila) pneumoniae* in that event. It has been shown that almost half of aortic aneurysm specimens contained this pathogen. Moreover, a high prevalence of *C. pneumoniae* seropositivity and the presence of *C. pneumoniae*-reactive T lymphocytes in aortic aneurysm-suffering individuals, seemed to further support this hypothesis. Strong evidence was also provided by the results of experimental studies indicating, that in animal models *C. pneumoniae* antigens stimulated an elastin degradation followed by dilatation of aorta (Petersen et al., 2002). It is plausible that *C. pneumoniae* infection may reveal such destructive influence on the aortic wall due to activation of inflammatory reaction, mainly by stimulation of tissue macrophages with *C. pneumoniae* heat shock protein 60. This stimulation could lead to the release of a variety of pro-inflammatory molecules, eicosanoids, cytokines and several MMPs. Thus, although the exact role of *C. pneumoniae* in pathogenesis of aortic aneurysm remains to be clarified, the results of several prospective clinical trials could provide some contribution to this matter. It has been proven, that antibiotics effective against *C. pneumoniae* - tetracyclines (doxycyclin) and macrolides (roxithromycin, but not azithromycin), may reduce the progression of small aortic aneurysm (Høgh et al., 2009, see also chapter 3.5.2.2). Based on mentioned observations one can expect a direct correlation between the presence of *C. pneumoniae* and tissue levels of MMPs in aneurismal aortic wall specimens. This hypothesis was tested by Petersen and coauthors (Petersen et al., 2002). Surprisingly, the authors found, that mean levels of MMP-2 and MMP-9 in *C. pneumoniae*-positive aortic wall specimens were lower, than in *C. pneumoniae*-negative samples. This astonishing result was explained by the authors as a consequence of possible irregular distribution of bacteria in the aortic wall. Since the *C. pneumoniae* detection and determination of MMPs activity were done using specimens from different locations, some of them could possibly display false negative results. It is noteworthy, that problems with detection of *C. pneumoniae* DNA in tissue specimens of *Chlamydia*-seropositive patients with abdominal aortic aneurysms have also been reported by other authors (Falkensammer et al., 2007). An additional cause behind such results in Petersen's study could be the relatively small patient groups (28 individuals, divided into 4 groups, 7 patients in each). Moreover, the results of gelatin zymography could be affected by components of the extraction buffer used for analysis of MMP activity, especially EDTA and potent proteinase inhibitor - phenyl methylsulphonylfluoride (PMSF). Finally, authors suggested that *C. pneumoniae* infection may result in activation of some other, different from MMP-2 or MMP-9, proteolytic enzymes, e.g. neutrophil- or mast cells-derived proteinases, like cathepsins G, or chymase. These enzymes can also reveal elastolytic activity, and therefore may directly contribute to the aortic wall destruction (Miyake & Morishita, 2009; Michel et al., 2011). Furthermore, it has been demonstrated, that mast cell-derived chymase could activate pro-enzyme forms of MMP-2 and -9 in aneurysm tissue. However, although these observations could confirm the association of *C. pneumoniae* with MMPs activation in pathogenesis of aortic aneurysm, this issue still requires further studies.

3. Matrix metalloproteinases – the dark side of the Force…

Matrix metalloproteinases (MMPs), also known as matrix metallopeptidases, or matrixins, belong to the large and still expanding family of zinc endoproteinases. The members of this evolutionarily ancient group were found in various organisms, from bacteria and plants, through hydra and worms, to humans. So far, at least 25 distinct MMPs have been identified in vertebrates. In humans a presence of 23 proteins, encoded for 24 distinct genes, has been confirmed. This discrepancy is due to the fact that human MMP-23 was found to be encoded by two identical genes located on chromosome 1. Together with the astacins, the adamalysins, and large bacterial proteinases - serralysins, MMPs constitute a huge superfamily of enzymes, called metzincins, which are characterized by the presence of the zinc-binding motif, with a conserved methionine nearby.

MMPs play a crucial role in extracellular matrix (ECM) turnover. They are able to cleave main ECM components, including collagens, elastin, fibronectin, gelatin and aggrecan, as well as a variety of non-ECM molecules - transforming growth factor (TGF)-β, pro-IL-1β, pro-IL-8, Fas ligand, and pro-TNF. Moreover, MMPs are responsible for the release of cryptic fragments and neo-epitopes from extracellular matrix and non-ECM macromolecules, which may reveal bioactivities different from those of the parent molecules. Furthermore, MMPs may liberate numerous growth factors (e.g. vascular endothelial growth factor - VEGF and TGF-β) and cytokines, which are embedded in extracellular matrix and require proteolytic release from binding proteins for their activation. Finally, MMPs may modify cells' attachment to the ECM by processing of syndecans, dystroglycan and other adhesion molecules (Endo et al., 2003; Yamada et al., 2001; Mott & Werb, 2004). These properties of MMPs make them key players in the majority of physiological conditions (e.g. pregnancy, embryogenesis, wound healing), but also in various pathologies, including cancer progression with metastases, liver fibrosis, periodontal disease, multiple sclerosis and vascular diseases, especially atherosclerosis and aortic aneurysm (Hadler-Olsen et al., 2011).

As mentioned previously, MMPs should not only be recognized as typical effector/"executioner" molecules, but also, at least in some circumstances, they may be considered as real causative factors/"executors". This status may be supported by results of studies concerning the genetic polymorphisms of MMP genes. The polymorphisms are natural differences in DNA sequence that occur in more than 1% of the entire population. The vast majority of them concern variability of single nucleotides and are known as single nucleotide polymorphisms (SNPs). The effect of particular SNP is determined by its position in a gene structure. Most SNPs are functionally neutral. However, some of them may lead to an amino acid substitution, thus influencing the structure and properties of encoded protein. Furthermore, some SNPs located in a promoter region may alter the level of gene transcription. There is the reason, for which functional SNPs may contribute to the individual susceptibility to common diseases, including aortic aneurysms. In this chapter authors will shortly review several polymorphisms of selected MMP genes, which have been suspected of being involved in aortic aneurysm development.

3.1 MMPs structure

The overall scheme of a protein structure is common among all MMPs, with more or less significant differences between particular groups (Fig. 1).

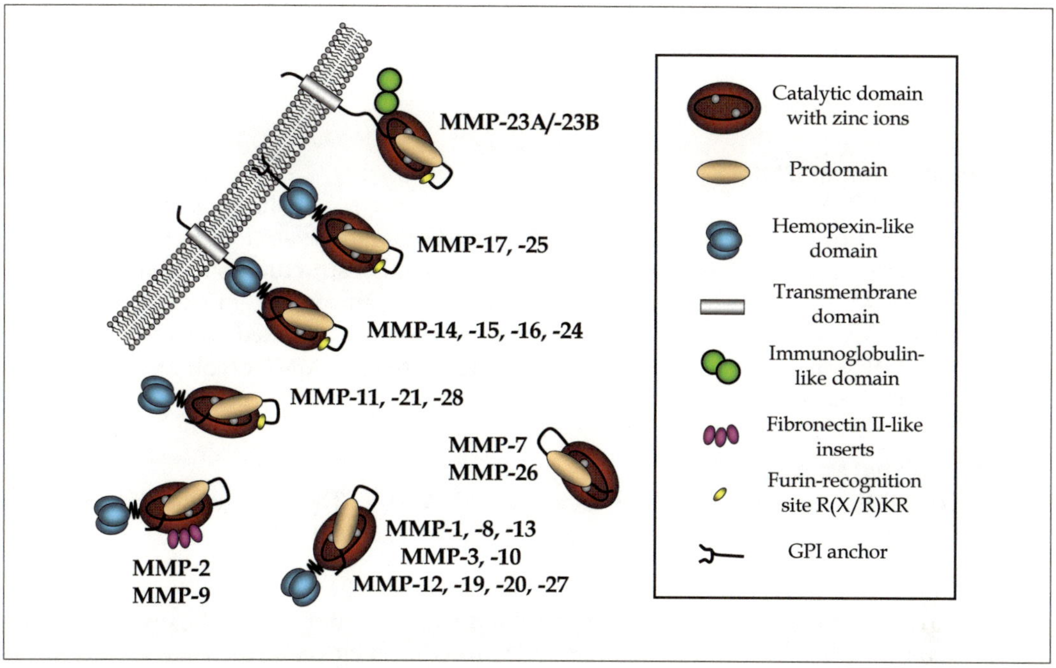

Fig. 1. The schematic structure of MMPs family

In general, on its N-terminus the MMP molecule contains a signal sequence, which directs the protein to the secretory pathway, and is removed during insertion of the protein into an endoplasmic reticulum. The signal sequence is followed by the propeptide composed of approximately 80 amino acid residues, that contains a characteristic conserved PRCGXPD motif, known as "cysteine-switch". The role of this sequence is to block a catalytic zinc and thus maintain the latent form of an enzyme. The next, the catalytic domain, has a sphere-like shape with an active site containing two atoms of zinc inside a large, shallow cleft. The catalytic domain is composed of approximately 160-170 amino acids, with a unique HEXXHXXGXXH sequence, that binds zinc ions. The last, approximately 200 amino acid residues-long C-terminal domain, called the hemopexin-like domain is found in all MMPs except for MMP-7, -23 and -26. In most MMPs the hemopexin-like domain is linked to a catalytic domain through a short, approximately 10-30 amino acid residues-containing hinge region. Exceptionally, the hinge region of MMP-9 is 64 amino acids-long, and is strongly O-glycosylated. Furthermore, six representatives of the membrane type (MT) MMPs subgroup hold either a type I transmembrane domain with a short intracellular segment (MT1, -2, -3 and -5-MMP) or a cell membrane-anchoring glycosylphosphatidylinositol (GPI) moiety (MT4- and -6-MMP).

Unlike other MMPs, in the MMP-23 molecule, a cystein-rich segment with an immunoglobulin-like domain is present, instead of the hemopexin-like domain on C-terminus, whereas the N-terminal signal peptide has been replaced by an N-terminal type II transmembrane domain. In addition to the previously mentioned common components, other elements, attached to the catalytic domain are fibronectin II-like inserts, which are found in MMP-2 and -9 molecules exclusively. Furthermore, three of the secreted MMPs (MMP-11, -21 and -28), as well as all the membrane-anchored MMPs, have a unique sequence R(X/R)KR between the prodomain and the catalytic domain. This motif is recognized and cleaved by a serine proteinase – furin, that results in removal of prodomain from the active site of the catalytic domain, followed by intracellular activation of mentioned MMPs (Fanjul-Fernandez et al., 2010).

3.2 Classification of MMPs

Traditionally, MMPs were classified into 6 main groups – collagenases, gellatinases, stromelysins, matrilysins, membrane type MMPs and others, unclassified to former groups. However, increasing knowledge, concerning the molecular structure, substrate specificity and mechanism of MMPs activation contributed to an arrangement of their new classification. According to this classification, MMPs are divided into four groups: archetypal MMPs, matrilysins, gelatinases and furin-activated MMPs (Fanjul-Fernandez et al., 2010, Hadler-Olsen et al., 2011)

3.2.1 Archetypal MMPs

Archetypal MMPs have the structure typical for all MMPs. They are further divided into three subgroups: collagenases, stromelysins and other archetypal MMPs.

3.2.1.1 Collagenases

This subgroup of archetypal MMPs is represented by three enzymes: collagenase-1 (MMP-1), collagenase-2 (MMP-8), and collagenase-3 (MMP-13). Their main common feature is the ability to cleave native collagens into characteristic N-terminal ¾ and C-terminal ¼ fragments (Fanjul-Fernandez et al., 2010). Since the triple helix conformation of native collagens is highly resistant to cleavage mediated by other proteinases, collagenases are crucial enzymes for initiation of collagen degradation. After the cleavage mediated by collagenases, the native collagens rapidly denature to gelatin and thus they become susceptible to degradation by other MMPs.

Besides the native fibrillar collagens (types I, II, III, V, and XI), the other targets for collagenases are numerous extracellular matrix components, as well as non-ECM molecules, including IL-8, pro-TNF, protease-activated receptor-1, several insulin-like growth factor-binding proteins (IGFBPs), etc... (Gearing et al., 1994; Boire et al., 2005; Amalinei et al., 2007).

The activation of MMP-1 requires a presence of active MMP-3 or plasminogen activator/plasmin system. The main sources of collagenases are stimulated fibroblasts (MMP-1), neutrophils (MMP-8) and VSMC (MMP-1 and MMP-13). Increased levels of mRNA and proteins for collagenases were found in aortic aneurysm tissue (Kadoglou & Liapis, 2004). Moreover, they are supposed to be involved in aneurysm rupture.

The studies focused on a presumable connection between aortic aneurysm formation and known SNPs in genes encoding for collagenases, including potentially clinically relevant SNP in MMP-1 promoter region (-1607 G/GG), did not reveal any significant correlation (Ogata et al., 2004; Sandford et al., 2007; Saratzis et al., 2011).

3.2.1.2 Stromelysins

The members of this group are stromelysin-1 (MMP-3) and stromelysin-2 (MMP-10). Both stromelysins have a structure analogous to that of collagenases, however, in contrast to those enzymes, stromelysins are not able to cleave native collagen. Their substrates include processed collagen types III, IV, V, IX and X, laminin, gelatin, fibronectin, proteoglycans and several other molecules, e.g. plasminogen, fibrinogen and IL-1β (Amalinei et al., 2007). Although both stromelysins display similar substrate specificity, MMP-3 reveals a grater proteolytic activity, as compared to MMP-10. Furthermore, MMP-3 is known to activate various pro-MMPs (collagenases and gelatinases) by removal of their pro-domain, and therefore it is crucial for their activation (Suzuki et al., 1990; Visse & Nagase, 2003). Stromelysins may be produced by fibroblasts and epithelial cells, however, in aortic aneurysm tissue their main source seem to be macrophages (Fanjul-Fernandez et al., 2010).

The possible clinical relevance of nucleotide polymorphism in promoter region of genes encoding for both, MMP-3 and MMP-10, has been studied by several authors (Sandford et al., 2007; Saratzis et al., 2011). It has been found, that in the MMP-3 promoter, at the position -1171, corresponding to the transcriptional start site, two variants - one of them, containing 5 adenosines (5A) and the other one with 6 adenosines (6A), may be present. *In vitro* tests have shown, that the 5A allele has nearly two fold higher activity, than the 6A variant. Presumably, this could be due to the higher affinity of the transcriptional repressor p50/p50 to 6A, than to the 5A allele. Epidemiological studies have shown, that the mentioned 5A/6A polymorphism of MMP-3 promoter may be associated with various cardiovascular diseases. It was revealed that 5A/5A homozygotic individuals are significantly more susceptible to hypertension, myocardial infarction and coronary artery aneurysms.

Interestingly, the 6A/6A variant carriers displayed a higher growth rate of atherosclerotic plaque, which, on the other hand, was more stable, than in patients with the 5A allele. Yoon and coauthors have observed a trend (p=0.06) for a higher 5A allele frequency in a small cohort of 47 Finnish patients with abdominal aortic aneurysm (Yoon et al., 1999). The higher 5A allele frequency among aortic aneurysm-suffering patients compared to a control group was also confirmed in a British population (Ye, 2006).

In contrast to MMP-3, studies concerning the presumable role of MMP-10 gene polymorphisms, including -180 A/G SNP, have failed to reveal any significant correlation with a prevalence of aortic aneurysm (Ogata et al., 2005).

3.2.1.3 Other archetypal MMPs

This subgroup of archetypal MMPs includes four enzymes: MMP-12, MMP-19, MMP-20 and MMP-27. The representative of this subgroup - MMP-12, also known as macrophage metalloelastase, is mainly expressed and secreted by activated macrophages and is necessary for its migration (Visse & Nagase, 2003; Kadoglou & Liapis, 2004). The main substrate for MMP-12 is elastin, but the enzyme may cleave some other ECM molecules, including aggrecan, fibronectin, laminin, and type IV collagen.

The increased expression of MMP-12 was found exclusively in aortic aneurysm wall, but not in the control, or atherosclerotic aorta specimens. Immunohistochemical studies have localized MMP-12 within the media of aortic aneurysms, predominantly in zones adjacent to non-dilated aorta. However, although MMP-12 is recognized as a key player in aneurysm formation, its prominent role has been neglected in the elastase-induced aneurysm animal model. Interestingly, it has been found that MMP-12-deficient mice revealed aortic dilatation similar to that of wild type animals, whereas mice lacking MMP-9 were resistant to aneurysm induction. Therefore, it was suggested that MMP-12 role is restricted rather to supporting other MMPs in aneurysm formation (Kadoglou & Liapis, 2004).

The analysis of polymorphic sites in the MMP-12 gene and *in vitro* studies suggested the possible connection between A to G substitution in -82 position of the promoter and the aortic aneurysm expansion. However, none of the clinical trials have confirmed the expected correlation to date (Sandford et al., 2007; Saratzis et al., 2011).

Group	Subgroup	MMP	Common name	Substrates	
				ECM	Non-ECM
Archetypal MMPs	Collagenases	MMP-1	Collagenase-1	Collagens (I, II, III, VII, VIII and X), gelatin, proteoglycan link protein, aggrecan, veriscan, tenacin, entactin	α1-PI, ILb-1, pro-TNF, IGFBP-3, MMP-2, MMP-9
		MMP-8	Collagenase-2	Collagens (I, II, III, V, VII, VIII and X), gelatin, aggrecan	α1-PI, α2-antiplasmin, fibronectin
		MMP-13	Collagenase-3	Collagens (I, II, III, IV, IX, X, XIV), gelatin, aggrecan, perlecan, large tenascin-C, fibronectin, osteonectin	MMP-9, plasminogen activator inhibitor-2
	Stromelysins	MMP-3	Stromelysin-1	Collagens (III, IV, V and IX), gelatin, aggrecan versican, hyaluronidase-treated versican, perle-can, decorin, proteoglycan link protein, large tenascin-C, fibronectin, laminin, entactin, osteonectin	α1-PI, antithrombin-III, ovosstatin, substance P, IL-1β, serum amyloid A, IGFBP-3, fibrinogen and cross- linked fibrin, plasminogen, MMP-2/TIMP-2 complex MMP-1,-7,-8,-9,-13
		MMP-10	Stromelysin-2	Collagens (III, IV and V), gelatin, casein, aggrecan, elastin, proteoglycan link protein	MMP-1,-8
	Other Archetypal	MMP-12	Metalloelastase	Collagen IV, gelatin, elastin, casein, laminin, proteoglycan monomer, fibronectin, vitronectin, enactin	α1-PI, fibrinogen, fibrin, fibrin, plasminogen, myelin basic protein
		MMP-19	RASI	Gelatin	ND
		MMP-20	Enamelysin	Amelogenin	ND
		MMP-27	-	ND	
Matrilysins		MMP-7	Matrilysin	Collagens IV and X, gelatin, aggrecan, decorin, proteoglycan link protein, fibronectin, laminin, insoluble fibronectin fibrils, entactin, large and small tenascin-C, osteonectin, β4 integrin, elastin, casein, transferrin	MMP-1,-2,-9 α1-PI, MMP-9/TIMP-1 complex, plasminogen
		MMP-26	Matrilysin-2	Collagen IV, gelatin, fibronectin	ProMMP-9, fibrinogen, α1-PI

ND-not determined

3.2.2 Matrilysins

Matrilysins are represented by matrilysin-1 (MMP-7) and matrilysin-2 (MMP-26, or endometase). The most prominent feature of matrilysins group members is the lack of the hemopexin domain. MMP-26 is the smallest known MMP; it is composed of only 261 amino acids and may activate itself by autocatalysis. Matrilysins play an important role in degradation of ECM molecules, including type IV collagen, laminin, entactin, as well as several cell surface molecules, e.g. Fas ligand, E-cadherin and syndecan-1 (Fanjul-Fernandez et al., 2010). Due to a shedding of membrane-bound Fas ligand and generation of its soluble form, matrilysins may stimulate apoptosis. Furthermore, while cleaving plasminogen to produce an angiostatin fragments, matrilysins are involved in inhibition of angiogenesis. Interestingly, MMP-26 has an ability to activate pro-MMP-9 in a specific site, that results in better stability of MMP-9 (Zhaoet al., 2003; Amalinei et al., 2007). Moreover, intracellular MMP-26 was found to process the estrogen receptor β, therefore in patients with breast cancer an increased MMP-26 level was found to correlate with longer survival (Hadler-Olsen et al., 2011)

3.2.3 Gelatinases

The group of gelatinases consists of two members: gelatinase A (MMP-2) and gelatinase B (MMP-9). Both of them are constitutively expressed by many cells, including fibroblasts, keratinocytes, endothelial cells, polymorphonuclear leukocytes, monocytes, alveolar macrophages and osteoclasts. When compared to other MMPs, the most significant difference in the structure of gelatinases is the presence of three type II fibronectin-like repeats within the catalytic domain. They are responsible for recognition and binding of denatured collagen and gelatin molecules (Visse & Nagase, 2003). Gelatinases may cleave various extracellular matrix molecules, e.g. collagen types I, IV, V, VII, IX, X, elastin, fibronectin, aggrecan, vitronectin, laminin, as well as numerous non-ECM molecules, including pro-TNF, TGF-β, pro-IL-1β and pro-IL-8 (Fanjul-Fernandez et al., 2010). Moreover, they are involved in generation of several pro- and anti-angiogenic factors, which may originate from both, ECM and non-ECM substrates (Mott & Werb, 2004).

Gelatinases are considered the most important members of the MMPs family, involved in pathogenesis of aortic aneurysm. The amounts of mRNA and specific proteins in the aneurysm wall, as well, as plasma levels of both, MMP-2 and MMP-9, were statistically significantly higher in patients with aortic aneurysms, as compared to healthy controls. Moreover, it has been found that plasma levels of gelatinases noticeably correlate with aneurysm expansion rate and therefore they were suggested as presumable predictors of the aneurysm rupture risk. In an animal experimental study it was proven, that infusion of gelatinases resulted in development of aortic aneurysms. Interestingly, MMP-2- and/or MMP-9-deficient mice were resistant to aneurysm formation in this model (Longo et al., 2002; Baxter, 2004; Kadoglou & Liapis, 2004).

Recently, it has been postulated, that, in addition to elastin degradation, gelatinases may also be engaged in the pathogenesis of aortic aneurysm in a proteolysis-independent fashion. This hypothesis is based on the observation, that both, MMP-2 and MMP-9, may display some inhibitory influence on the calcium-dependent contraction of VSMC isolated from the aortic wall (Raffetto & Khalil, 2008). In addition to maintenance of aortic wall integrity, the contraction of those cells is considered as a counterbalance of hemodynamic forces, that protects the aorta against dilatation during each cardiac cycle. Thus, the MMP-mediated reversible inhibition of vascular myocytes contraction could promote aneurysm progression. However, this issue requires further elucidation.

3.2.3.1 MMP-2 (Gelatinase A)

MMP-2, or gellatinase A, is constitutively expressed by vascular myocytes, however, it may be produced in small amounts by macrophages and fibroblasts, too. As described in chapter 3.4, the activation of MMP-2 occurs mainly by its interaction with MT1-MMP/TIMP-2. Due to its elastolytic activity, MMP-2 is believed to play a pivotal role in aortic aneurysm development. It was found, that VSMC isolated from aortic aneurysm tissue produced higher amounts of MMP-2, as compared to those from atherosclerotic, or normal aortic wall. Surprisingly, the activity of MMP-2 negatively correlated with aneurysms diameter. This observation could support the opinion, that MMP-2 may be essential in the early stages of aneurysm development. Besides weakness of the aortic wall, MMP-2-mediated degradation of elastic fibers may lead to production of elastin-derived peptides, which have a great chemotactic potential. These peptides may promote recruitment of inflammatory cells and enhance further proteolysis. Moreover, MMP-2 liberates TGF-β from an inactive extracellular complex consisting of TGF-β, latent TGF-β binding protein and TGF-β-latency associated protein, which may stimulate various MMPs expression and results in further progression of the disease (Rizas et al., 2009).

Among 18 polymorphisms found in the MMP-2 gene, the SNP located in a promoter (-1306 C/T) was initially considered as clinically relevant. The studies focusing on the influence of this particular SNP on promoter function have shown, that the presence of C allele was associated with a higher promoter activity (Price et al., 2001). However, none of clinical studies, addressed at verifying a possible correlation between -1306 C/T SNP and aortic aneurysm prevalence, has revealed such a connection (Eriksson et al., 2005; Ogata et al., 2005; Sandford et al., 2007; Saratzis et al., 2011).

3.2.3.2 MMP-9 (Gelatinase B)

MMP-9, or gellatinase B, is mainly produced by macrophages and neutrophils. Subsequently to proteolytic activation by a variety of factors, including plasminogen activators and other MMPs (MMP-2, -3, -12), MMP-9 displays elastolytic, collagenolytic and gelatinolytic activity. The leader position of MMP-9 in the pathogenesis of aortic aneurysm may be confirmed by several observations. Animal studies have shown, that MMP-9-deficient mice were resistant to experimentally induced aortic dilation and they did not reveal elastin degradation despite the presence of inflammatory cell in the aortic wall (Kadoglou & Liapis, 2004; Baxter, 2004). On the other hand, among all metalloproteinases, MMP-9 is the most abundantly expressed enzyme in aortic aneurysm wall, in contrast to normal aortic tissue, where it was not present. Also, huge amounts of MMP-9 are released by neutrophils trapped in the intraluminal thrombus (see also chapter 2.1). Furthermore, high MMP-9 concentrations were detected in ruptured aneurysms. However, although patients with an aortic aneurysm have significantly higher levels of MMP-9, than control individuals, there is no consensus regarding a direct correlation between MMP-9 plasma levels and aneurysm progression and rupture risk to date (Takagi et al., 2009; Eugster et al., 2005). Therefore, this issue still requires further elucidation.

Several polymorphisms have been found in the MMP-9 gene. Most of the studies have focused on -1562 C/T polymorphism in a promoter region. It has been proven that a common T to C substitution in -1562 position of the MMP-9 promoter is associated with approximately 50% increase of the promoter activity. A clinical study by Medley and coauthors has shown that mRNA level, protein concentration, as well as enzymatic activity of MMP-9 in aortic aneurysm tissues of -1562 T allele carriers were significantly higher, as compared to those with the -1562 C variant. Also, plasma levels of MMP-9 were much higher in -1562 T carriers, than in patients with -1562 C allele (Medley et al., 2004). Furthermore, Jones and coauthors have also reported a higher frequency of the -1562 T variant in a group of patients with aortic aneurysm (n=414), in comparison to individuals with atherosclerotic peripheral vascular disease (n=172, adjusted odds ratio 2.94), or healthy control subjects (n=203, adjusted odds ratio 2.41) (Jones et al., 2003).

Interestingly, subsequent studies, independently conducted by Ogata and Eriksson on large groups of aortic aneurysm-suffering individuals (n=387 and n=455, respectively) have failed to confirm this association (Ogata et al., 2005; Eriksson et al., 2005). In a large study by Smallwood and coauthors, carried out on 678 patients with aortic aneurysms and 659 healthy controls, no statistically significant association between occurrence of the -1562 T allele and development of aortic aneurysm was found (Sandford et al., 2007; Smallwood et al., 2008; Saratzis et al., 2011).

It is noteworthy, that although recent studies have negated the direct involvement of -1562 C/T polymorphism in pathogenesis of aortic aneurysm, the potential importance of other functional polymorphisms in the MMP-9 gene cannot be excluded. Presumably, two additional functional SNPs - the first located in the exon encoding for catalytic domain (Q279R), and the next relating to the sequence encoding for hemopexin domain (P574R), could be considered as attractive candidates for further studies.

3.2.4 Furin-activated MMPs

The members of this group are characterized by the presence of an unique RXKR or RRKR sequence, inserted between the prodomain and the catalytic domain. This site is recognized and cleaved by pro-protein convertases or serine proteinases - furins, thus resulting in an activation of enzyme. The furin-activated MMPs are further divided into small subgroups: secreted MMPs, membrane-type I and type II MMPs and GPI-anchored MMPs (Fu et al., 2008; Fanjul-Fernandez et al., 2010).

The furin-activated secreted MMPs include MMP-11, MMP-21 and MMP-28. In contrast to other secreted MMPs, members of this subgroup undergo intracellular processing by furin, or furin-like proteases and therefore they are secreted already in active form (Fanjul-Fernandez et al., 2010).

3.2.4.1 Membrane type MMPs

All the membrane type MMPs (MT-MMPs) contain a hydrophobic component that enables their insertion in the cell membrane. They control the close neighborhood of both, normal and pathological cells, thus being involved in promoting of cell migration, invasion, experimental metastasis and angiogenesis (Hernandez-Barrantes et al., 2002).

Type I transmembrane MMPs include: MT1-, MT2-, MT3-, and MT5-MMP (MMP-14, -15, -16, and -24, respectively). They are characterized by a long hydrophobic transmembrane sequence followed by a short cytoplasmic tail, which could participate in several signaling pathways. The main representative of this subgroup, MT1-MMP (MMP-14) may be expressed on the cell surface of various cells, however, activated macrophages and VSMC are considered as its most important producers. It may cleave native type I collagen into ¾ - ¼ fragments in a collagenase-specific fashion. Apart from collagen I, MT1-MMP is able to process various components of extracellular matrix, including collagens type II and III, gelatin, fibronectin, as well, as non-ECM molecules, e.g. hyaluronan receptor (CD44), myelin-inhibitory protein and α-2 macroglobulin (Fanjul-Fernandez et al., 2010). Furthermore, as previously mentioned, MT1-MMP plays a key role in the proteolytic activation of pro-MMP-2 (see chapter 3.4).

Group	Subgroup	MMP	Common name	Substrates	
				Extracellular matrix (ECM)	Non-ECM
Gelatinases		MMP-2	Gelatinase A	Collagens (I, IV, V, VII, X, XI and XIV), gelatin, elastin, fibronectin, laminin-1, laminin-5, galectin-3, aggrecan, decorin, hyaluronidase-treated versican, proteoglycan link protein, osteonectin	IL-1b, α1-PI, prolysyl oxidase fusion protein, MMP-1, MMP-9, MMP-13
		MMP-9	Gelatinase B	Collagens (IV, V, VII, X and XIV), gelatin, elastin, galectin-3, aggrecan, fibronectin, hyaluronidase-treated versican, proteoglycan link protein, entactin, osteonectin	α1-PI, IL-1β, plasminogen
Furin-activated MMPs	Secreted	MMP-11	Stromelysin-3	Casein, laminin, fibronectin, gelatin, collagen IV and carboxymethylated transferrin	α1-PI, casein, IGFBP-1
		MMP-21	XMMP	ND	
		MMP-28	Epilysin	ND	
	Type I transmembrane	MMP-14	MT1-MMP	Collagens (I, II and III), casein, elastin, fibronectin, gelatin, laminin, vitronectin, large tenascin-C, entactin, proteoglycans	α1-PI, MMP-2,-13
		MMP-15	MT2-MMP	Large tenascin-C, fibronectin, laminin, entactin, aggrecan, perlecan	MMP-2
		MMP-16	MT3-MMP	Collagen-III, gelatin, casein, fibronectin	MMP-2
		MMP-24	MT5-MMP	ND	
	GPI-anchored	MMP-17	MT4-MMP	ND	
		MMP-25	MT6-MMP	ND	
	Type II transmenbrane	MMP-23A	-	ND	
		MMP-23B	-	ND	

ND – not determined

Recently, it was found, that mRNA and protein levels of MT-MMP-1 were significantly higher among patients with an aortic aneurysm, than in healthy controls or atherosclerosis-suffering subjects. Therefore, it is suggested, that MT-MMP-1 may also be important in pathogenesis of aortic aneurysm, especially due to its multidirectional action. Besides direct destruction of extracellular matrix components, MT1-MMP activates MMP-2 and facilitates migration of macrophages, thus promoting inflammatory infiltration of the aortic wall (Kadoglou & Liapis, 2004).

Type II transmembrane MMPs are represented by enzymes: MMP-23A and MMP-23B, which, despite being encoded by two different genes, actually have an identical amino acid sequence. Their structure is significantly distinct from other MMPs, since they lack the signal peptide, the cysteine-switch motif and the hemopexin domain. Moreover, opposite to type I MT-MMPs, they have a transmembrane domain located in their N-terminal tail, whereas C-terminus contains a cysteine array and immunoglobulin-like domains (Fanjul-Fernandez et al., 2010).

The last subgroup of MT-MMPs includes MT4-MMP and MT6-MMP (MMP-17 and -25, respectively). Both of them have the glycosylphosphatidylinositol (GPI) anchor instead of a transmembrane domain on their C-terminus, that enables binding of the MMP molecule to the cell membrane. To date, little is known about the presumable role of other MT-MMPs in pathogenesis of aortic aneurysm, with the exception of MT1-MMP, therefore, this subject still requires further studies.

3.3 Regulation of expression

The critical role of MMPs in physiology, as well as their involvement in various pathological conditions decipher the tight control of production and activation of these enzymes. Among all MMPs, only MMP-2 and MMP-9 were found to be expressed constitutively, whereas the expression of the remaining members of the MMP family has to be induced, e.g. in response to a tissue remodeling, or inflammatory reaction. Numerous factors, including pro-inflammatory cytokines (IL-1β, IL-6, TNF, etc.), growth factors (platelet-derived growth factor - PDGF; epidermal growth factor - EGF; TGF-β; etc.) and corticosteroids are involved in the control of MMPs gene expression Kadoglou & Liapis, 2004; Diehm et al., 2007). The common feature of the majority of inducible genes, including these encoding for MMPs, is the presence of the binding sites for transcription factors AP-1 and/or NF-κB in their promoter region. AP-1 transcription factors are heterodimer complexes, composed of two proto-oncogene family proteins - Jun and Fos. Together with NF-κB, a p50/p65 heterodimer, which controls the expression of numerous immune response- and inflammation-engaged molecules, AP-1 complexes interconnect a number of growth factor- and cytokine-mediated pathways. Another group of transcription factors involved in regulation of MMPs expression are members of Ets family. They recognize and bind to the conserved polyomavirus enhancer activator protein-3 (Pea3) binding site, which is found in MMP promoters. Since the Pea3 binding site is located contiguously to at least one AP-1 element, the interaction between both transcription factors will presumably modulate promoter response to various stimuli. Most recently, it was suggested that, in addition to the formerly discussed, the modification of chromatin structure through its acetylation-deacetylation could be another mechanism, involved in the regulation of MMP genes expression. Interestingly, it has been found that inhibition of histone deacetylase (HDAC) results in enhanced MMP-3, but decreased MMP-1 and MMP-9 expression in response to stimulation with IL-1β or TNF (Clark et al., 2007; Clark et al., 2008). Therefore, this aspect of MMPs expression control remains unclear and requires further studies. The next issue to be clarified is the role of mechanotransduction and the involvement of putative mechanoreceptors or mechano-responsive elements in MMPs expression control. This pathway seems to be of great importance especially in tissues permanently exposed to dynamic stress, like joint cartilage chondrocytes or VSMC in blood vessels (Blain, 2007). Finally, it is noteworthy, that besides transcriptional level, MMPs expression in response to various stimuli, including cytokines and growth factors, may also be controlled by the modulation of specific mRNA stability (Chakraborti et al., 2003).

Most recently, it has been found that MMP-2 activity may also be modulated by protein kinase C–mediated phosphorylation at the post-translational level (Sariahmetoglu et al., 2007). This modification may involve at least 5 amino acid residues from active site of catalytic domain and may result in modulation of its activity. Possibly, 3'-5' cyclic adenosine monophosphate (cAMP) pathway may be involved in this step, too.

3.4 Activation of MMPs

As mentioned previously, all MMPs are produced and secreted in an inactive zymogen form. This status is maintained due to the presence of the "cysteine-switch", the particular interaction between the thiol group of the prodomain cysteine and the zinc ion from the catalytic domain. The disruption of this interaction is essential for enzyme activation and may occur in two different manners (Fig. 2).

The first mode is an alteration of the cysteine thiol group by some physiological factors, including disulfides, oxidants and electrophiles, as well as non-physiological compounds, among them denaturing surfactants with sodium dodecyl sulphate (SDS), alkylating agents, organomercurials with 4-aminophenylmercuric acetate (APMA), and heavy metal ions. This alteration results in some allosteric changes in MMP structure, followed by an exposure of the catalytic site of the enzyme. It may lead to the auto-cleavage and removal of prodomain, and thus is associated with reduction of enzyme molecular size. On the other hand, the prodomain may stay attached to the active enzyme and thus the molecular weight of activated MMP remains unchanged (Fu et al., 2008; Hadler-Olsen et al., 2011) (Fig. 2A).

The second mechanism of MMPs activation is direct cleavage of their prodomain by another proteolytic enzyme. It has been shown that proteolytic activation of MMPs may be conducted by other MMPs, as well as a broad spectrum of extracellular serine-, cysteine- or aspartate-proteinases. Moreover, this mechanism is also utilized during an intracellular activation of MMPs by furin, the subtilisin-like serine proteinase from the trans-Golgi network (Fig. 2A).

An interesting combination of both, allosteric and proteolytic mode of action, represents activation of MMP-2 by the membrane type 1-MMP (MT1-MMP, or MMP-14) in the presence of the endogenous MMP inhibitor – the tissue inhibitor of MMPs (TIMP)-2. The TIMP-2 molecule serves as a link between MMP-2 and MMP-14, where the N-terminal part of TIMP-2 inactivates MMP-14 and its C-terminal part binds to the hemopexin domain of pro-MMP-2 (Fig. 2B). The prodomain of immobilized MMP-2 is then cleaved by another recruited MMP-14 molecule, thus resulting in proteolytic activation of MMP-2. Remarkably, other membrane type MMPs: MT2-MMP and MT3-MMP are able to activate pro-MMP-2 without involvement of TIMP (Hadler-Olsen et al., 2011, Klein & Bischoff, 2010).

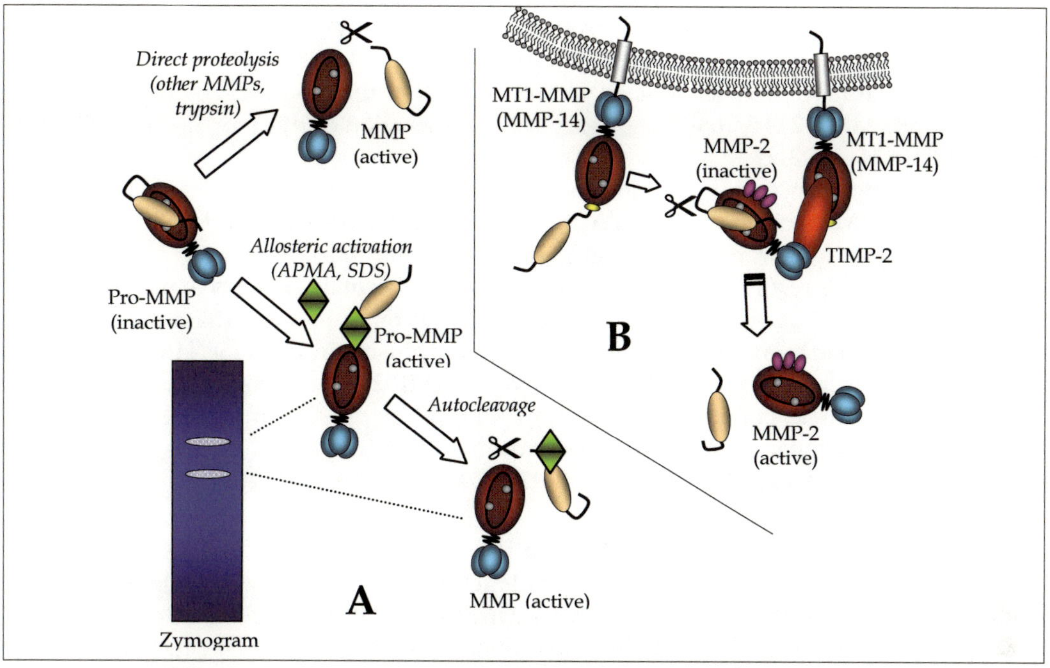

Fig. 2. The MMP activation pathways (a detailed description in text)

3.5 Inhibition of MMPs

When firmly supervised, matrix metalloproteinases control various physiological reactions very precisely. However, if this supervision appears incompetent, MMPs reveal their "dark side of the Force" and become highly dangerous molecules, which are engaged in many pathologies, including the development of an aortic aneurysm. Therefore, mechanisms responsible for this regulation and factors participating in these mechanisms are potentially useful in some therapeutic approaches.

Standard mechanisms of MMPs silencing include interaction with the specific tissue inhibitors of metalloproteinases and other endogenous inhibitors, such as α2-macroglobulin, reversion-inducing cysteine-rich protein with Kazal motifs (RECK) and tissue-factor-pathway-inhibitor 2 (TFPI2) (Maskos & Bode, 2003).

Surprisingly, although reactive oxygen species are known to activate autolytic cleavage of MMPs due to disruption of their "cysteine switch", it has been suggested that oxidants may also inactivate MMPs by modification of some amino acids critical for their catalytic activity (Fu et al., 2008).

3.5.1 TIMPs

Tissue inhibitors of metalloproteinases are secreted by different types of cells, including macrophages, VSMC and platelets. The basically defined function of TIMPs is a suppression of the MMPs activity by biding to their catalytic domain and blocking enzymatic activity. Based on *in vitro* studies, TIMPs are recognized as highly efficient MMPs inhibitors (with K_i at the level of 10^{-11} M for TIMP-1/MMP-1 interaction). The affinity of various TIMPs to specific MMPs differs among them, e.g. TIMP-1 preferably binds to MT-MMPs, whereas other TIMPs are generally less selective. However, a direct interaction between TIMPs and active MMPs may be difficult to observe *in vivo*, mainly due to a presence of α2-macroglobulin, a common MMP-neutralizing agent (Fu et al., 2008). On the other hand, as clearly shown for TIMP-2, as well as for other TIMPs, their binding to the hemopexin domain of pro-MMP-2 is actually necessary for the activation of this enzyme by MT1-MMP (Hadler-Olsen et al., 2011).

It is plausible, that functional polymorphisms in genes encoding for TIMPs could influence the activity of MMPs in the aneurysm wall. Thus, several SNPs supposed to affect the level of TIMP transcription, were assessed in patients with aortic aneurysms. It is noteworthy, that the genotyping results were analyzed for male and female patients separately due to the fact, that TIMP-1 gene is located on the X chromosome. To date, the association with aortic aneurysm has been suggested for two polymorphisms in gene for TIMP-1 (434 C/T and rs2070584 T/C) (Ogata et al., 2005) and two in TIMP-2 (a promoter SNP -479 C/T, and 573 G/A, but in male patients group only) (Wang et al., 1999; Hinterseher et al., 2007). Nevertheless, since the mentioned analyses concerned relatively small groups, this issue still requires additional investigation (Sandford et al., 2007; Saratzis et al., 2011).

3.5.2 Pharmacological modulation of MMPs

Since the modulation of MMPs activity by endogenous inhibitors in pathology seems to be inefficient, several strategies with exogenous MMP modulators have been developed. It is noteworthy, that some of these modulators are already used in clinical practice, although the primary indication for their application did not concern inhibition of MMPs.

An interesting approach may be the use of MMP-specific antibody-based inhibitors. The experimental model with neutralizing antibodies directed against MMP-2 has shown their protective influence on a heart exposed to ischemia/reperfusion injury (Cheung et al., 2000). However, the verification, whether this procedure would be useful in management of aortic aneurysms, needs further studies. Apart from endogenous inhibitors, various pharmacological agents may reveal inhibitory activity against MMPs. The small hydroxamate-based zinc-chelating synthetic agents, such as batimastat, marimastat or ilomastat (galardin), were first used in oncology, to suppress MMPs-dependent metastasis and tumor invasion. However, due to non-selective, generalized inhibition of MMPs activity with numerous adverse events, accompanied by relatively poor effectiveness, their clinical career was ended very soon (Baxter, 2004).

3.5.2.1 Tetracyclines

Tetracyclines are natural antibiotics derived from *Streptomyces*. They are known for many non-antibiotic properties, including inhibition of proteolysis, or anti-apoptotic and anti-inflammatory activity. The most intensively tested representative of tetracyclines - doxycycline, has been shown to prevent formation of aortic aneurysm in several animal models. Also, the results of three small clinical trials in humans have shown that doxycycline in a well tolerated dose 150-200 mg/day significantly reduced aneurysm expansion rate. It has been suggested, that doxycycline inhibits MMPs directly, by binding to their catalytic site. Furthermore, it may reduce the MMP expression attenuating the inflammatory cascade. However, the results of the studies on putative effects of tetracyclines on MMP-9 are not fully consistent. The first published study by Cruci and coauthors has shown that doxycycline treatment in a dose 200 mg/day resulted in a 2.5-fold reduction of MMP-9 protein levels and 82% reduction of MMP-9 mRNA expression (Cruci et al., 1998).

Surprisingly, in a subsequent placebo-controlled study Ding and colleagues did not observe any effect of 1 month 100 mg/day doxycycline therapy on MMP-9 mRNA, or protein expression (Ding et al., 2005). Finally, Lindeman and coauthors have shown that 2-weeks doxycycline treatment decreased MMP-9 protein levels ($p<0.0026$), but did not affect mRNA expression level ($p=0.206$). The authors have concluded, that the beneficial effect of doxycycline on aneurysm progression might be due to the reduction of aneurysm wall infiltration by neutrophils and T CD8-positive lymphocytes rather, than the decrease of MMP-9 gene expression (Lindeman et al., 2009).

3.5.2.2 Macrolides

The beneficial influence of tetracyclines on aneurysm expansion rate may be multidirectional, including their antimicrobial activity against *Chlamydia pneumoniae,* and thus, indirect MMPs modulation (also discussed in chapter 2.2). This concept led to the introduction of macrolides, other antibiotics with potent *Chlamydia*-killing activity, to the arsenal of anti-aneurysm agents. In a randomized trial by Vammen and coauthors, the aortic aneurysm expansion rate in patients treated with roxithromycin was 1.56 mm/year, in comparison to 2.75 mm/year in the placebo-receiving control group. Interestingly, no significant correlation between *C. pneumoniae* titers and roxithromycin ability to suppress the aneurysm expansion was observed (Vammen et al., 2001) .

The mechanism of anti-aneurysm protective action of macrolides remains unclear. Recently, another macrolide derivative, rapamycin, was tested in animal aortic aneurysm model. Due to its strong anti-inflammatory and immunosuppressive properties, rapamycin is commonly used to prevent transplanted organ rejection. It has been found, that rapamycin administration in experimentally induced aortic aneurysms in rat significantly inhibits activation of NF-κB and, subsequently, MMP-9 expression thus resulting in 40% decrease of aneurysm expansion rate, as compared to control animals (Lawrence et al., 2004).

3.5.2.3 Statins

The inhibitors of hydroxymetylglutaryl-coenzyme A reductase, better known as statins, are widely used in a treatment of patients with cardiovascular diseases. Apart from their main activity, which decreases atherogenic lipoproteins, statins reveal various pleiotropic effects, including an augmentation of pro-apoptotic properties of some anticancer drugs, or an inhibition of inflammatory cell activity. Possibly, these anti-inflammatory properties of statins result from suppression of NF-κB, that is also involved in regulation of MMPs expression. Indeed, *in vitro* studies have demonstrated, that simvastatin and cerivastatin may decrease the production of MMPs, especially MMP-9, in VSMC, macrophages and neutrophils. A subsequent small clinical study by Nagashima, and a randomized prospective trial by Evans group independently showed, that statins were potent inhibitors of inflammatory cells *in vivo,* and they effectively suppressed the MMP-9 production in the aortic aneurysm wall (Nagashima et al., 2002; Evans et al., 2007). Also, Wilson and his colleagues observed, that simvastatin, pravastatin and atorvastatin decreased local concentrations of MMP-3 and MMP-9 in the anterior wall of aortic aneurysms in patients undergoing open heart surgery. Furthermore, as shown by Schouten and coauthors, statin use resulted in lower aneurysm expansion rate with 2.0 mm/year in statin-treated versus 3.6 mm/year in the placebo control group (Schouten et al., 2006). Interestingly, in contrast to reports mentioned previously, Hurks and coauthors did not observe any statistically

significant differences in MMP-9 level between patients treated with statins and a control group. Moreover, they have found, that a level of active MMP-9 in patients treated with pravastatin was higher, than in control subjects (Hurks et al., 2010). This may suggest, that a pleiotropic actions profile of these drugs may differ among the various statins.
Unfortunately, the issue concerning statins influence on aortic aneurysm progression seems unlikely to be resolved in the near future, because of two reasons at least. Firstly, the prevalence of statin use in aortic aneurysm-suffering patients is very high, mainly due to other concomitant cardiovascular diseases. Therefore, it may be difficult to assemble a control group for a large randomized study. Secondly, according to current recommendations, statins should be used as perioperative protection during open surgical, as well as endovascular aneurysm repair (Diehm et al. 2007). Thus, such a study, additionally to being difficult to design, appears to be ethically controversial.

3.5.2.4 Low molecular weight heparin

As was discussed previously (chapter 2.1), the aortic aneurysm is usually accompanied by an intraluminal thrombus, that is always associated with more or less clinically overt coagulation abnormalities. It has been shown, that these coagulopathies may be successfully treated with small doses of low molecular weight heparin (LMWH) (Jelenska et al., 2004). Moreover, our subsequent studies revealed, that in addition to the attenuation of coagulation abnormalities, a LMWH treatment resulted in statistically significant decrease of circulating MMP-9 plasma activity. Interestingly, the *in vitro* studies did not show any direct influence of LMWH on MMP-9 production by activated leucocytes, or enzyme activity, either. Therefore, the most plausible explanation seems to be an indirect mechanism of LMWH action. According to our concept, the stabilized thrombus does not capture any new leukocytes. In such circumstances the number of MMP-9-producing cells, which are already entrapped in fibrin clot, decreases slowly. Finally, theses conditions lead to the decrease of MMP-9 amounts, released from intraluminal thrombus to the circulating blood. However, the verification of this hypothesis, as well as further clinical studies, concerning LMWH influence on aneurysm progression, are necessary.

3.5.2.5 JNK inhibitor

Based on results of studies focused on molecular aspects of aortic aneurysm pathophysiology, the c-Jun N-terminal kinase (JNK) has been selected as a new target for therapy. Using pharmacological JNK inhibitor Yoshimura and coauthors prevented the development, or induced the regression of already formed aneurysm in calcium-, or angiotensin II-induced aortic aneurysm mouse models. This effect was associated with decreased MMP-9 activity, but also with restoration of aortic tissue architecture, mainly due to the upregulation of various extracellular matrix proteins synthesis. Obviously, the results of further studies are expected highly impatiently (Yoshimura et al., 2005; Miyake & Morishita, 2009).

3.5.2.6 Renin-angiotensin system modulators

Recently, it has been suggested, that the renin-angiotensin system and its main effector molecule – angiotensin II, may also be involved in the initiation of inflammatory reaction in the aortic wall and, thus, it significantly contributes to the development of aneurysm. Therefore, antagonists of the angiotensin II receptor were tested for their presumable protective effect on aneurysm progression. Indeed, it was shown, that losartan and valsartan, two representatives of the group, were effective in preventing aneurysm formation. Interestingly, although they do not appear to influence MMPs activity directly, their beneficial influence was associated with decrease of MMPs expression in aneurismal tissue, possibly due to the suppression of NF-κB-controlled inflammatory reaction (Fujiwara et al., 2008; Miyake & Morishita, 2009). However, since the career of angiotensin II receptor antagonists in a management of cardiovascular diseases is rather short, their value in aortic aneurysm treatment still remains to be verified.

The next group of pharmaceuticals, addressed to interfere with the renin-angiotensin system are angiotensin converting enzyme (ACE) inhibitors. In contrast to the previously described angiotensin II receptor antagonists, they bind to the active site of MMPs and directly block their enzymatic activity in a dose dependent manner. Using animal models, it has been shown, that ACE inhibitors, including captopril, enalapril, lisinopril and perindopril, reduced the aortic wall degeneration and aneurysm progression. Surprisingly, data provided by several clinical trials are highly inconsistent. Reports by Lederle and Taylor, or Hackam group suggested independently, that patients with aortic aneurysms, which received ACE inhibitors, displayed lower aneurysm expansion rate and were better protected from aneurysm rupture, as compared to individuals treated without convertase inhibitors (Hackam et al., 2006; Lederle & Taylor, 2006). On the other hand, Schouten and colleagues did not find any correlation between aneurysm dilatation rate and ACE inhibitors (Schouten et al., 2006; Baxter et al., 2008; Miyake & Morishita, 2009). Moreover, the abdominal aortic aneurysm screening program in UK revealed an increasing aneurysm growth rate, that was apparently associated with ACE inhibitors intake (Sweeting et al., 2010). Therefore, this approach urgently needs further elucidation in multicenter prospective randomized trials, although, due to the common use of ACE inhibitors in cardiovascular diseases, the study design will possibly meet similar obstacles, as in statins case.

3.5.2.7 Decoy oligodeoxynucleotides

Recently, the novel strategy based on targeting transcription factors, which are known to be involved in regulation of inflammatory reaction and MMPs expression, appears to be highly promising approach in the management of aortic aneurysm. A principle of this strategy is the use of synthetic oligodeoxynucleotides (ODNs), referred as "decoy" ODNs, which specifically recognize and bind to respective transcription factors and thus competitively block their binding to promoter of gene of interest.

This decoy strategy was used to inhibit two transcription factors – NF-κB and ets-1, which are suggested to control gene expression of several MMPs, including MMP-1, -2, -3 and -9. Using elastase-induced aneurysm rat and rabbit models, and chimeric anti-NF-κB/ets-1 decoy ODNs, Miyake and colleagues have analyzed the effects of the simultaneous suppression of both, NF-κB and ets-1. They found, that this approach resulted in marked decrease of aortic aneurysm progression, that was accompanied by significant decrease of MMP-1 and MMP-9 expression in the aneurysm wall. Moreover, in the rabbit model the application of the mentioned decoy system onto already formed aneurysms led to their significant regression, which in addition to MMPs inhibition, was possibly due to induction of collagen and elastin synthesis, that is negatively controlled by ets-1. Hopefully, this strategy will be effective also in human, since the anti-NF-κB/ets-1 ODNs decreased MMPs expression in *ex vivo* experiments with cultured human aortic tissue (Miyake & Morishita, 2009). It is noteworthy, that the decoy ODNs-based therapy has some limitations, too. The main problem is the rapid degradation and relatively short half-life of therapeutic ODNs, that require their local application. This in turn raises the problem with an effective delivery system. In experiments by Miyake and coauthors the cellulose-based ODNs delivery system was applied intraoperatively on the outer surface of dilated aorta. In clinical practice this could be done using low-invasive procedures, such as laparoscopy, or more likely by endovascular access. However, this issue remains to be resolved.

3.6 Methods of MMP detection and analysis

The increasing evidence concerning the involvement of MMPs in various pathologies, including aortic aneurysm, results in the necessity to develop methods of analysis that would be sufficiently sensitive and specific enough to detect minute amounts of MMPs.

3.6.1 ELISA

The above mentioned main requirements are met by an enzyme-linked immunosorbent assay (ELISA). Despite its high sensitivity (picograms per ml) and availability for all known MMPs, the ELISA method provides data reflecting only the specific protein amount, without any information about its enzymatic activity. This obstacle is partially resolved by a new generation of ELISA kits, that can discriminate between full length pro-enzyme and proteolytically activated MMP (Fig. 3A). Obviously, similar data could be obtained using the western-blot method with respective anti-MMP antibodies. Nevertheless, the previously mentioned non-proteolytic activation of full-length molecules may result in false negative, or at least, underestimated results of MMP measurement. Thus, the studies focusing on MMPs require another method that would enable convenient analysis of their enzymatic activity.

3.6.2 Substrate-specific zymography

Currently, the standard method used for the analysis of MMPs activity is a substrate-specific zymography with sodium dodecyl sulphate (SDS)-polyacrylamide gel electrophoresis (PAGE). The method is based on a molecular size-dependent electrophoretic separation of tested samples in a polyacrylamide gel, containing substrate specific for MMP being analyzed, e.g. gelatin for MMP-2 and MMP-9, casein for MMP-1, -3, -7, -10, -12 and -13 or collagen for MMP-1 and -13 (Kupai et al., 2010). Then, the gel is incubated in zinc- and calcium-rich reaction buffer to re-activate enzyme particles separated in the gel. The high local concentration of enzyme molecules results in a substrate digestion, that is restricted to the area close to the position of respective MMP in the gel. The visualization of enzymatic activity of assayed samples occurs after incubation of the whole gel with the staining solution, e.g. Coomassie blue. The presence of an unstained area in a gel corresponds to a substrate cleavage, due to enzymatic activity of respective MMP, whereas the size of this area directly correlates with amount and/or activity of the enzyme. Thus, the standard SDS-PAGE zymography allows a semi-quantitative comparison of respective MMP amount, or more precisely – activity between various samples. When used with known amounts of recombinant MMP, as a reference, the method permits the quantitative assessment of respective MMP. Furthermore, due to the gel electrophoresis of analyzed samples, this method enables the molecular size-based identification and individual measurement of both, full length pro-MMP and its short processed form, too (Fig. 3D, also Fig.2). It has been proven that sensitivity of standard SDS-PAGE zymography is sufficient to detect similar amounts of active MMP, as those using ELISA method (Table 1).

Substrate	Enzyme	Detection limit
gelatin	MMP-2	10 pg
casein	MMP-7	1 ng
collagen	MMP-1	0.1 pg

Table 1. Examples of SDS-PAGE zymography detection limits (Kupai et al., 2010)

It is noteworthy, that the standard SDS-PAGE zymography is not free of some problems, either. The important issue is the unspecific, SDS-mediated activation of pro-MMP, that may occur during electrophoresis. Obviously, this event affects the results, and is usually associated with an overestimation of MMP activity. Additional difficulty with the use of this method is the long, time-consuming procedure. Therefore, although the SDS-PAGE zymography is sensitive enough and relatively inexpensive, in some circumstances the better choice for a fast MMP assessment could be the fluorescent zymography.

3.6.3 Fluorescent zymography

The fluorescent zymography is based on a technology known as the fluorescence resonance energy transfer (FRET). Briefly, the tested sample is incubated in small volume (10-20 µl) of reaction mixture containing the substrate, that is labeled with fluorochrome and quencher tags. When a substrate remains intact, the energy emitted by fluorochrome is entirely absorbed by the quencher, therefore no fluorescence is detected. The substrate degradation abolishes the suppressive effect of the quencher on fluorochrome, thus resulting in increase of fluorescence in the reaction mixture. The intensity of fluorescence corresponds to the amount of digested substrate, that, in turn, reflects the amount of active enzyme in a sample (Fig. 3B).

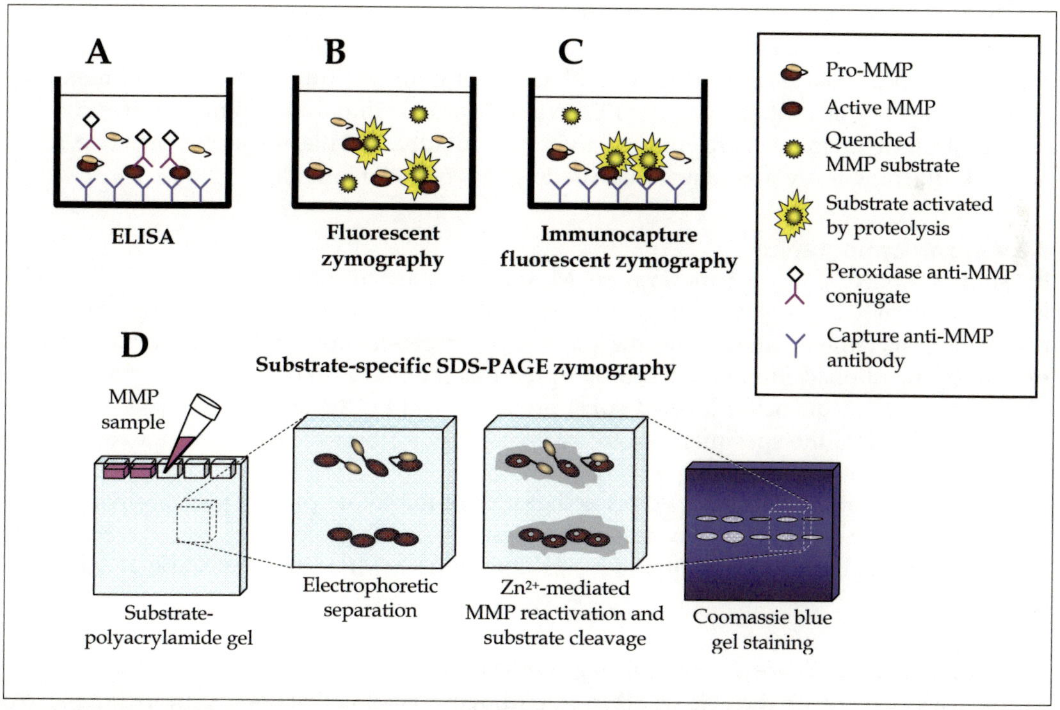

Fig. 3. Schematic representation of main methods of MMPs detection (description in text).

Oppositely to standard SDS-PAGE zymography, this method is very fast and enables the measurement of proteolytic activity in analyzed samples within several minutes. In contrast to the previously mentioned ELISA and SDS-PAGE zymography, the fluorescent zymography allows an assessment of the direct influence of various factors on MMP activity. However, the outcome of the analysis is highly sensitive to sample preparation and the reaction conditions. The samples should be prepared without addition of EDTA or other metal-ion chelators, and without addition of protease inhibitors. This step may be of great importance for final results of analysis, especially since the extraction procedures themselves may induce MMPs activation or lead to release of natural MMP inhibitors. After tissue disruption during sample preparation, these inhibitors, although initially localized in different compartments, can interact with active enzymes, and thus, may affect the results of assay. Another important issue may be the concentration of non-ionic detergents in the reaction mixture, which may "neutralize" small molecules that potentially could interfere with MMP activity (Kupai et al., 2010).

The most significant disadvantage of the fluorescent zymography is, that it does not determine MMP, that directly contributes to the observed substrate degradation. This obstacle may be omitted by the use of respective, MMP-specific, monoclonal antibodies, which block the proteolytic activity of the selected enzyme. With a panel of blocking antibodies, this modification allows the quantitative assessment of each constituent of MMP-mediated proteolytic activity in the analyzed sample.

Another solution to this problem may be the method that combines the idea of both, ELISA and fluorescent zymography. Briefly, the plate is coated with specific anti-MMP antibodies, which capture molecules of the respective enzyme from the sample being assessed. Then, non-captured, unspecific proteins are washed out and the fluorochrome/quencher-labeled substrate is added to the plate followed by incubation. Finally, since the intensity of MMP-mediated fluorescence corresponds to the activity of specific MMP, it may be measured using the fluorescence plate reader. This solid-phase, or immunocapture fluorescent zymography represents the key advantages of both, ELISA and "normal" fluorescent zymography (Fig. 3C). It enables a measurement of enzymatic activity of individual MMPs, is specific, sensitive, rapid and lacks the previously mentioned main deficiencies of both methods.

3.6.4 *In situ* zymography

In studies concerning distribution of MMPs in affected tissues, the use of *in situ* zymography may be very advantageous. This test allows the detection of MMPs activity in histological specimens, directly on the place of their production or activation. Similarly to previously mentioned fluorescent zymography, this method also exploits FRET technology. The fluorochrome/quencher-labeled substrate is applied on the surface of a specimen, and is incubated. Then, the specimen can be assessed with a fluorescent microscope, or using a confocal laser scanning microscope.

The main disadvantage of this method is that it does not allow precise measurement of the amount of active MMP. Moreover, similarly to "normal" fluorescent zymography, it is necessary to use neutralizing antibodies, to determine MMPs that contribute to substrate cleavage.

3.6.5 Reverse zymography - detection of MMP inhibition

The studies concerning the role of MMP in pathogenesis of aortic aneurysm include also a method that enables assessment of the natural tissue inhibitors of MMP (TIMPs). This method, known as reverse zymography, utilizes polyacrylamide gel with specific substrate, that is additionally supplemented with respective MMP. After electrophoresis of tested samples the gel is subjected to the same processing as in routine zymography. Then, the MMP, which is equally distributed in the whole gel, cleaves the substrate with the exception of those places, where TIMPs inhibit its proteolytic activity. Those places are visible as Coomassie blue-stained bands, whereas the other parts of the gel remain unstained.

In addition to reverse zymography, the expected interaction between MMPs and their tissue inhibitors can also be analyzed using a modified western blotting (SDS-PAGE and immunoblotting) method. The formation of higher molecular weight complex by interacting molecules results in its slower migration during polyacrylamide gel electrophoresis, and thus reveals a band shift of specific MMP or its inhibitor, depending on the antibody used for detection.

3.6.6 Possible applications

Currently, the methods of MMPs analysis in aortic aneurysm clinics described above are predominantly used for research purpose. However, due to an increasing interest in the monitoring of MMPs level and/or activity in aneurysm-suffering patients, it is plausible that some of these methods will become the standard diagnostic tools in the near future.

The first postulated indication for clinical use could be the screening of plasma MMPs activity in patients with newly recognized aortic aneurysm. Although there is no consent, whether low plasma levels of MMPs may be considered as a low risk indicator of aneurysm progression and/or rupture, it is nevertheless widely accepted that the higher concentration, or more precisely, their higher activity should at least encourage more frequent monitoring of aneurysm diameter. The second, important clinical application for MMP assessment seems to be the periodic monitoring of MMPs activity in patients with small aneurysms and subjected to pharmacological treatment. Obviously, the method selected for monitoring should depend on the mechanism of action of controlled MMP modulator. Thus, the monitoring of pharmacological treatment of aortic aneurysm using compounds displaying indirect influence on MMP amount and/or activity, including statins, heparins or ODNs, may engage a broad spectrum of methods mentioned above. However, in regimens using potent direct MMP inhibitors, e.g. tetracycline-derivatives, or angiotensin converting enzyme-inhibitors, the fluorescent zymography rather, than other methods, including substrate-specific SDS-PAGE zymography, should be used preferentially.

It has been found that open aneurysm repair leads to transient (usually within first 3 moths) MMP-9 increase, followed by its later significant reduction. Nevertheless, in some patients high levels of MMPs may still persist even a very long time after surgery (Kadoglou & Liapis, 2004). An interesting example of this condition may by the case of a 50-year old men with an abdominal aortic aneurysm, subjected to successful open aneurysm repair. Surprisingly, after 4 years the patient was qualified again for surgical treatment due to the significant enlargement of the thoracic aorta, remaining suprarenal part of abdominal aorta and common iliac arteries. The plasma level of MMP-2 was similar to those observed in other aortic aneurysm-suffering individuals. However, his MMP-9 plasma activity was extraordinarily (almost 10-fold) higher, than mean MMP-9 level, observed in other patients bearing an aortic aneurysm.

In contrast to open repair, patients subjected to endovascular aneurysm exclusion usually reveal a gradual decrease of circulating MMP-3 and -9, whereas the persisting high concentration and/or activity of circulating MMP-9 actually correlates with some postoperative complications. They include graft migration, or presence of endo-leak, where both conditions are accompanied by the contact of circulating blood with the thrombus still existing in the aneurysm lumen (Kadoglou & Liapis, 2004). Therefore, the temporary monitoring of MMP activity may be an important diagnostic procedure also in patients after both, open surgical, but also endovascular intervention.

4. Conclusion

Despite numerous studies, the role of MMPs in pathogenesis of aortic aneurysm remains unclear. Also, the question, whether they are "executors", or "executioners", is still unanswered. Since MMPs are obviously engaged in all stages of the aneurysm development, from the beginning, till the fatal aneurysm rupture, they are very attractive targets in approaches, concerning pharmacological treatment of this pathology. However, due to some discrepancies between results of experimental, as well as clinical studies conducted so far, this issue still requires intensive research. Nevertheless, it is plausible that in the near future the majority of patients with aortic aneurysms might simply require regular drug intake, without the necessity for surgical intervention, which would be reserved for particular cases only. Since it is very similar to the history of management of gastric ulcers, this vision seems to be quite realistic in the near future…

5. References

Amalinei, C.; Caruntu, I.D. & Balan, R.A. (2007). Biology of metalloproteinases. *Romanian Journal of Morphology and Embryology*, Vol.48, No.4, (October), pp. 323–334, ISSN 1220-0522

Baxter, B.T. (2004). Could medical intervention work for aortic aneurysms? *American Journal of Surgery*, Vol.188, No.6, (December), pp. 628-632, ISSN 0002-9610

Baxter, B.T.; Terrin, M.C. & Dalman, R.L. (2008). Medical management of small abdominal aortic aneurysms. *Circulation*, Vol.117, No.14, (April), pp. 1883-1889, ISSN 0009-7322

Blain, E.J. (2007). Mechanical regulation of matrix metalloproteinases *Frontiers in Bioscience*, Vol.12, No.2 (January), pp. 507-527, ISSN 1093-4715

Boire, A.; Covic, L.; Agarwal, A.; Jacques, S.; Sherifi, S. & Kuliopulos, A. (2005). PAR1 is a matrix metalloprotease-1 receptor that promotes invasion and tumorigenesis of breast cancer cells. *Cell*, Vol.120, No.3, (February), pp. 303-313, ISSN 0092-8674

Chakraborti, S.; Mandal, M.; Das, S.; Mandal, A. & Chakraborti, T. (2003). Regulation of matrix metalloproteinases: An overview. *Molecular and Cellular Biochemistry*, Vol.253, No.1-2, (November), pp. 269-285, ISSN 0300-8177

Cheung, P.Y.; Sawicki, G.; Wozniak, M.; Wang, W.; Radomski, M.W. & Schulz, R. (2000). Matrix metalloproteinase-2 contributes to ischemia-reperfusion injury in the heart. *Circulation*, Vol.101, No.15, (April), pp. 1833-1839, ISSN 0009-7322

Clark, I.M.; Swingler, T.E. & Young D.A. (2007). Acetylation in the regulation of metalloproteinase and tissue inhibitor of metalloproteinases gene expression. *Frontiers in Bioscience*, Vol.12, No.2, (January), pp. 528-535, ISSN 1093-4715

Clark, I.M.; Swingler, T.E.; Sampieri, C.L. & Edwards D.R. (2008). The regulation of matrix metalloproteinases and their inhibitors *International Journal of Biochemistry and Cell Biology*, Vol.40, No.6-7, pp. 1362–1378, ISSN 1357-2725

Curci, J.A.; Petrinec, D.; Liao, S.; Golub, L.M. & Thompson, R.W. (1998). Pharmacologic suppression of experimental abdominal aortic aneurysms: acomparison of doxycycline and four chemically modified tetracyclines. *Journal of Vascular Surgery*, Vol.28, No.6, (December), pp. 1082–93, ISSN 0741-5214

Diehm, N.; Dick, F.; Schaffner, F.; Schmidli, J.; Kalka, C.; Di Santo, S.; Voelzmann, J. & Baumgartner, J. (2007). Novel insight into the pathobiology of abdominal aortic aneurysm and potential future treatment concepts. *Progress in Cardiovascular Diseases*, Vol. 50, No. 3 (November-December), pp. 209-217, ISSN 0033-0620

Ding, R.; McGuinness, C.L.; Burnand, K.G.; Sullivan, E. & Smith, A. (2005). Matrix metalloproteinases in the aneurysm wall of patients treated with low-dose doxycycline, *Vascular*, Vol.13, No.5, (September-October), pp. 290–297, ISSN 1708-5381

Endo, K.; Takino, T.; Miyamori, H.; Kinsen, H.; Yoshizaki, T.; Furukawa, M. & Sato, H. (2003). Cleavage of syndecan-1 by membrane type matrix metalloproteinase-1 stimulates cell migration. *Journal of Biological Chemistry*, Vol.278, No.42, (October), pp. 40764-40770, ISSN 0021-9258

Eriksson, P.; Jormsjo-Pettersson, S.; Brady, A.R.; Deguchi, H.; Hamsten, A. & Powell, J.T. (2005). Genotype-phenotype relationships in an investigation of the role of proteases in abdominal aortic aneurysm expansion. *British Journal of Surgery*, Vol.92, No.11, (November), pp. 1372-1376, ISSN 1365-2168

Eugster, T.; Huber, A.; Obeid, T.; Schwegler, I.; Gürke, L. & Stierli, P. (2005). Aminoterminal propeptide of type III procollagen and matrix metalloproteinases-2 and -9 failed to serve as serum markers for abdominal aortic aneurysm. *European Journal of Vascular and Endovascular Surgery*, Vol.29, No.4, (April), pp. 378-382, ISSN 1078-5884

Evans, J.; Powell, J.T.; Schwalbe, E.; Loftus, I.M. & Thompson, MM. (2007). Simvastatin Attenuates the activity of matrix metalloprotease-9 in aneurysmal aortic tissue. *European Journal of Vascular and Endovascular Surgery*, Vol.34, No.3, (September), pp. 302–303, ISSN 1078-5884

Falkensammer, B.; Duftner, C.; Seiler, R.; Pavlic, M.; Walder, G.; Wilflingseder, D.; Stoiber, H.; Klein-Weigel, P.; Dierich, M.; Fraedrich, G.; Würzner, R. & Schirmer, M. (2007). Lack of microbial DNA in tissue specimens of patients with abdominal aortic aneurysms and positive *Chlamydiales* serology. *European Journal of Clinical Microbiology and Infectious Disease*, Vol.26, No.2, (February); pp. 141-145, ISSN 0934-9723

Fanjul-Fernández, M.; Folgueras, A.R.; Cabrera, S. & López-Otín, C. (2010). Matrix metalloproteinases: evolution, gene regulation and functional analysis in mouse models. *Biochimica et Biophysica Acta*, Vol.1803, No.1, (January), pp. 3-19, ISSN 0304-4165

Fu, X.; Parks, W. & Heinecke, J.W. (2008). Activation and silencing of matrix metalloproteinases. *Seminars in Cell and Developmental Biology* Vol.19, No.1, (February), pp. 2-13, ISSN 1084-9521

Fujiwara, Y.; Shiraya, S.; Miyake, T.; Yamakawa, S.; Aoki, M. & Makino, H. (2008). Inhibition of experimental abdominal aortic aneurysm in a rat model by an angiotensin receptor blocker, valsartan. *International Journal of Molecular Medicine*, Vol.22, No.6, (December), pp. 703-708, ISSN 1107-3756

Gearing, A.J.; Beckett, P.; Christodoulou, M.; Churchill, M.; Clements, J.; Davidson, A.H.; Drummond, A.H.; Galloway, W.A.; Gilbert, R.; Gordon, J.L.; Leber, T.M.; Mangan, M.; Miller, K.; Nayee, P.; Owen, K.; Patel, S.; Thomas, W.; Wells, G.; Wood, L.M. & Woolley, K. (1994). Processing of tumour necrosis factor-alpha precursor by metalloproteinases. *Nature*, Vol.370, No.6490, (August), pp. 555-557, ISSN 0028-0836

Hackam, D.G.; Thiruchelvam, D. & Redelmeier, D.A. (2006). Angiotensin-converting enzyme inhibitors and aortic rupture: a population-based case-control study. *Lancet*, Vol.368, No.9536, (August), pp. 659-665, ISSN 0140-6736

Hadler-Olsen, E.; Fadnes, B.; Sylte, I.; Uhlin-Hansen, L. & Winberg, J.O. (2011). Regulation of matrix metalloproteinase activity in health and disease. *FEBS Journal*, Vol.278, No.1, (January), pp. 28–45, ISSN 0014-5793

Hernandez-Barrantes, S.; Bernardo, M.; Toth, M. & Fridman, R. (2002). Regulation of membrane type-matrix metalloproteinases. *Seminars in Cancer Biology* Vol.12, No.2, (April), pp. 131-138, ISSN 1044-579x

Hinterseher, I.; Krex, D.; Kuhlisch, E.; Schmidt, K.G.; Pilarsky, C.; Schneiders, W.; Saeger, H.D. & Bergert, H. (2007). Tissue inhibitor of metalloproteinase-1 (TIMP-1) polymorphisms in a Caucasian population with abdominal aortic aneurysm, *World Journal of Surgery*, Vol.31, No.11 (November), pp. 2248-2254, ISSN 1432-2323

Høgh, A.; Vammen, S.; Ostergaard, L.; Joensen, J.B.; Henneberg, E.W. & Lindholt, J.S. (2009). Intermittent roxithromycin for preventing progression of small abdominal aortic aneurysms: long-term results of a small clinical trial. *Vascular and Endovascular Surgery*; Vol.43, No.5, (October-November); pp. 452-456; ISSN 1078-5884

Hurks, R.; Hoefer, I.E.; Vink, A.; Pasterkamp, G.; Schoneveld, A.; Kerver, M.; de Vries, J-P.P.M.; Tangelder, M.J. & Moll, F.L. (2010). Different effects of commonly prescribed statins on abdominal aortic aneurysm wall biology. *European Journal of Vascular and Endovascular Surgery*, Vol.39, No.5, (May), pp. 569-576, ISSN 1078-5884

Jelenska, M.M.; Szmidt, J.; Bojakowski, K.; Grzela, T. & Palester-Chlebowczyk, M. (2004) Compensated activation of coagulation in pateints with abdominal aortic aneurysm: effects of heparin treatment prior to elective surgery. *Thrombosis and Haemosthasis*, Vol.92, No.5, (November), pp. 997-1002, ISSN 0340-6245

Jones, G.T.; Phillips, V.L.; Harris, E.L.; Rossaak, J.L. & van Rij, A.M. (2003). Functional matrix metalloproteinase-9 polymorphism (C -1562 T) associated with abdominal aortic aneurysm. *Journal of Vascular Surgery,* Vol.38, No.6, (December), pp. 1363-1367, ISSN 0741-5214

Kadoglou, N.P. & Liapis, C.D. (2004). Matrix metalloproteinases: contribution to pathogenesis, diagnosis, surveillance and treatment of abdominal aortic aneurysms. *Current Medical Research and Opinion,* Vol.20, No.4, (April), pp. 419-32, ISSN 0300-7995

Klein, T. & Bischoff, R. (2010). Physiology and pathophysiology of matrix metalloproteases. *Amino Acids,* (July); Available on: http://www.ncbi.nlm.nih.gov/pubmed/20640864

Kupai, K.; Szucs, G.; Cseh, S.; Hajdu, I.; Csonka C.; Csont, T. & Ferdinandy, P. (2010). Matrix metalloproteinase activity assays: Importance of zymography. *Journal of Pharmacological and Toxicological Methods,* Vol.61, No.2, (March-April), pp. 205-209, ISSN 1056-8719

Lawrence, D.M.; Singh, R.S.; Franklin, D.R.; Carey, D.J. & Elmore, J.R. (2004). Rapamycin suppresses experimental aortic aneurysm growth. *Journal of Vascular Surgery,* Vol.40, No.2, (August), pp.334-338, ISSN 0741-5214

Lederle, FA. & Taylor, B.C. (2006). ACE inhibitors and aortic rupture, *Lancet,* Vol.368, No.9547, (November), pp. 1571, ISSN 0140-6736

Lindeman, J.H.; Abdul-Hussien, H.; van Bockel, J.H.; Wolterbeek, R. & Kleemann, R. (2009). Clinical trial of doxycycline for matrix metalloproteinase-9 inhibition in patients with an abdominal aneurysm: Doxycycline selectively depletes aortic wall neutrophils and cytotoxic T cells. *Circulation,* Vol.119, No.16, (April), pp. 2209-2216, ISSN 0009-7322

Longo, G.M.; Xiong, W.; Greiner, T.C.; Zhao, Y.; Fiotti, N. & Baxter, B.T. (2002). Matrix metalloproteinases 2 and 9 work in concert to produce aortic aneurysms. *Journal of Clinical Investigation,* Vol.110, No.5, pp. 625-632, ISSN 0021-9738

Maskos, K. & Bode, W. (2003). Structural basis of matrix metalloproteinases and tissue inhibitors of metalloproteinases. *Molecular Biotechnology,* Vol.25, No.3, (November), pp. 241-266, ISSN 1073-6085

Medley, T.L.; Cole, T.J.; Dart, A.M.; Gatzka, C.D. & Kingwell, B.A. (2004). Matrix metalloproteinase-9 genotype influences large artery stiffness through effects on aortic gene and protein expression. *Arteriosclerioslerosis Thrombosis and Vascular Biology,* Vol.24, No8, (August), pp. 1479-1484, ISSN 1079-5642

Michel, J.B.; Martin-Ventura, J.L.; Egido, J.; Sakalihasan, N.; Treska, V.; Lindholt, J.; Allaire, E.; Thorsteinsdottir, U.; Cockerill, G. & Swedenborg, J. (2011). Novel aspects of the pathogenesis of aneurysms of the abdominal aorta in humans. *Cardiovascular Research,* Vol.90, No.1, pp. 18-27, ISSN 1755-3245

Miyake, T. & Morishita, R. (2009). Pharmacological treatment of abdominal aortic aneurysm. *Cardiovascular Research,* Vol.83, No.3, (August), pp. 436-443, ISSN 1755-3245

Mott, J. & Werb, Z. (2004). Regulation of matrix biology by matrix metalloproteinases. *Current Opinion in Cell Biology*. Vol.16, No.5, (October), pp. 558–564, ISSN 0955-0674

Nagashima, H.; Aoka, Y.; Sakomura, Y.; Sakuta, A.; Aomi, S.; Ishizuka, N.; Hagiwara, N.; Kawana, M. & Kasanuki, H. (2002). A 3-hydroxy-3-methylglutaryl coenzyme A reductase inhibitor, cerivastatin, suppresses production of matrix metalloproteinase-9 in human abdominal aortic aneurysm wall. *Journal of Vascular Surgery*, Vol.36, No.1, (July), pp. 158 –163, ISSN 0741-5214

Ogata, T.; Shibamura, H. & Tromp, G. (2005). Genetic analysis of polymorphisms in biologically relevant candidate genes in patients with abdominal aortic aneurysms. *Journal of Vascular Surgery*, Vol.41, No.6, (June), pp. 1036-1042, ISSN 0741-5214

Petersen, E.; Boman, J.; Wågberg, F. & Ängquist K.-A. (2002). Presence of *Chlamydia pneumoniae* in abdominal aortic aneurysms is not associated with increased activity of matrix metalloproteinases. *European Journal of Vascular and Endovascular Surgery*, Vol.24, No.4, (October), pp. 365-369, ISSN 1078-5884

Price, S.J.; Greaves, D.R. & Watkins, H. (2001). Identification of novel, functional genetic variants in the human matrix metalloproteinase-2 gene. *Journal of Biological Chemistry*, Vol.276, No.10, (March), pp. 7549-7558, ISSN 0021-9258

Raffetto, J.D. & Khalil, R.A. (2008). Matrix metalloproteinases and their inhibitors in vascular remodeling and vascular disease. *Biochemical Pharmacology*, Vol.75, No.2, (January), pp. 346-359, ISSN 006-2952

Rizas, K.D.; Ippagunta, N. & Tilson, M.D. 3rd. (2009). Immune cells and molecular mediators in the pathogenesis of the abdominal aortic aneurysm. *Cardiology Reviews*, Vol.17, No.5, (September-October), pp. 201-210, ISSN 1573-403x

Sandford, R.M.; Bown, M.J.; London, N.J. & Sayers, R.D. (2007). The genetic basis of abdominal aortic aneurysms: a review. *European Journal of Vascular and Endovascular Surgery*, Vol.33, No.4, (April), pp. 381-390, ISSN 1078-5884

Saratzis, A.; Abbas, A.; Kiskinis, D.; Melas, N.; Saratzis, N. & Kitas, G.D. (2011). Abdominal aortic aneurysm: a review of the genetic basis. *Angiology*, Vol.62, No.1, (January), pp. 18-32, ISSN 0003-3197

Sariahmetoglu, M.; Crawford, B.D.; Leon, H.; Sawicka, J.; Li, L.; Ballermann, B.J.; Holmes, C.; Berthiaume, L.G.; Holt, A.; Sawicki, G. & Schulz, R. (2007). Regulation of matrix metalloproteinase-2 (MMP-2) activity by phosphorylation *FASEB Journal*, Vol.21, No.10, (August), pp. 2486-2495, ISSN 1530-6860

Schouten, O.; van Laanen, J.H.; Boersma, E.; Vidakovic, R.; Feringa, H.H.; Dunkelgrun, M.; Bax, J.J.; Koning, J.; van Urk, H. & Poldermans, D. (2006). Statins are associated with a reduced infrarenal abdominal aortic aneurysm growth. *European Journal of Vascular and Endovascular Surgery*, Vol.32, No.1, (July), pp. 21–26, ISSN 1078-5884

Smallwood, L.; Allcock, R.; van Bockxmeer, F.; Warrington, N.; Palmer, L.J.; Iacopetta, B.; Golledge, J. & Norman, P.E. (2008). Polymorphisms of the matrix metalloproteinase 9 gene and abdominal aortic aneurysm. *British Journal of Surgery*, Vol.95, No.10, (October), pp. 1239-1244, ISSN 1365-2168

Suzuki, K.; Enghild, J.J.; Morodomi, T.; Salvesen, G. & Nagase H. (1990). Mechanisms of activation of tissue procollagenase by matrix metalloproteinase 3 (stromelysin). *Biochemistry,* Vol.29, No.44, (November), pp. 10261- 10270, ISSN 0006-2960

Sweeting, M.J.; Thompson, S.G.; Brown, L.C.; Greenhalgh, R.M. & Powell, J.T. (2010). Use of angiotensin converting enzyme inhibitors is associated with increased growth rate of abdominal aortic aneurysm. *Journal of Vascular Surgery,* Vol.52, No.1, (July), pp. 1-4, ISSN 0741-5214

Takagi, H.; Manabe, H.; Kawai, N.; Goto, S.N. & Umemoto, T. (2009). Circulating matrix metalloproteinase-9 concentrations and abdominal aortic aneurysm presence: a meta-analysis. *Interactive Cardiovascular and Thoracic Surgery,* Vol.9, No.3, (September), pp. 437-440, ISSN 1569-9293

Tsuruda, T.; Kato, J.; Hatakeyama, K.; Kojima, K.; Yano, M.; Yano, Y.; Nakamura, K.; Nakamura-Uchiyama, F.; Matsushima, Y.; Imamura, T.; Onitsuka, T.; Asada, Y.; Nawa, Y.; Eto, T. & Kitamura, T. (2008). Adventitial mast cells contribute to pathogenesis in the progression of abdominal aortic aneurysm. *Circulation Research,* Vol.102, No11, (June), pp. 1368-1377, ISSN 0009-7300

Vammen, S.; Lindholt, JS.; Ostergaard, L.; Fasting, H. & Henneberg, EW. (2001). Randomized double-blind controlled trial of roxithromycin for prevention of abdominal aortic aneurysm expansion. *British Journal of Surgery,* Vol.89, No.1 (January), pp. 1066 –1072, ISSN 1365-2168

Visse, R. & Nagase, H. (2003). Matrix Metalloproteinases and Tissue Inhibitors of Metalloproteinases. Structure, function, and biochemistry. *Circulation Research.* Vol.92, No.8, (May), pp. 827-839, ISSN 0009-7300

Wang, X.; Tromp, G.; Cole, C.W.; Verloes, A.; Sakalihasan, N.; Yoon, S. & Kuivaniemi, H. (1999). Analysis of coding sequences for tissue inhibitor of metalloproteinases 1 (TIMP1) and 2 (TIMP2) in patients with aneurysms. *Matrix Biology,* Vol.18, No.2, (April), pp. 121-124, ISSN 0945-053X

Yamada, H.; Saito, F.; Fukuta-Ohi, H.; Zhong, D.; Hase, A.; Arai, K.; Okuyama, A.; Maekawa, R.; Shimizu, T. & Matsumura, K. (2001). Processing of beta-dystroglycan by matrix metalloproteinase disrupts the link between the extracellular matrix and cell membrane via the dystroglycan complex. *Human Molecular Genetics,* Vol.10, No.15, (July), pp. 1563-1569, ISSN 0964-6906

Ye, S. (2006). Influence of matrix metalloproteinase genotype on cardiovascular disease susceptibility and outcome. *Cardiovascular Research,* Vol.69, No.3, (February), pp. 636–645, ISSN 1755-3245

Yoon, S.; Tromp, G.; Vongpunsawad, S.; Ronkainen, A.; Juvonen, T. & Kuivaniemi, H. (1999). Genetic analysis of MMP-3, MMP-9 and PAI-1 in Finnish patients with abdominal aortic or intracranial aneurysms. *Biochemical and Biophysical Research Communication,* Vol.265, No2, (November), pp. 563-568, ISSN 0006-291X

Yoshimura, K.; Aoki, H.; Ikeda, Y.; Fujii, K.; Akiyama, N.; Furutani, A.; Hoshii, Y.; Tanaka, N.; Ricci, R.; Ishihara, T.; Esato, K.; Hamano, K. & Matsuzaki, M. (2005). Regression of abdominal aortic aneurysm by inhibition of c-Jun N-terminal kinase. *Nature Medicine,* Vol.11, No.12, (December), pp. 1330-1338, ISSN 1078-8956

Zhao Y.G.; Xiao, A.Z.; Newcomer, R.G.; Park, H.I.; Kang, T.; Chung, L.W.; Swanson, M.G.; Zhau, H.E.; Kurhanewicz, J. & Sang Q.X. (2003). Activation of pro-gelatinase B by endometase/matrilysin-2 promotes invasion of human prostate cancer cells. *Journal of Biological Chemistry,* Vol.278, No.17, (April), pp. 15056-15064, ISSN 0021-9258

3

Mast Cell Density and Distribution in Human Abdominal Aortic Aneurysm

Sumiharu Sakamoto[1], Toshihiro Tsuruda[1], Kinta Hatakeyama[2], Yoko Sekita[1], Johji Kato[3], Takuroh Imamura[1], Yujiro Asada[2] and Kazuo Kitamura[1]
[1]Department of Internal Medicine, Circulatory and Body Fluid Regulation, Faculty of Medicine,
[2]Department of Pathology, Faculty of Medicine,
[3]Frontier Research Center, University of Miyazaki, Japan

1. Introduction

Atherosclerosis exhibits many inflammatory characteristics, in which macrophages and T-lymphocytes are found at the shoulder region of atherosclerotic plaque, and are associated with its rupture and thrombosis (Libby et al. 2010). On the other hand, abdominal aortic aneurysm (AAA) shows distinct histological features; inflammatory cell infiltration was observed predominantly at the outer media and adventitia (Michel et al. 2010). Several experimental studies have suggested important roles of inflammatory cells (macrophages, T-lymphocytes and neutrophils) in AAA development (Longo et al. 2002; Xiong et al. 2004; Eliason et al. 2005). Mast cell, unique effector components of the immune system, play a critical role in defending hosts against pathogens by releasing a number of immunoregulatory mediators (Marshall & Jawdat 2004). Mast cells synthesize a number of substances, which include histamine, heparin, tryptase, chymase, carboxypeptidase, cathepsin G, leukotriene C_4, prostaglandin D_2, tumor necrosis factor-α and interleukin (IL)-4,-5,-6,-13, some of which are stored in secretory vesicles (Krishnaswamy et al. 2006). Recently, mast cells have been recognized not only to be involved in host defense but also to initiate the inflammatory response by recruiting macrophages and T-lymphocytes (von Stebut et al. 2003; Henz et al. 2001) and by releasing pro-inflammatory cytokines, growth factors, angiogenic mediators and proteases (Krishnaswamy et al. 2006). Specifically, tryptase and chymase have been examined for their unique biological actions to modulate extracellular matrix formation and induce apoptosis of vascular smooth muscle cells (Cairns & Walls 1997; Leskinen et al. 2001; Tchougounova et al. 2005). In this chapter, we characterize mast cell density and distribution in the human aneurysmal abdominal aorta, compared with atherosclerotic abdominal aorta, and discuss the potential role of this type of cell to understand the pathophysiology of AAA.

2. Materials and methods

This study was approved by the Human Investigation Review Committee of the University of Miyazaki (No. 99) and conformed with the principles outlined in the Declaration of Helsinki (World Medical Association Declaration of Helsinki. 1997).

2.1 Human tissue preparation
Aneurysmal tissues were obtained from the anterior side of aortic walls of 60 Japanese suffering from AAA associated with atherosclerosis during elective repair surgery. AAA tissues were fixed in 10 % formalin or frozen in liquid nitrogen immediately after resection. Aortic tissues with various degrees of atherosclerosis were collected from the anterior side of the aorta at autopsy performed within 6 hours postmortem: 26, early stage atherosclerosis including diffuse intimal thickening or fatty streak; 30, advanced atherosclerosis formed by an extracellular lipid core (Stary et al. 1995). Hypertension was defined as a blood pressure >140/90 mm Hg or the need for antihypertensive medication. Diabetes mellitus was defined as fasting plasma glucose 126 mg/dL or higher and/or two-hour postprandial plasma glucose readings of 200 mg/dL or higher and/or the need for medicine in the medical records.

2.2 Immunohistochemistry
Single Staining: Aortic tissues fixed in 10% formalin were embedded in paraffin wax. The tissue sections (3 μm thick) were microwaved at 95 °C for one hour in 10 mmol/L citrate buffer (pH 6.0) to stain mast cell tryptase, prior to incubation with the primary antibody. The sections were incubated at 4 °C overnight with the monoclonal antibody against tryptase (80 μg/mL, Clone AA1; DAKOcytomation), followed by incubation with horseradish peroxidase-labeled polymer conjugated secondary antibody (Dako Envision+ System) for 30 min at room temperature. Immunoreactivity was visualized with 3,3'-diaminobenzidine (Dako), counterstained with Mayer's hematoxylin. For IL-4 staining, frozen sections of AAA tissues were fixed in acetone and incubated with the monoclonal antibody against human IL-4 (10 μg/mL, clone 3007.11; R&D Systems, Inc.).
Double Staining: To identify the phenotype of mast cells in aortic tissues, double staining was performed using a Histofine kit (Nichirei, Tokyo, Japan) according to the manufacturer's instructions. In double staining of tryptase (80 μg/mL, Clone AA1; DAKOcytomation) and chymase (1:100, Clone CC1; abcam), enzymatic activity of alkaline phosphatase for tryptase was visualized with new fuchsin in red (New Fuchsin Kit; Nichirei) and for chymase with 3, 3', 5, 5'-tetramethylbenzidine in blue (TMB substrate kit; Vector Laboratories).

2.3 Morphometric analysis
Mast cell numbers in at least 10 microscopic fields were counted at a magnification of x400 and expressed as a density (cells per mm^2) in the intima, outer media and adventitia of early (diffuse intimal thickening and fatty streak), advanced atherosclerotic abdominal aorta and AAA. In counting the cell number, the intima was defined as the region of the arterial wall from the endothelial surface to the luminal margin of the media;(Stary et al. 1992) however, the internal elastic lamina becomes unclear or absent in the advanced atherosclerotic aorta, so we counted mast cells located on the luminal side of atheromatous plaques. On the other hand, the adventitia was defined as the area outside the external elastic lamina and inside the border of inner dense and outer loose connective tissues, and the number of cells in the outer media and adventitia was combined because the external elastic lamina was mostly unclear in AAA specimens. Capillary vessel number positive for CD34 antigen was also evaluated in the outer media and adventitia, and was expressed as a density (/mm^2).

2.4 Western blot
Denatured protein extract (30 μg) from the AAA and non-dilated atherosclerotic aorta was subjected to sodium dodecyl sulfate-polyacrylamide gel as described (Tsuruda et al. 2008).

The separated proteins electrically transferred onto polyvinylidene difluoride (PVDF) membranes were incubated with anti-mouse monoclonal IL -4 antibody (2 μg/mL, clone 3007.11; R&D Systems, Inc.), followed by incubation with horseradish peroxidase-coupled second antibody. Immunoreactive bands were visualized by the ECL Plus detection kit (Amersham), and intensities of the bands were analyzed densitometrically (Chemi Doc™ Documentation System; BIO-RAD).

3. Statistical analysis

All data were analyzed with JMP 7.0.1 and GraphPad prism 5. Comparisons between groups were assessed with the chi-square test or Kruskal-Wallis test, and the mast cell density and capillary number were correlated with the Spearman rank correlation coefficient test. Protein expression between the two groups was analyzed with Student's t-test. The data are expressed as the mean ± SEM or as the median with the quartile range, 1.5 interquartile and outlying values. Statistical significance was accepted at $p<0.05$.

4. Results

4.1 Patients' characteristics

Clinical parameters of the patients enrolled in this study are shown in the Table 1. The advanced atherosclerosis and AAA groups were significantly older than the early stage atherosclerosis group, but there was no difference in age between AAA patients and those with advanced atherosclerosis. The AAA group showed a significantly higher rate of hypertension than the early or advanced atherosclerosis group, whereas the ratio of diabetes mellitus was equivalent in advanced atherosclerosis and AAA groups.

	Early (n=26)	Advanced (n=30)	Aneurysm (n=60)
Age	40±4	77±2 **	76±1 **
Sex (M/F)	19 / 7	24 / 6	46 / 14
Smoking (%)	34.6	53.3	66.7
Hypertension (%)	6.7	63.3	90.0 ** ##
Diabetes mellitus (%)	7.7	13.3	11.7 *

Table 1. Patients' characteristics. Data are expressed as the mean ±SEM. *$p<0.01$, **$p<0.0001$ vs. early stage of atherosclerosis, ##$p<0.0001$ vs. advanced atherosclerosis

4.2 Mast cell density in atherosclerotic abdominal aorta and AAA

Figure 1 shows representative pictures of tryptase-positive mast cells at the intima and outer media and adventitia of early atherosclerosis (diffuse intimal thickening, DIT), advanced atherosclerosis and AAA. As shown in Figure 2A, the density of mast cells at the intima tended to decrease according to the degree of atherosclerosis, and was further diminished in AAA. On the other hand, the cell number significantly increased at the outer media and adventitia of the AAA group, compared with those in the early or advanced atherosclerotic aorta (Figure 2B).

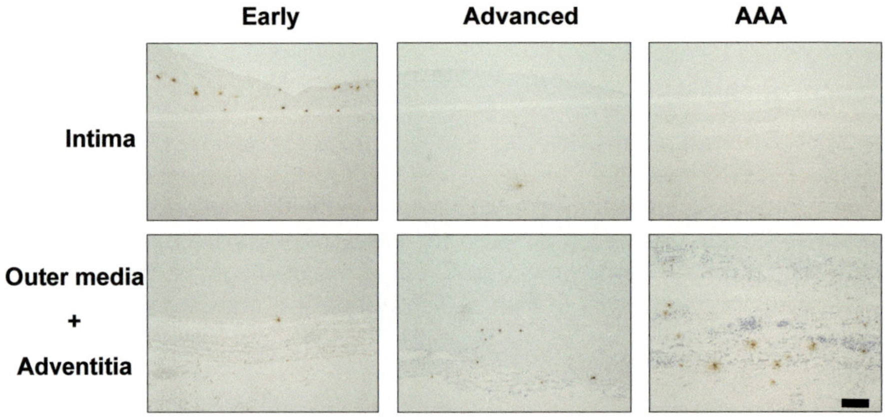

Fig. 1. Representative pictures of tryptase-positive mast cells at intima and outer media and adventitia of early atherosclerosis (diffuse intimal thickening, DIT), advanced atherosclerosis and AAA. Scale bar, 200 μm.

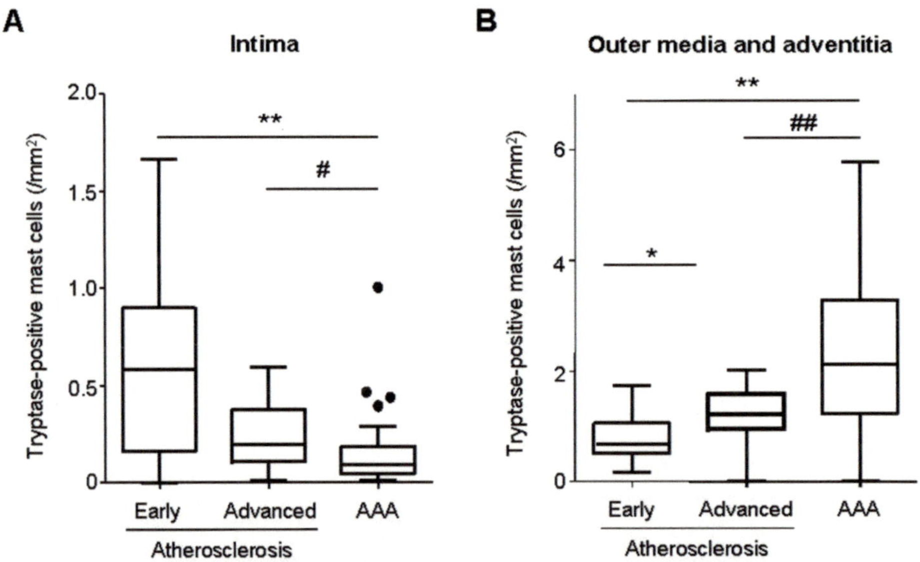

Fig. 2. Mast cell density in early or advanced atherosclerosis and AAA. Number of tryptase-positive mast cells was counted at intima **(A)** and outer media and adventitia **(B)**, respectively in early (n=26) or advanced (n=30) atherosclerosis and AAA (n=60). Data are expressed as the median with the quartile range, 1.5 interquartile and outlying values. *p<0.05, **p<0.01 vs. early stage atherosclerosis, #p<0.05, ##p<0.01 vs. advanced atherosclerosis.

4.3 Phenotype of mast cells in AAA

Figure 3A-C illustrate the representative pictures of the mast cell phenotype in the AAA specimens. As shown in Figure 3D, most of the mast cells distributed at the outer media and adventitia of AAA were positive both for tryptase and chymase (97.9%), while the remainder of the mast cell subtypes, tryptase-positive/chymase-negative (0.27%) or tryptase-negative/chymase-positive (1.9%) were a minor population. The proportion of mast cell phenotypes was similar in early or advanced atherosclerotic aortae.

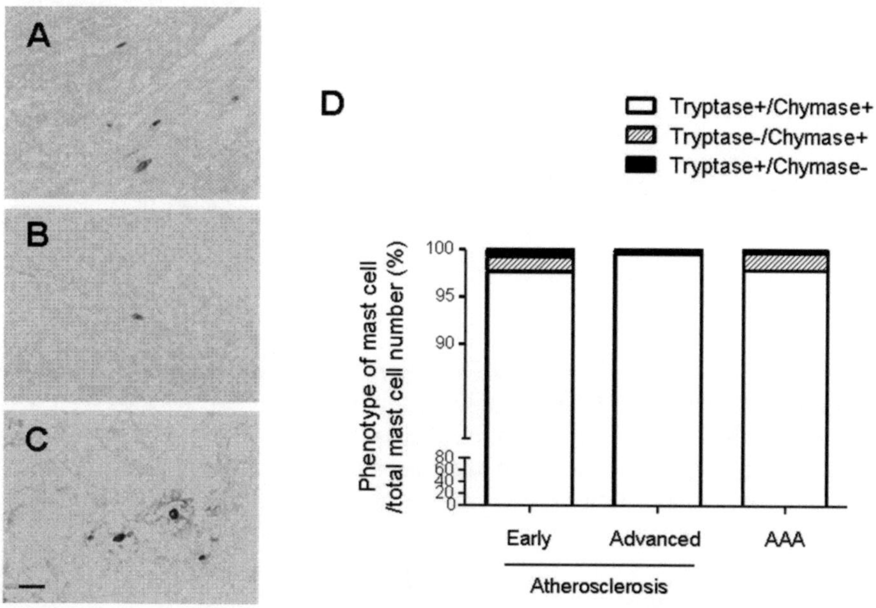

Fig. 3. Phenotype of mast cells in early or advanced atherosclerosis and AAA. Representative pictures of tryptase-positive/chymase-negative **(A)**, tryptase-negative/chymase-positive **(B)** and tryptase-positive/chymase-positive mast cells **(C)**. Scale bar, 20 µm. **D,** Percentage of mast cell phenotype in early (n=10) or advanced (n=5) atherosclerosis and AAA (n=26).

4.4 Expression and distribution of IL-4 in AAA

Figure 4A illustrates that the protein expression of IL-4 was significantly increased in AAA compared to the atherosclerotic aorta. The immunoreactivity of IL-4 was widely distributed in the endothelial cells of microvessels and fibroblast-like cells at the outer media and adventitia of AAA (Figure 4B).

4.5 Correlation between numbers of capillary vessel and mast cell

Figure 5A shows that the number of capillary vessels distributed at the outer media and adventitia (so called "vasa vasorum") was significantly increased in the advanced atherosclerotic aorta group compared with the early stage of atherosclerosis; however, the number did not change significantly between advanced atherosclerosis and AAA. As shown in Figure 5B, mast cell density correlated with the capillary vessel number at the outer media and adventitia of all cases (n=116, r=0.349, p=0.0001).

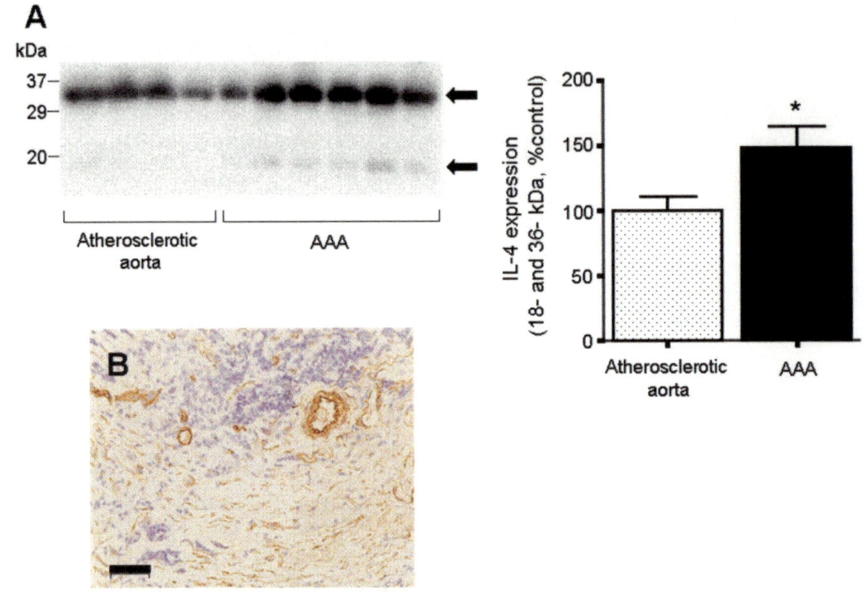

Fig. 4. Protein expression of IL-4 and its distribution in AAA specimen. **A,** Western blot for IL-4 in non-dilated atherosclerotic aorta (n=5) and AAA (n=6). Arrows indicate the mono-form (18 kDa) and dimer (36 kDa) of IL-4, respectively. The two forms of IL-4 expression were combined to present the data. Data are expressed as the mean ± SEM. *p<0.05 vs. non-dilated atherosclerosis. **B,** Immunolocalization of IL-4 in AAA. Scale bar, 50 μm.

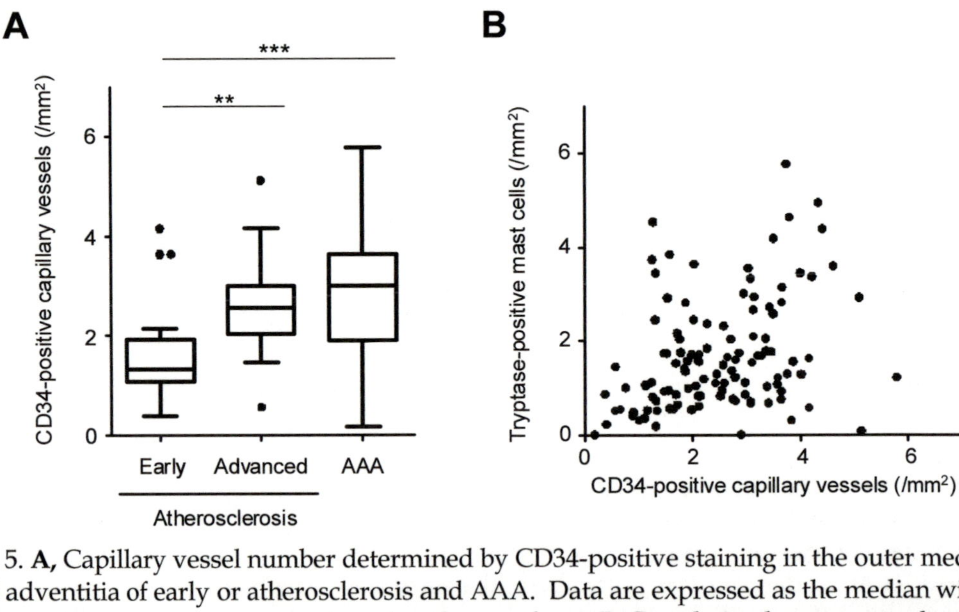

Fig. 5. **A,** Capillary vessel number determined by CD34-positive staining in the outer media and adventitia of early or atherosclerosis and AAA. Data are expressed as the median with the quartile range, 1.5 interquartile and outlying values. **B,** Correlation between numbers of mast cells and capillary vessels in the outer media and adventitia in early or advanced atherosclerosis and AAA (n=116, r=0.3494, p=0.0001).

5. Discussion

Up to 8 % of men older than 65 years harbor AAA, and it is associated with several risk factors, such as smoking and hypertension (Nordon et al. 2010). AAA progresses asymptomatically and patients with AAA eventually die due to rupture. At the tissue level, inadequate remodeling of the extracellular matrix in aortic walls appears to be involved in the development, progression or rupture of AAA (Kadoglou & Liapis 2004; Choke et al. 2005; Longo et al. 2002; Xiong et al. 2004; Daugherty & Cassis 2004; Brown & Powell 1999; Singh et al. 2001; Freestone et al. 1995); however, to date, the underlying mechanism is not fully understood and there is no effective pharmacological therapy to inhibit/reverse enlargement of the aneurysmal aorta in humans. The immune system is assumed to participate because of the inflammatory infiltration of macrophages and T lymphocytes that can produce enzymes degrading the extracellular matrix at the outer media and adventitia of human and experimental AAA (Longo et al. 2002; Ocana et al. 2003; Xiong et al. 2004).

As a component of the immune system, mast cells are widely distributed throughout the body and have an important role in defending hosts against pathogens. In the cardiovascular tissues, this type of cell is present at the intima of normal/fatty streak (Kaartinen et al. 1994), whereas it is more prominent at the adventitia of atherosclerotic aorta (Atkinson et al. 1994) and in the vulnerable plaques of atherosclerotic coronary and carotid arteries (Kaartinen et al. 1998; Jeziorska et al. 1997). Our data support a previous study (Kaartinen et al. 1994) which shows that mast cells at the intima decreased according to the degree of atherosclerosis, assuming that a loss of endogenous heparin production by mast cells stimulates pro-coagulant activity on atherosclerotic plaques. More importantly, we demonstrated that the cell number was significantly increased at the outer media and adventitia of AAA, compared with either the early or advanced stage of atherosclerosis. The proportion of activated mast cells (seen as "degranulation") has been reported to be frequently observed in the adventitia of AAA compared to in advanced atherosclerosis (15±2 % vs. 0.4±0.3% total number of mast cells) (Tsuruda et al. 2008). Thus, mast cells distributed "outside of aortic wall" appear to be associated with the AAA pathogenesis.

Mast cells mature with tissue-specific phenotypes from circulating multipotent haematopoietic progenitor cells in response to signals communicated by quiescent microvascular environment cells where they become resident (Krishnaswamy et al. 2006). Stem cell factor (SCF), a ligand for the proto-oncogene c-kit, is widely produced in various types of cells, such as fibroblasts (Nocka et al. 1990), endothelial cells and stromal cells (Heinrich et al. 1993), and is the main factor for the growth and differentiation of mast cells (Zsebo et al. 1990). Circulating mast cell precursor has been reported to mature in tissues by SCF (Zsebo et al. 1990) and other cytokines such as IL-4 (Conti et al. 2003; Yanagida et al. 1995). In accordance with the report (de Paulis et al. 1999), we have shown that the immunoreactivity of SCF was detected in the cytoplasm of mast cells (Tsuruda et al. 2008), suggesting autocrine or paracrine regulation of differentiation and maturation of cells in aortic tissues. Schönbeck et al. (2002) showed the augmented expressions of IL-4 and IL-10 in inflammatory cells of AAA tissues. Importantly, these cytokines enhanced the growth-promoting effect of SCF on mast cells (Conti et al. 2003; Yanagida et al. 1995), and we further demonstrated that IL-4 was widely present in the endothelial cells of microvessels and fibroblast-like cells in AAA specimens. In contrast, we could not detect IL-10 expression in AAA tissues in this study (data not shown). It seems likely that mast cells can mature or differentiate in the aneurysmal aortic wall, at least partly through SCF and IL-4 stimulation.

Human mast cells exhibit tissue-specific functional heterogeneity; they are divided conventionally into two different phenotypes depending on the proteases in their secretory vesicles. In this study, the majority of mast cells distributed at the outer media and adventitia of AAA were positive both for tryptase and chymase. One of the histopathological features of AAA is the degeneration of the media by apoptosis of smooth muscle cells (Lopez-Candales et al. 1997) and fragmentation of elastic fibers digested by matrix metalloproteinase (MMP) (Baxter et al. 1994), resulting in loss of integrity to maintain the architecture of the aortic wall. Mast cell tryptase stimulates fibroblast proliferation (Cairns & Walls 1997) as well as MMP-1,-3 activation (Johnson et al. 1998). On the other hand, mast cell chymase may have a wide range of actions in AAA tissues: induction of apoptosis of smooth muscle cells (Leskinen et al. 2001), conversion of angiotensin I to angiotensin II (Takai et al. 1999) and of pro-MMP-2 and -9 to the mature forms (Tchougounova et al. 2005), whereas mast cells themselves are found to express MMPs-2 and 9 (Fang et al. 1999). We have reported that interferon-γ produced from mast cells stimulated MMP-9 synthesis by macrophages in the co-culture (Tsuruda et al. 2008). Angiogenesis appears to be another important histopathological characteristic of AAA (Paik et al. 2004; Reeps et al. 2009). Mast cells are capable of synthesizing factors associated with angiogenesis (Hiromatsu & Toda 2003), and indeed, are often positioned around capillary vessels. We found a positive correlation between mast cell density and capillary number at the adventitial layer, speculating that mast cells might contribute to initiate the inflammatory response by stimulating the growth of the vasa vasorum, and thereby recruit macrophages and T-lymphocytes from outside the aortic wall (Satta et al. 1998; Reeps et al. 2009). However, it remains to be elucidated whether angiogenesis itself is relevant to AAA development, because the vessel number was statistically insignificant between AAA and advanced atherosclerosis in this study. Based upon the observation in human tissues, we propose that mast cells infiltrating at the outer media and adventitia of the AAA wall contribute to the development or progression of aneurysm formation, coordinating with other inflammatory cells. Furthermore, the inhibition of mast cell accumulation, maturation and activation in the aortic wall with a mast cell stabilizer would be a potential pharmacological target for preventing/attenuating the development of AAA (Tsuruda et al. 2008; Sun et al. 2007).

6. Conclusion

Mast cells are predominantly present at the outer media and adventitia, and are susceptible to maturation/activation by interaction with cytokines in AAA tissues. In addition, the mediators expressed by mast cells and neovascularization might contribute to enhance the inflammatory response in AAA. These results underline the pathophysiological role of this type of immune cell in the development/progression of aneurysm formation.

7. Acknowledgements

We are greatly indebted to Ms. Ritsuko Sotomura for her expert technical assistance. This study was supported by grants-in-aid for Scientific Research (C) (20590830) from the Ministry of Education, Culture, Sport, Science and Technology, Japan; grants-in-aids for the Japan Cardiovascular Research Foundation; Mitsubishi Pharma Research Foundation; Takeda Science Foundation.

8. References

Atkinson, J.B., Harlan, C.W., Harlan, G.C., & Virmani R. (1994). The association of mast cells and atherosclerosis: a morphologic study of early atherosclerotic lesions in young people. *Hum Pathol* 25 (2):154-159.

Baxter, B.T., Davis, V.A., Minion, D.J., Wang, Y.P., Lynch, T.G., & McManus, B.M. (1994). Abdominal aortic aneurysms are associated with altered matrix proteins of the nonaneurysmal aortic segments. *J Vasc Surg* 19 (5):797-802.

Brown, L.C., & Powell, J.T. (1999). Risk factors for aneurysm rupture in patients kept under ultrasound surveillance. UK Small Aneurysm Trial Participants. *Ann Surg* 230 (3):296-297.

Cairns, J.A., & Walls, A.F. (1997). Mast cell tryptase stimulates the synthesis of type I collagen in human lung fibroblasts. *J Clin Invest* 99 (6):1313-1321.

Choke, E., Cockerill, G., Wilson, W.R., Sayed, S., Dawson, J., Loftus, I., & Thompson, M.M. (2005). A review of biological factors implicated in abdominal aortic aneurysm rupture. *Eur J Vasc Endovasc Surg* 30 (3):227-244.

Conti, P., Kempuraj, D., Kandere, K., Di Gioacchino, M., Barbacane, R.C., Castellani, M.L., Felaco, M., Boucher, W., Letourneau, R., & Theoharides, T.C. (2003). IL-10, an inflammatory/inhibitory cytokine, but not always. *Immunol Lett.* 86 (2):123-129.

Daugherty, A., & Cassis, L.A. (2004). Mouse models of abdominal aortic aneurysms. *Arterioscler Thromb Vasc Biol* 24 (3):429-434.

de Paulis, A., Minopoli, G., Arbustini, E., de Crescenzo, G., Dal Piaz, F., Pucci, P., Russo, T., &. Marone, G. (1999). Stem cell factor is localized in, released from, and cleaved by human mast cells. *J Immunol* 163 (5):2799-2808.

Eliason, J.L., Hannawa, K.K., Ailawadi, G., Sinha, I., Ford, J.W., Deogracias, M.P., Roelofs, K.J., Woodrum, D.T., Ennis, T.L., Henke, P.K., Stanley, J.C., Thompson, R.W., & Upchurch, G.R. Jr. (2005). Neutrophil depletion inhibits experimental abdominal aortic aneurysm formation. *Circulation* 112 (2):232-240.

Fang, K.C., Wolters, P.J., Steinhoff, M., Bidgol, A., Blount, J.L., & Caughey, G.H. (1999). Mast cell expression of gelatinases A and B is regulated by kit ligand and TGF-β. *J Immunol* 162 (9):5528-5535.

Freestone, T., Turner, R.J., Coady, A., Higman, D.J., Greenhalgh, R.M., & Powell. J.T. (1995). Inflammation and matrix metalloproteinases in the enlarging abdominal aortic aneurysm. *Arterioscler Thromb Vasc Biol* 15 (8):1145-1151.

Heinrich, M.C., Dooley, D.C., Freed, A.C., Band, L., Hoatlin, M.E., Keeble, W.W., Peters, S.T., Silvey, K.V., Ey, F.S., Kabat, D., Maziarz, R.T. &. Bagby, G.C. Jr. (1993). Constitutive expression of steel factor gene by human stromal cells. *Blood* 82 (3):771-783.

Henz, B.M., Maurer, M. Lippert, U. Worm, M. & Babina, M. (2001). Mast cells as initiators of immunity and host defense. *Exp Dermatol* 10 (1):1-10.

Hiromatsu, Y., & Toda, S. (2003). Mast cells and angiogenesis. *Microsc Res Tech* 60 (1):64-69.

Jeziorska, M., McCollum, C. & Woolley, D.E. (1997). Mast cell distribution, activation, and phenotype in atherosclerotic lesions of human carotid arteries. *J Pathol* 182 (1):115-122.

Johnson, J.L., Jackson, C.L., Angelini, G.D., & George, S.J. (1998). Activation of matrix-degrading metalloproteinases by mast cell proteases in atherosclerotic plaques. *Arterioscler Thromb Vasc Biol* 18 (11):1707-1715.

Kaartinen, M., Penttilä, A., & Kovanen, P.T. (1994). Mast cells of two types differing in neutral protease composition in the human aortic intima. Demonstration of tryptase- and tryptase/chymase-containing mast cells in normal intimas, fatty streaks, and the shoulder region of atheromas. *Arterioscler Thromb* 14 (6):966-972.

Kaartinen, M., van der Wal, A.C., van der Loos, C.M., Piek, J.J., Koch, K.T., Becker, A.E., & Kovanen, P.T. (1998). Mast cell infiltration in acute coronary syndromes: implications for plaque rupture. *J Am Coll Cardiol* 32 (3):606-612.

Kadoglou, N.P., & Liapis, C.D. (2004). Matrix metalloproteinases: contribution to pathogenesis, diagnosis, surveillance and treatment of abdominal aortic aneurysms. *Curr Med Res Opin* 20 (4):419-432.

Krishnaswamy, G., Ajitawi, O., & Chi, D.S. (2006). The human mast cell: an overview. *Methods Mol Biol* 315:13-34.

Leskinen, M., Wang, Y., Leszczynski, D., Lindstedt, K.A., & Kovanen, P.T. (2001). Mast cell chymase induces apoptosis of vascular smooth muscle cells. *Arterioscler Thromb Vasc Biol* 21 (4):516-522.

Libby, P., Okamoto, Y., Rocha, V.Z., & Folco, E. (2010). Inflammation in atherosclerosis: transition from theory to practice. *Circ J* 74 (2):213-220.

Longo, G.M., Xiong, W., Greiner, T.C., Zhao, Y., Fiotti, N., & Baxter, B.T. (2002). Matrix metalloproteinases 2 and 9 work in concert to produce aortic aneurysms. *J Clin Invest* 110 (5):625-632.

Lopez-Candales, A., Holmes, D.R., Liao, S., Scott, M.J., Wickline, S.A., & Thompson, R.W. (1997). Decreased vascular smooth muscle cell density in medial degeneration of human abdominal aortic aneurysms. *Am J Pathol* 150 (3):993-1007.

Marshall, J.S., & Jawdat, D.M. 2004. Mast cells in innate immunity. *J Allergy Clin Immunol* 114 (1):21-27.

Michel, J.B., Martin-Ventura, J.L., Egido, J., Sakalihasan, N., Treska, V., Lindholt, J., Allaire, E., Thorsteinsdottir, U., Cockerill, G., & Swedenborg, J. (2010). Novel aspects of the pathogenesis of aneurysms of the abdominal aorta in humans. *Cardiovasc Res* [Epub ahead of print].

Nocka, K., Buck, J., Levi, E., & Besmer, P. (1990). Candidate ligand for the c-kit transmembrane kinase receptor: KL, a fibroblast derived growth factor stimulates mast cells and erythroid progenitors. *EMBO J* 9 (10):3287-3294.

Nordon, I.M., Hinchliffe, R.J., Loftus, I.M., & Thompson, M.M. (2011). Pathophysiology and epidemiology of abdominal aortic aneurysms. *Nat Rev Cardiol* 8(2):92-102.

Ocana, E., Bohórquezb, JC., Pérez-Requenac, J., Brieva, J.A., & Rodríguez, C. (2003). Characterisation of T and B lymphocytes infiltrating abdominal aortic aneurysms. *Atherosclerosis* 170 (1):39-48.

Paik, D.C., Fu, C., Bhattacharya, J., & Tilson, M.D. (2004). Ongoing angiogenesis in blood vessels of the abdominal aortic aneurysm. *Exp Mol Med* 36 (6):524-533.

Reeps, C., Pelisek, J., Seidl, S., Schuster, T., Zimmermann, A., Kuehnl, A., & Eckstein, H.H. (2009). Inflammatory infiltrates and neovessels are relevant sources of MMPs in abdominal aortic aneurysm wall. *Pathobiology* 76 (5):243-252.

Satta, J., Soini, Y., Mosorin, M., & Juvonen, J. (1998). Angiogenesis is associated with mononuclear inflammatory cells in abdominal aortic aneurysms. *Ann Chir Gynaecol* 87 (1):40-42.

Schönbeck, U., Sukhova, G.K., Gerdes, N., & Libby, P. (2002). T_H2 predominant immune responses prevail in human abdominal aortic aneurysm. *Am J Pathol* 161 (2):499-506.

Singh, K., Bønaa, K.H., Jacobsen, B.K., Bjørk, L., & Solberg, S. (2001). Prevalence of and risk factors for abdominal aortic aneurysms in a population-based study. The Tromsø Study. *Am. J. Epidemiol.* 154 (3):236-244.

Stary, H.C., Blankenhorn, D.H., Chandler, A.B., Glagov, S., Insull, W, Jr., Richardson, M., Rosenfeld, M.E., Schaffer, S.A., Schwartz, C.J., Wagner, W.D., & Wissler, R.W. (1992). A definition of the intima of human arteries and of its atherosclerosis-prone regions. A report from the Committee on Vascular Lesions of the Council on Arteriosclerosis, American Heart Association. *Circulation* 85 (1):391-405.

Stary, H.C., Chandler, A.B., Dinsmore, R.E., Fuster, V., Glagov, S., Insull, W, Jr., Rosenfeld, M.E., Schwartz, C.J., Wagner, W.D., & Wissler, R.W. (1995). A definition of advanced types of atherosclerotic lesions and a histological classification of atherosclerosis. A report from the Committee on Vascular Lesions of the Council on Arteriosclerosis, American Heart Association. *Circulation* 92 (5):1355-1374.

Sun, J., Sukhova, G.K., Yang, M., Wolters, P.J., Macfarlane, L.A., Libby, P., Sun, C., Zhang, Y., Liu, J., Ennis, T.L., Knispel, R., Xiong, W., Thompson, R.W., Baxter, B.T., & Shi, G.P. (2007). Mast cells modulate the pathogenesis of elastase-induced abdominal aortic aneurysms in mice. *J Clin Invest* 117 (11):3359-3368.

Takai, S., Jin, D., Sakaguchi, M., & Miyazaki, M. (1999). Chymase-dependent angiotensin II formation in human vascular tissue. *Circulation* 100 (6):654-658.

Tchougounova, E., Lundequist, A., Fajardo, I., Winberg, J.O., Abrink, M., & Pejler, G. (2005). A key role for mast cell chymase in the activation of pro-matrix metalloprotease-9 and pro-matrix metalloprotease-2. *J Biol Chem* 280 (10):9291-9296.

Tsuruda, T., Kato, J., Hatakeyama, K., Kojima, K., Yano, M., Yano, Y., Nakamura, K., Nakamura-Uchiyama, F., Matsushima, Y., Imamura, T., Onitsuka, T., Asada, Y., Nawa, Y., Eto, T., & Kitamura, K. (2008). Adventitial mast cells contribute to pathogenesis in the progression of abdominal aortic aneurysm. *Circ Res* 102 (11):1368-1377.

World Medical Association Declaration of Helsinki (1997). Recommendations guiding physicians in biomedical research involving human subjects. *Cardiovasc Res* 35(1):2-3.

von Stebut, E., Metz, M., Milon, G., Knop, J., & Maurer, M. (2003). Early macrophage influx to sites of cutaneous granuloma formation is dependent MIP-1α/β released from neutrophils recruited by mast cell-derived TNFα. *Blood* 101 (1):210-215.

Xiong, W., Zhao, Y., Prall, A., Greiner, T.C., & Baxter, B.T. (2004). Key roles of $CD4^+$ T cells and IFN-γ in the development of abdominal aortic aneurysms in a murine model. *J Immunol* 172 (4):2607-2612.

Yanagida, M., Fukamachi, H., Ohgami, K., Kuwaki, T., Ishii, H., Uzumaki, H., Amano, K., Tokiwa, T., Mitsui, H., Saito, H., Iikura, Y., Ishizaka, T., & Nakahata, T. (1995). Effects of T-helper 2-type cytokines, interleukin-3 (IL-3), IL-4, IL-5, and IL-6 on the survival of cultured human mast cells. *Blood* 86 (10):3705-3714.

Zsebo, K.M., Williams, D.A., Geissler, E.N., Broudy, V.C., Martin, F.H., Atkins, H.L., Hsu, R.Y., Birkett, N.C., Okino, K.H., & Murdock, D.C. (1990). Stem cell factor is encoded at the Sl locus of the mouse and is the ligand for the c-kit tyrosine kinase receptor. *Cell* 63 (1):213-224.

4

The Role of Complement in the Pathogenesis of Artery Aneurysms

Fengming Liu[1], Annie Qin[2], Lining Zhang[1] and Xuebin Qin[3,4]
[1]*Department of Immunology, Shandong University School of Medicine, Shandong,*
[2]*Department of Life Sciences, Harvard College, Cambridge,*
[3]*Laboratory for Translational Research, Harvard Medical School, Cambridge,*
[4]*Department of Medicine, Brigham and Women's Hospital,*
Harvard Medical School, Boston,
[1]*PR China*
[2,3,4]*USA*

1. Introduction

Aneurysm is an abnormal widening or ballooning of a portion of an artery due to weakness in the wall of the blood vessel. Although venous aneurysms do occur, arterial aneurysms are much more common and severe than venous aneurysms. Aneurysmal degeneration of the abdominal aortic and iliac arteries is a common and frequently lethal age-related disease process (Baxter et al., 2008; Weintraub, 2009). Arterial aneurysm is a potentially lethal vascular disorder, much more common in older men with estimates of prevalence ranging up to 10 percent (Thompson et al., 2002). Death from a ruptured aneurysm accounts for about 1 percent of all the deaths in the Western world (Collin et al., 1988). Extensive evidence indicates that mediators of immunity and inflammation participate in the development of aneurysm formation (Duftner et al., 2006; Shimizu et al., 2006). However, the pathogenesis of the aneurysm formation and rupture remains unclear. Recent results obtained from clinical and experimental studies suggest that complement, an important mediator for immune and inflammatory responses may contribute to the pathogenesis of artery aneurysms. Here, we will extensively review the potential roles of complement in artery aneurysm formation and rupture.

2. Artery aneurysms

Artery aneurysms such as aortic, cerebral and ventricular aneurysms develop as a result of weakening of the vascular wall in response to the initiation of a complex extracellular matrix remodeling process that culminates in alterations in artery compliance and resilience (Powell and Greenhalgh, 1989; Schneiderman et al., 1995). Aortic aneurysm is located within the wall of the aorta. Typically, the widened part of the aorta is considered to be an aneurysm when it is more than 1.5 times its normal size. Cerebral aneurysm, also known as a berry aneurysm, occurs in the wall of a blood vessel in the brain. Ventricular aneurysm is a ballooning out of part of the wall of the heart. Most aneurysms are asymptomatic and undiagnosed and the rupture of aneurysms is associated with a systemic inflammatory

response and multiple organ dysfunctions, which remain a primary cause of death in patients who survive the initial surgery (Harkin et al., 2004). Aneurysm rupture has an overall mortality rate of 80–90 percent, and an operative mortality rate of 50 percent. Other than relatively high risk and costly open surgical repair, few interventional modalities are available to treat patients with AAA (Baxter et al., 2008; Krishna et al., 2010). This mainly stems from little understanding of the underlying mechanism of aortic aneurysms. Therefore, better understanding of the pathogenesis of artery aneurysms and developing more effective therapies for the treatment and prevention of artery aneurysms is imperative.
Extensive evidence indicates that the mediators of immunity and inflammation participate in the development of aneurysm formation (Duftner et al., 2006; Shimizu et al., 2006). The aneurysm is characterized by chronic adventitial and medial inflammatory cell infiltration, extracellular matrix degeneration, and apoptosis of smooth muscle cells, which lead to vessel wall weakening, aortic dilatation and aneurysm formation (Jagadesham et al., 2008). Inflammatory cells accumulate in aortic aneurysm lesions with a predominance of CD4+ T ,B cells and macrophage, which secrete various inflammatory factors, including cytokines, chemokines, leukotrienes, reactive oxygen species, and immunoglobulins, contributing to the immune response in aneurysm lesions (Shimizu et al., 2006). Macrophages promote aneurysm development by secreting collagenases and elastases, which could degrade elastic lamellae and extracellular matrix (ECM) proteins, constituting the underlying characteristics of the aneurysm (Kadoglou and Liapis, 2004). Consistently, extensive evidence indicates that MMP2 and MMP9 play critical roles in the pathogenesis of artery aneurysms, and macrophages are the primary source of MMP-9 production in human and mouse aneurysm tissues (Longo et al., 2002; Thompson et al., 1995). The excessive local production of the matrix metalloproteinases (MMPs), which are mainly secreted from macrophages, results in the damaging of smooth muscle cells (SMC) and thinning of the artery wall (Allaire et al., 1998; Caird et al., 2006; Eliason et al., 2005; Hannawa et al., 2009; Newman et al., 1994; Palombo et al., 1999; Tanaka et al., 1995). Moreover, the development of aneurysms is suppressed by pharmacologic inhibition of MMPs, such as the use of tetracycline derivatives, or genetic alterations that eliminate the expression of either MMP 9 or MMP 2 (Curci et al., 2000; Mosorin et al., 2001; Pyo et al., 2000). Elastolytic cysteine proteases, including cathepsin, also play a critical role in the development of aneurysms (Shi et al., 1999). In addition, endothelial and smooth muscle cells in aneurysm lesions may release an array of growth factors and cytokoines to attract inflammatory cells recruitment, which contributes to aneurysm development (Nicholson-Weller and Halperin, 1993). Nevertheless, the exact underlying mechanism and cause of aneurysms are unclear. The risk factors for aneurysms include advanced age, male gender, smoking, hypertension, diabetes, obesity, high cholesterol, genetic predisposition, and atherosclerosis (Wassef et al., 2007). Among these factors, the most common culprits are atherosclerosis and high blood pressure (Daugherty and Cassis, 2004; Wassef et al., 2007). Most of the abdominal aortic aneurysms (AAA) in humans are associated with atherosclerosis (Daugherty and Cassis, 2004; Wassef et al., 2007).
Although both atherosclerosis and aneurysm are immune and inflammatory diseases, they have different pathogeneses. The hallmark pathologic feature of atherosclerosis is foam-cell formation, whereas aneurysms are typified by intense oxidative stress, inflammation, matrix degradation, and apoptosis of smooth-muscle cells (Miller et al., 2002; Weintraub, 2009). In aneurysm development, first, inflammatory leukocytes play an important role in the degradation of elastin and collagen in the vessel wall. Subsequent dilation of the vessel will trigger the vascular cells to remodel and repair to prevent vessel rupture (de Waard et al.,

2010). Most aortic aneurysms occur in association with advanced atherosclerosis (Nordon et al., 2009). Atherosclerosis may induce AAA formation by causing mechanical weakening of the aortic wall with loss of elastic recoil, along with degenerative ischemic changes, through obstruction of the vasa vasorum. Many patients with advanced atherosclerosis do not develop artery aneurysms, while some patients for which there is having no evidence of atherosclerosis do develop artery aneurysms. The observed association between atherosclerosis and aneurysm is probably not causative; however, atherosclerosis may represent a nonspecific secondary response to vessel wall injury that is induced by multiple factors. These facts clearly indicate that aneurysm has a different pathogenesis and consequences for aortic walls vs. atherosclerosis. Although increasing emerging evidence obtained from clinical and experimental studies indicates that complement system plays a critical pathogenic role in the development of atherosclerosis (An et al., 2009; Halas et al., 2005; Hansson et al., 1984; Lewis et al., 2009; Meuwissen et al., 2006; Niculescu et al., 1999b; Nijmeijer et al., 2003; Ross, 1999; Seifert and Kazatchkine, 1988; Vlaicu et al., 1985; Wu et al., 2009; Yun et al., 2008), the role of complement system in the pathogenesis of aneurysm remains unclear.

3. Complement activation and regulation

3.1 Complement activation

The complement system consists of about 30 soluble and membrane-bound proteins, and is activated by three distinct pathways: classical, mannose-binding lectin (MBL) and alternative pathways, either on pathogen surfaces or in plasma (Yu et al., 2010; Zhou et al., 2008). Activation of these pathways depends on different molecules for their initiation (Qin and Gao, 2006; Zhou et al., 2008). All three activation pathways converge at the level of C3 to form C5 convertase such as the C4bC2bC3b from classical and MBL pathways and (C3b)2Fbb from alternative pathway. The C5 convertase then cleaves C5 to form C5b and C5a. The terminal complement activation pathway is induced initially by C5b, followed by the sequential condensation of C6 form to C5b6, and then C7, C8, and C9. Polymerization of C9 bound to the C5b-8 complex forms the MAC, an end-product of the complement activation pathway. The MAC forms a lytic pore in the lipid bilayer membrane that allows the free passage of solutes and water across the membrane and destroys membrane integrity, followed by killing of foreign pathogens and cells (Mayer, 1984).

The liver (mainly hepatocytes) is the main source of complement proteins, accounting for 80%~90% of plasma complement components and their soluble regulators (Qin and Gao, 2006). Many other non-hepatic cells including macrophage, endothelial, neutrophil and lymphocytes could produce complement proteins. This local synthesis of complement occurs in the brain, heart, lung, joints, intestine, skeletal muscle and bone marrow (Morgan and Gasque, 1997). It has been demonstrated that the absence of locally synthesized complement component C3 is capable of modulating the rejection of renal allografts in vivo and regulating T-cell responses in vivo and in vitro (Pratt et al., 2002). The result indicates that the local complement production also plays a critical role in the pathogenesis of human diseases such as organ rejection.

3.2 Biological functions of complement activation byproducts

The byproducts produced in complement activation, such as C1q, C3b, iC3b, and C4b, are critical opsonins for host defense against pathogen and for disposal of immune complexes and dead cell debris by the phagocytosis/lysis effect of the immune cells (macrophages, neutrophils, natural killer [NK] cells, etc.) through their surface receptor binding to these byproducts. On the other hand, the small fragment byproducts such as C3a, C4a, and C5a, termed anaphylatoxins, also play an important role in inflammation and especially in host defense against parasites. These anaphylatoxins can cause mast cell and basophil degranulation, with the release of histamine and other substances that increase vascular permeability and stimulate smooth muscle constriction. C3a and C5a are potent leukocyte chemoattractants, and can also activate these immune effector cells by binding to cell surface receptors (Haas and van Strijp, 2007). Among these anaphylatoxins, C5a has the most potent biological activity (Guo and Ward, 2005).

3.3 MAC function

The cellular response to MAC formation can be classified into two groups along a response continuum: lytic and sublytic. Lytic MAC formation results in colloidoosmotic swelling and lysis of the target (Mayer, 1984; Yu et al., 2010). Normally, MAC attacks homologous nucleated cells mainly through sublytic MAC because nucleated cells possess several protective mechanisms against the cytolytic effect of the MAC, including CD59, anti-apoptotic genes and endocytosis/shedding of MAC (Haskard et al., 2008; Zhou et al., 2008). The sublytic MAC can mediate non-lethal physiological and/or pathological responses in autologous cells (Nicholson-Weller and Halperin, 1993).

Biological functions of sublytic MAC include insertion into the membrane of endothelial cells resulting in the release of: a) bFGF and PDGF (Benzaquen et al., 1994; Halperin et al., 1993; Shankland et al., 1999); b) interleukin-1, which stimulates the expression of pro-inflammatory adhesion molecules such as VCAM-1 and E-selectin, and of prothrombotic tissue factor (Acosta et al., 1996); and c) MCP-1, which attracts monocytes and macrophages that contribute to the pathogenesis of the atherosclerotic plaque (Fosbrink et al., 2006; Torzewski et al., 1996). Consistently, we have demonstrated that sublytic MAC up-regulated the transcripts of these growth factors and cytokines in the plaques of the deficient CD59 mice as well as of targeted macrophages and endothelial cells. However, the role of MAC-induced growth factors and cytokines in the aneurysms is unclear.

In vitro studies have shown that sublytic MAC induces following cellular signaling pathways (Niculescu et al., 1999a; Niculescu and Rus, 1999, 2004), which may contribute to the increase of the release of these growth factors and cytokines. These cellular signaling pathways include 1) elevated Ca^{2+} via Ca^{2+} influx through transient pore in cells, which partially activates PKC and other cellular signaling pathways (Carney et al., 1990; Papadimitriou et al., 1991); 2) G protein coupled-activation of Ras, Raf-1, MEK, ERK-1 pathway and increased activities of ERK-1, c-jun NH2-terminal kinase JNK1 and p38 MAPK in many cells including endothelial cells and smooth muscle cells (Niculescu et al., 1999a; Niculescu and Rus, 1999; Niculescu et al., 1997); 3) activation of the PI3/Akt kinase pathway (Fosbrink et al., 2006; Hila et al., 2001; Niculescu et al., 1999a; Soane et al., 2001); 4) activation of the nuclear factors NF-κB and activator protein-1 (AP-1), which may be responsible for MAC-induced release of IL-6 in smooth muscle cells and IL-8 and MCP-1 in endothelial cells (Viedt et al., 2000) (Kilgore et al., 1996; Kilgore et al., 1997); and 5) activation of the JAK1/STAT3 pathway (Niculescu and Rus, 1999). These in vitro experimental results strongly suggest that MAC is an important mediator of cellular signals that may trigger cell mitogenic effects, which could explain MAC-mediated growth factor and cytokine release. Their activations may result from the secondary effects from the released inflammatory mediators by transiently sublytic MAC and/or the direct effect from sublytic MAC, which have not been addressed so far.

3.4 Complement regulation

To prevent the potentially harmful effect of complement activation on autologous cells, about 10 plasma- and membrane-bound inhibitory proteins have evolved to restrict complement activation at different stages of activation pathways (Yu et al., 2010; Zhou et al., 2008). The soluble plasma complement regulatory proteins include C1 inhibitor, which regulates C1; factor H and factor I, which regulate the cleavage of C3b and C3/C5 convertases; C4 binding protein, which splits C4 convertase and assists factor I in the cleavage of C4b; and S-protein, clusterin, and serum lipids, which compete with membrane lipids to react with nascent C5b67 (Yu et al., 2010; Zhou et al., 2008). Moreover, three membrane proteins that are expressed on the surface of almost all cell types inhibit autologous complement activation, thereby protecting self cells from complement-mediated injury (Morgan, 1999). These regulators include decay-accelerating factor (DAF or CD55), membrane cofactor protein (MCP or CD46), and membrane inhibitor of reactive lysis (CD59). DAF inactivates the C3 (C4b2a and C3bBb) and C5 (C4b2a3b and C3bBb3b) convertases by accelerating the decay of these enzymes (Davitz et al., 1986; Medof et al., 1987; Nicholson-Weller et al., 1985). MCP acts as a cofactor for the cleavage of cell-bound C4b and C3b by the serum protease factor (Brodbeck et al., 2000). CD59 restricts MAC formation by preventing C9 incorporation and polymerization (Sugita et al., 1989).

3.4.1 Anti-MAC regulator CD59

Several lines of evidence indicate that CD59 is much more relevant than DAF, MCP and other complement regulators in protecting cells from MAC formation and MAC-induced phenomena (reviewed in (Acosta et al., 2004; Fisicaro et al., 2000)): 1) an isolated deficiency of DAF has been described in four families that had an unusual blood group phenotype termed Inab (Lin et al., 1988; Telen and Green, 1989). Although DAF was completely absent from all circulating cells (Reid et al., 1991), none of the propositi had symptoms suggestive of paroxysmal nocturnal hemoglobinuria (PNH), a complement-mediated hemolytic disease due to the deficiency of complement regulators such as CD59 and DAF; 2) a mDAF knockout mouse did not show any evidence of intravascular hemolysis (Sun et al., 1999); and 3) an index case report from Japan described a man who had a global deficiency of hCD59 due to single nucleotide deletions in the CD59 gene, which placed the gene product out of frame and introduced a premature stop codon. This subject expressed a severe PNH phenotype from the unusually young age of thirteen and also had a stroke that left him with permanent neurological damage (Yamashina et al., 1990). Not only does the Cd59 knockout out mouse exhibit a full PNH-like anemia as well as platelet activation, but it also exhibits progressive loss of fertility (Holt et al., 2001; Qin et al., 2009; Qin et al., 2003). Also, although the role of S-protein as an inhibitor of MAC formation in tissues has been suggested, the S-protein knockout mouse did not show any detectable phenotype and instead developed normally and was fully fertile (Zheng et al., 1995). This indicates that, at least in mice, the S-protein is not essential for survival nor does it play a major role in restricting complement activation or MAC formation. In addition to the anti-MAC role, CD59 has a complement-independent function in regulating NK, B, and T cell activities (Longhi et al., 2007; Sivasankar et al., 2007).

3.4.2 The delicate balance between complement activation and regulation

There is a delicate balance between complement activation and regulation on autologous cells, which is subject to perturbation by either increased complement activation or decreased regulation. The perturbation may cause a variety of immune diseases and chronic diseases (Yu et al., 2010). It is very likely that this delicate balance between complement activity and regulation differs in the different tissues because of differential expression of complement regulatory proteins and focal activation of complement proteins (Acosta et al., 2004). Indeed, extensive study has shown an offset balance between complement activation and complement regulation, which contributes to the pathogenesis of inflammatory or immune diseases, such as systemic lupus erythematosus (Abe et al., 1998), rheumatoid arthritis (Breitner et al., 1995),Alzheimer's disease (Gasque et al., 1995), and acute renal transplant rejection (Pratt et al., 2002). In the case of the development of aneurysms, there may be an offset balance between complement activation and regulation in the vascular walls, thereby leading to the development of aneurysm formation and rupture, which will be discussed below.

4. Clinical evidence indicates that complement may contribute to the development of aneurysms

There are a few clinical studies examining the role of complement and MAC in the pathogenesis of aneurysms. The results obtained from human studies only provide indirect evidence supporting the role of complement and highlighting the possible involvement of each complement activation pathway in the development and rupture of artery aneurysms like cerebral and aortic aneurysms.

4.1 Complement activation and complement deposition in autoimmune disease-associated aneurysms

The potential role of complement in the artery aneurysms was first recognized by the study of autoimmune disease-associated aneurysms. Early demonstration that there is a negative correlation between serum immunoglobin level and complement activity in the Kawasaki disease patients with aneurysm provides the clinical evidence to link the potential role of complement to the formation of artery aneurysms (Miyata et al., 1984). Kawasaki disease (KD), is an autoimmune disease that manifests as a systemic necrotizing medium-sized vessel vasculitis and is largely seen in children under five years of age (Ozkan et al., 2007). It affects many organ systems, mainly those including the blood vessels, skin, mucous membranes and lymph nodes; however, its most serious effect is on the heart, where it can cause severe coronary artery aneurysms in untreated children. In 1984, Miyata et al (Miyata et al., 1984) conducted a study to measure the serum immunoglobin level and complement activity in 32 Kawasaki disease patients with or without coronary aneurysm. They (Miyata et al., 1984) demonstrated that the group of patients with coronary aneurysm showed relatively higher levels of IgG. Regardless of the presence of coronary aneurysm, the level of IgE in the acute phase was higher than that in the convalescent phase. In addition, the level of immune complexes was higher in the group of patients with coronary aneurysm. There was a low negative correlation between immune complexes and CH50, a clinical measurement for total complement activity.

Another clinical study demonstrates that there is an extensive complement deposition in Behcet's disease-related aneurysm (Yamana et al., 1988). Behçet's disease is a multisystem disorder of probable autoinflammatory etiology with manifestations that can affect many organ systems (Gul, 2005). Its classical presentation includes recurrent oral and genital ulcers and skin inflammatory reactivity. Neurologic involvement is rare, as is the development of peripheral arterial aneurysms (1990). In 1988, Yamana et al (Yamana et al., 1988) reported two patients with vasculo-Behçet's disease who had femoral and popliteal aneurysms. They found that the most interesting histological features in these patients were prominent fibrosis of the adventitia, including the surrounding tissue, venous occlusion, perivasculitis and deposits of C3, C4 and immunoglobulins (IgA, IgG and IgM) in the arterial wall and surrounding tissue. These findings indicate that the formation of aneurysm in vasculo-Behçet's disease is caused by destruction of the intimal and outer side of the arterial wall. Complement may participate in this destruction. Therefore, the complement activation/consumption from increased immune complexes in the circulation of autoimmune diseases may be involved in the development of aneurysms associated with autoimmune diseases.

Extensive clinical and experimental evidence indicates that inflammatory aortic aneurysm is associated with increased incidence of autoimmune disease (Haug et al., 2003; Jagadesham et al., 2008). Complement plays a critical role in the pathogenesis of a variety of autoimmune diseases. However, the role of complement in the autoimmune-associated aneurysms remains unclear and requires further investigation.

4.2 Immunoglobins and C3 deposition in aneurysms

Gregory et al used immunoblotting techniques to compare the reactivity of IgG (detected with secondary goat antihuman antibody) from fourteen patients with abdominal aortic aneurysm (AAA) with soluble proteins extracted from normal and aneurysmal aortas (Gregory et al., 1996). Immunoglobulins G purified from extracts obtained from nine patients with no AAA were used for control experiments. They demonstrated that a unique band at approximately 80 kd was visualized when the filters were probed with IgG from eleven (79 percent) of fourteen patients with AAA compared with only one (11 percent) of nine control subjects. Immunoglobulins G from patients with AAA co-distributed with matrix fibers in normal aortic sections, particularly in the adventitia (suggestive of a microfibrillar component). These findings suggest that these IgGs may participate in the development and progression of AAA because these IgGs binding to the matrix fibers in artery may initiate local classical pathway activation and mediate complement attack on the artery wall, leading to initiation of the formation of artery aneurysms associated with autoimmune disease.

This prediction was further confirmed by increased C3 deposition, along with IgG content in the AAA (Capella et al., 1996). In 1996, Capella et al further demonstrated that compared to the amounts of IgG by subclass in normal aorta, AAA had increases of 193-fold in IgG1, 160-fold in IgG2, 389-fold in IgG3, and 627-fold in IgG4. There was a 125-fold increase in immunoreactive C3 by ELISA in AAA vs normal aorta. Western immunoblotting techniques revealed the presence of multiple C3 degradation products in AAA. Increases in IgG1, 2, and 3 may be responsible for activation of complement in AAA by the classical pathway (Capella et al., 1996). Consistent with this finding, Stella et al (Stella et al., 1991) demonstrated that the interstitial matrix contained deposits of IgG, IgM and C3c together with an increase in type III collagen and a reduction in elastin which appeared fragmented and swollen. The degree of activation shown by these cell elements and the activation of complement suggest that the relevant antigen may have been localized in the aneurysm wall at the time of observation. Taken together, the presence of complement-fixing IgG subclasses along with increased C3 in the aneurysm wall may be an important mechanism promoting matrix proteolysis in AAA.

Moreover, in addition to C3 and IgG deposits in aneurysm, C9 were also found to deposit in aneurysm (Chyatte et al., 1999). Chyatte et al. conducted immunohistochemistry studies with aneurysm tissue collected at the time of microsurgical repair from 23 unruptured and two ruptured aneurysms (25 patients) and compared with 11 control basilar arteries harvested at autopsy. Immunohistochemistry revealed the localization of complement (C3c, C9) and immunoglobulins (IgG, IgM) with inflammatory cells such as macrophages and monocytes (CD68), T lymphocytes (CD3), and B lymphocytes (CD20). Complement (C3c), immunoglobulin (IgG), macrophages (CD68), and T lymphocytes (CD3) were all frequently present in the wall of aneurysm tissue but were rarely identified in control basilar arteries. A few B lymphocytes (CD20) were found in aneurysm tissue, but none were found in the basilar arteries. Extensive inflammatory and immunological reactions are common in unruptured intracranial aneurysms and may be related to aneurysm formation and rupture. These results strongly suggest that the IgM and/or C3 and MAC deposits located in the endothelium of intracranial arteries may play a role in aneurysm-associated neurological complications.

4.3 Complement activation in ruptured aneurysm associated with hemorrhage

The roles of complement and complement activation in ruptured aneurysms were further investigated by several independent groups. In 1987, Ostergaard et al, (Ostergaard et al., 1987) monitored circulating immune complexes and complement activation (plasma C3d levels) during a two week period in patients with ruptured cerebral aneurysms and also in patients with cerebral hematoma unrelated to saccular aneurysms. They found that thirteen of eighteen aneurysm patients were found to have immune complexes on admission as compared to three of 21 healthy blood donors. The presence of immune complexes in aneurysm patients was associated with a poor prognosis. Patients with vasospasm showed a twofold increase in plasma C3d levels at the time when the spasm occurred, whereas no significant changes in the C3d concentration could be demonstrated in aneurysm patients without spasm or in patients with hematoma unrelated to aneurysm rupture. These findings suggest that complement-activation mediated by immune complex are involved in the pathogenesis of cerebral vasospasm following rupture of saccular aneurysms (Ostergaard, 1989).

Kawano et al. investigated serum complements (CH50, C3, C4) after aneurysmal subarachnoid hemorrhage in 21 patients over a two to three week period (Kawano and Yonekawa, 1990). Preoperative grading was well correlated with the C4 level but not the C3 level. C4 levels in patients without symptomatic vasospasm did not change markedly after subarachnoid hemorrhage over investigation. There were no remarkable changes of serum complements in the control patients. C3 and C4 levels of the patients without symptomatic vasospasm did not change markedly after subarachnoid hemorrhage, while they decreased severely in patients with severe vasospasm and majorneurological deficit. The patients with mild symptomatic vasospasm without major neurological deficit showed transient decrease of C3 and C4 levels within a period of five to ten days after subarachnoid hemorrhage. These results show that sequential determinations of serum complement (C3 and C4) levels after subarachnoid hemorrhage is a useful method for the choice of therapy and for the prognosis of aneurysmal patients after subarachnoid hemorrhage. The reduction of plasma C3 and C4 in patients with aneurysmal vasospasm indicates that complement have been activated before rupture of the aneurysm. These results further support the role of complement activation in the pathogenesis of aneurysmal hemorrhage (Kawano and Yonekawa, 1990).

4.4 Complement including MAC deposits in ruptured aneurysm associated with hemorrhage

Complement including MAC deposition in ruptured intracranial aneurysm has been extensively investigated in clinical samples. An intracranial aneurysm is an important acquired cerebrovascular disease that can cause a catastrophic subarachnoid hemorrhage. Despite modern therapy, most patients die or are left disabled as a direct result of a severe initial hemorrhage. The development of more effective treatment strategies depends on understanding the fundamental biology of cerebral aneurysms. The presence of IgM and/or C3 in the endothelium of intracranial aneurysms was demonstrated in five out of six patients with subarachnoid hemorrhage (SAH) (Ryba et al., 1992). In none of them were the immune deposits found in the gyrus rectus. Cortical tissue of four epileptic patients which served as a control gave negative results.

Complement activation associated with the rupture and subarachnoid hemorrhage of sacculare cerebral artery aneurysm (SCAA) was also examined by electromicroscopy and immunoelectron microscopy. Tulamo et al recently demonstrated that MAC localized consistently in a decellularized layer in the outer SCAA wall, and was found in all SCAA samples (Tulamo et al., 2006). The percentage of MAC-positive area relative to the total SCAA wall surface area was greater in ruptured than in unruptured SCAAs. It was also associated significantly with SCAA wall degeneration, de-endothelialization, and CD163+ macrophage and T-lymphocyte infiltrations. Apoptotic terminal deoxynucleotidyl transferase-mediated deoxyuridine triphosphate nick end-labeling-positive nuclei and MAC were located at the same wall areas in four out of 14 double-stained samples, but no double-positive cells were found. Electromicroscopy and immunoelectron microscopy of an unruptured SCAA showed cell death in the MAC-positive layers in the outer SCAA wall. These results suggest that complement activation and MAC formation are involved in SCAA wall degeneration and rupture (Tulamo et al., 2006).

4.5 Local classical complement activation may be involved in aneurysm formation and rupture

Tulamo et al further investigated initiators and the pathway of complement activation in unruptured and ruptured intracranial aneurysms (Tulamo et al., 2010a). Unruptured and ruptured intracranial aneurysm wall samples were studied in parallel sections by immunohistochemical and immunofluorescence stainings. Classical pathway components such as C1q, C3b/iC3b, C3d, C4b/iC4b and MAC were seen in all intracranial aneurysms, and they were located mostly in the extracellular matrix. The early pathway complement components co-localized with each other, but were present in larger areas than C5b-9. The areas positive for complement component accumulation were significantly broader in ruptured than in unruptured intracranial aneurysms. The potential complement activators IgG, IgM, CRP and OxLDL were found mostly in the extracellular matrix and in partial overlap with MAC. These results indicate that immunoglobulins, CRP, and OxLDL may locally activate classical complement pathway, thereby leading to complement and MAC deposits in the intracranial aneurysms wall, which participates in the formation and rupture of aneurysms (Tulamo et al., 2010a).

Furthermore, Tulamo et al also reported that the complement regulatory capacity of the complement system thus appears disturbed in the outer part of the intracranial aneurysms (IA) wall (Tulamo et al., 2010b). The outer part of the IA walls, where MAC is mainly localized in, lacked CD59 and cellular parts in comparison to normal controls. In contrast, complement inhibitors factor H, C4b binding protein, and CD59 as well as glycosaminoglycans were sufficient in the luminal part of the IA wall where MAC was lacking from (Tulamo et al., 2010b). Thus, these human studies indicate that dysregulation of the complement system, such as loss of CD59 in the outer intracranial aneurysm walls leads to an increased susceptibility to complement activation and MAC formation which may associate with inflammation and aneurysm formation. The insufficiency of complement regulation may be due to matrix remodeling and cell loss by mechanical hemodynamics and/or inflammatory stress (Tulamo et al., 2010b). Therefore, there is an imbalance between complement activation and regulation in the outer part of the intracranial aneurysms wall, which results from more complement activation and less complement regulation. This imbalance may allow full pro-inflammatory complement activation to occur before aneurysm rupture.

In contrast, whether alternative and lectin pathways are involved in the aneurysm formation and rupture remains unclear. Recently, Bradley et al (Bradley et al., 2010) demonstrated that there was no evidence for significant association between presence or size of aneurysm with 49 single nucleotide polymorphisms, including common putatively functional polymorphisms, in the genes of the alternative complement cascade (CFH, CFB, CFD, CFI, properdin, CR1, CR1L, CR2, CD46, vitronectin, C3, C5, C6, C7, C8A, C8B, C8G and C9). This study suggests that variation in the genes of the alternative pathway is not an important cause of AAA development. However, the relative role of each of the complement activation pathways in the pathogenesis of artery aneurysms still warrants further investigation. This is because 1) complement system is a critical mediator of the inflammatory process; and 2) the complement-mediated inflammatory process results from imbalance between complement activation and regulation, which highly depends on the sites and tissues of complement activation.

4.6 Complement participates in the ischemia-reperfusion injury of the patients undergoing the surgery for aneurysm repair

Although open surgical repair is highly costly and has high mortality rate, it still is a common approach for the treatment of aortic aneurysm because few interventional modalities are available to treat patients with aortic aneurysm (Baxter et al., 2008; Krishna et al., 2010). Since complement activation contributes to ischemia-reperfusion injury, it is conceivable that patients undergoing thoracoabdominal aortic aneurysm repair suffer extensive ischemia-reperfusion and considerable systemic inflammation. Consistent with this prediction, Odegard et al (Odegard et al., 2007) reported that preoperatively, the thoracic aortic aneurysms patients had significantly elevated concentrations of myeloperoxidase, neopterin and complement activation products compared to controls. Myeloperoxidase and lactoferrin increased after the first contrast dose and peaked at 8 h postoperatively. Platelet counts decreased, while soluble MAC increased from 8 h postoperatively. This result indicates that stent graft treatment induces further activation, and markers of endothelial, platelet, and complement activation were increased for several days after the procedure.

4.6.1 Lectin pathway activation participates in the ischemia-reperfusion injury of patients undergoing surgery for aneurysm repair

Norwood et al reported that there is the consumption of MBL during AAA repair (Norwood et al., 2006). They demonstrated that 23 patients undergoing AAA repair experienced a mean decrease in plasma MBL levels of 41 percent representing significant lectin pathway activation ($p = 0.003$). In contrast, no lectin pathway activation could be demonstrated in eight control patients. The consumption of MBL occurs during AAA repair and is indicative of an important role for the lectin pathway in the ischemia-reperfusion injury associated with aortic aneurysm repair.

The degree and mechanism of complement activation and its role in inflammation were further investigated in the patients undergoing thoracoabdominal aortic aneurysm (TAAA) repair by Fiane et al (Fiane et al., 2003). Substantial complement activation was seen in TAAA patients but not in controls. C1rs-C1-inhibitor complexes increased moderately, whereas C4bc, C3bBbP, C3bc, and the soluble C5b9 (MAC) increased markedly after reperfusion, reaching a maximum at eight hours after reperfusion. Interleukin (IL)-1, tumor necrosis factor α (TNF-α), and IL-8 increased significantly in TAAA patients but not in controls, peaking at 24 hours postoperatively and correlating closely with the degree of complement activation. IL-6 and IL-10 increased to a maximum 8 hours after reperfusion in the TAAA patients, were not correlated with complement activation, and increased moderately in the control subjects. Furthermore, no increase was observed in complement activation products, IL-1, TNF-α, or IL-8 in a MBL–deficient TAAA patient, whereas IL-6 and IL-10 increased as in the controls. Two other MBL-deficient TAAA patients receiving plasma attained significant MBL levels and showed complement and cytokine patterns identical to the MBL-sufficient TAAA patients. These results strongly suggest that complement activation during TAAA repair is MBL mediated, amplified through the alternative pathway, and responsible in part for the inflammatory response (Fiane et al., 2003).

Altogether, these clinical results suggest that complement contributes to the formation and rupture of artery aneurysm and plays a critical role in ischemia-reperfusion injuries associated with aortic aneurysm repair. However, the underlying molecular and cellular mechanisms, through which complement participates in the pathogenesis of artery aneurysm still remains unclear. Therefore, there is a strong need to experimentally dissect the mechanisms in animal models.

5. Animal studies

5.1 Current animal model of aneurysms

Experimental models of artery aneurysms played an important role in understanding the underlying mechanism of artery aneurysms. A number of chemically induced AAA mouse models have been used extensively for the study of aneurysm pathogenesis (Daugherty and Cassis, 2004). These chemical approaches include intraluminal infusion of elastase, periaortic incubations of calcium chloride, and subcutaneous infusion of angiotensin II (Ang II) in Apoe$^{-/-}$background (Daugherty and Cassis, 2004). These mouse models can recapitulate some pathological features of human aneurysms, including medial degeneration, inflammation, thrombus formation, and rupture (Daugherty and Cassis, 2004).

5.2 Complement-dependent neutrophil recruitment is critical for the development of elastase-induced AAA in mice

Transient perfusion of the abdominal aorta with a porcine elastase solution reproducibly leads to the formation of AAA in all C57BL/6 WT mice. In this elastase-induced model of AAA, Pagano, M.B et al reported that mice that were treated with cobra venom factor(CVF, a potent complement inhibitor with the ability to deplete serum C3), before or 24 hours after elastase perfusion, were resistant to elastase-induced AAA, characterized by smaller aortic dilatation, well-preserved elastic fibers, significantly less smooth muscle cell depletion, reduced numbers of macrophages, and activity of mast cells (Pagano et al., 2009). These results indicate that complement activation was involved in elastase-induced AAA development. Examination of mice deficient in factor B further indicated that the alternative pathway of complement played a major role in this process. Activation of the alternative pathway led to generation of the anaphylatoxins C3a and C5a, which recruited neutrophils to the aortic wall. Moreover, antagonism of both C3a and C5a activity was required to block AAA, which suggests that each can independently promote the aneurysmal phenotype. In addition, Pagano, M.B et al demonstrated that complement alternative-pathway involvement was not restricted to this experimental model, but was instead also evident in human AAA (Pagano et al., 2009). These results indicate that complement dependent neutrophile recruitment is critical for the development of AAA.

5.3 Complement may play a role in canine subarachnoid hemorrhage models

Gao et al (Gao et al., 2009) investigated the correlation between sympathetic nerve activation and inflammatory response in the acute stage of subarachnoid hemorrhage (SAH) in a canine perforating model. SAH was induced by perforation of the basilar artery with the use of a microcatheter via the femoral artery in twenty mongrel dogs. They demonstrated that the peak values of C3a and soluble MAC in plasma correlated positively with the peak value of noradrenaline. The peak values of IL-6 and IL-8 also correlated positively with the peak values of noradrenaline. These results suggest that a pronounced activation of the sympathetic nervous system and the inflammatory response occur in the acute stage of SAH and highlight that sympathetic activation and immune responses such as complement activation are quantitatively linked in the early stage after SAH (Gao et al., 2009). These results further support the potential role of complement activation in the aneurysm rupture.

5.4 C5a receptor antagonist attenuates multiple organ injury in a model of ruptured AAA in rats

The C5a-C5a receptor pathway may also play a critical role in multiple organ injuries after aneurysm rupture. Harkin et al (Harkin et al., 2004) examined the role of a novel complement factor 5a (C5aR) receptor antagonist, the cyclic peptide AcF-(OpdChaWR), in attenuation of pathologic complement activation and tissue injury in a model of AAA rupture. They demonstrated that C5aR antagonist AcF treatment significantly reduced lung and intestinal permeability index and myeloperoxidase activity and down-regulated lung TNF-alpha levels. These results indicate that a potent antagonist of C5a receptor protects the rat intestine and lung from neutrophil-associated injury in a model of AAA rupture. These data suggest that complement-mediated inflammation can be modulated at the C5a receptor level, independent of pro-inflammatory TNF-alpha production, and can prevent acute local and remote organ injury (Harkin et al., 2004).

5.5 Protective role of CD59 and potential pathogenic role of MAC in the AAA model

Extensive evidence from human and animal studies indicates a protective role of CD59 and an atherogenic role of MAC in the pathogenesis of atherosclerosis (Wu et al., 2009). In a well-accepted rabbit model of atherosclerosis induced by a 3 percent cholesterol diet, the deficiency of C6, a necessary complement for formation of MAC, protected against the development of atherosclerosis (Schmiedt et al., 1998; Seifert et al., 1989; Seifert and Kazatchkine, 1988). Recently, four independent groups defined the anti-atherogenic role of CD59 using mCd59 deficient mice (An et al., 2009; Lewis et al., 2009; Wu et al., 2009; Yun et al., 2008). Furthermore, we (Wu et al., 2009)* and Lewis et al (Lewis et al., 2009) have recently documented the in vivo atherogenic roles of MAC using anti-mouse C5 antibody (Ab) to block the formation of MAC in mCd59 deficient mice and using mC6 deficient mice to block the formation of MAC respectively. Moreover, MAC mediated endothelial damage and promoted foam cell formation (Wu et al., 2009). These combined results highlight the atherogenic role of MAC (Wu et al., 2009). Although atherosclerosis and AAA have different pathogeneses, they are all immune and inflammatory diseases. Atherosclerosis is considered to be a main cause of AAA, thus the atherogenic role of MAC shed light on its possible role in aortic aneurysm.

Moreover, human studies have suggested that MAC may play a role in the formation and rupture of aorta aneurysms as we discussed above. Taken together, this evidence prompted us to explore the role of MAC in the pathogenesis of AAA with our recent generation of both anti-MAC inhibitor CD59 deficient and overexpressing mice (Qin et al., 2009; Wu et al., 2010). In an angiotensin (Ang) II-induced AAA model, deficiency of both mouse Cd59a and Cd59b ($mCd59ab^{-/-}$) in ApoE-null mice accelerated the disease development, while transgenic over-expression of human CD59 in the endothelial and circulating cells(macrophages and platelets) ($hCD59^{ICAM\text{-}2+/-}$) attenuated AAA progression (Wu et al., 2010), these results suggest a protective role of CD59 in AAA development. Staining of the aneurysm sections with anti–C9-specific antibodies revealed that $mCd59ab^{-/-}$/$ApoE^{-/-}$ mice had significantly more extensive deposits of C9 than $ApoE^{-/-}$ mice and that $ApoE^{-/-}$ mice have significantly more deposits of C9 than $hCD59^{ICAM\text{-}2+/-}$/$ApoE^{-/-}$mice. The fact that deposition of MAC in the AAA Lesions correlated with the severity of AAA strongly supports a pathogenic role of MAC in the development of AAA (Wu et al., 2010).

Macrophage plays a critical role in the development of aorta aneurysms. Macrophages are the primary source of MMP-9 production in human and mouse AAA (Longo et al., 2002; Thompson et al., 1995). Consistent with the pathogenic role of MMPs, AAA aortic extracts from $mCd59ab^{-/-}$/$ApoE^{-/-}$ mice exhibited significantly higher MMP2 and MMP9 activities, whereas extracts from $hCD59^{ICAM\text{-}2+/-}$/$ApoE^{-/-}$ mice showed lower activities than $ApoE^{-/-}$ mice. Meanwhile, in the AAA lesions of $mCd59ab^{-/-}$/$ApoE^{-/-}$ mice, the macrophage content is significantly increased, which is consistent with higher levels of MMP2 and MMP9 and the severity of AAA in this model (Wu et al., 2010). Furthermore, in vitro study demonstrated that sublytic MAC treatment in mouse endothelial, macrophage, and smooth muscle cells (SMC) increased MMP2 and MMP9 activities (Wu et al., 2010). Twelve hours after MAC treatment on these cells, activities of MMP2 or MMP9 from the cell extracts significantly increased. Further studies demonstrate that MAC upregulates MMP2 and MMP9 activities through AP-1 and NF-κB signaling pathways. Western blot assay revealed significantly increased phosphorylation of c-Jun, c-Fos, IKK-a/b and p65 in lesions of $mCd59ab^{-/-}$/$ApoE^{-/-}$ mice, whereas decreased phosphorylation in $hCD59^{ICAM\text{-}2\text{-}/-}$/$ApoE^{-/-}$. Firefly luciferase reporter gene assay and RNA interference assay confirmed that MAC-activated c-Jun and NF-κB signaling pathways participate in the upregulation of MMP2 and MMP9, which may in turn contribute to the pathogenesis of AAA in Ang-II-induced AAA model.

It was previously demonstrated that MAC induced more severe endothelial dysfunction in mCd59ab-/-/ApoE-/- mice than in ApoE-/-, which contributes to atherogenesis (Wu et al., 2009). MAC also mediates endothelial cell apoptosis in vitro. MAC insertion into endothelial and other cell membranes releases an array of growth factors and cytokoines, which may participate in the development of aneurysms.

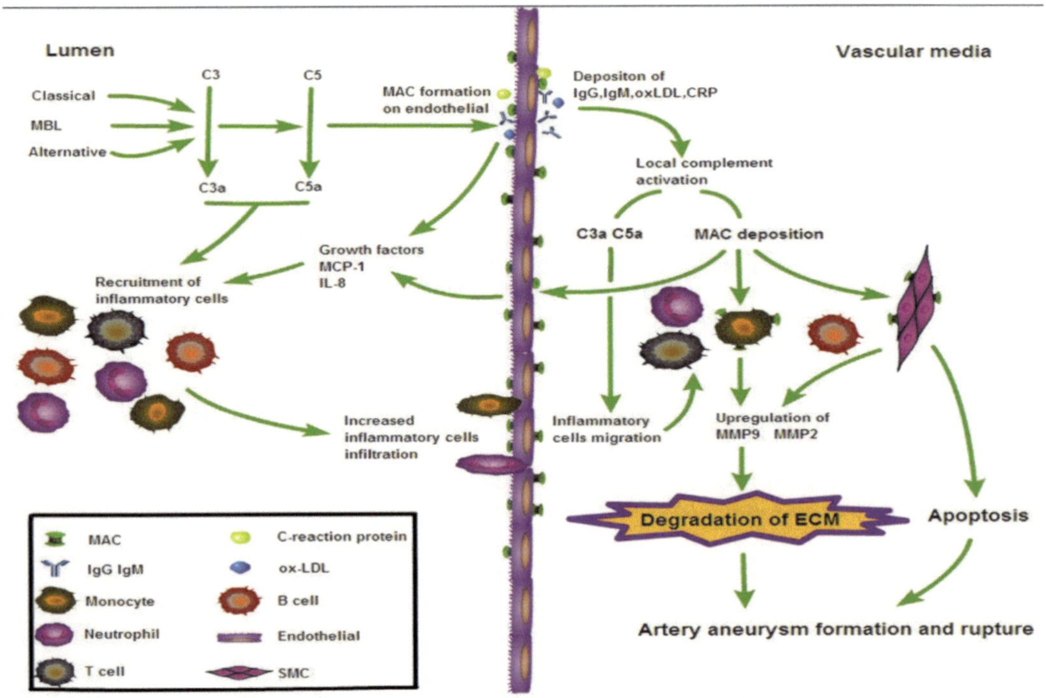

Fig. 1. Potential roles of complement in the pathogenesis of artery aneurysms
MBL: Mannose Binding lection pathway, oxLDL: Oxidized low density lipoprotein, CRP: ECM: extracellular matrix and MAC: Membrane attack complex.

Furthermore, the supernatant obtained from MAC-treated endothelial cells triggers the migration of both MAC-treated and non–MAC-treated macrophage in vitro. The increase in macrophage migration may result from the release of growth factors and cytokines induced by sublytic MAC assembly in endothelial cells. These findings suggest that MAC may promote AAA development through different target cells or signal pathways. In Ang-II induced AAA model, increased MMP expression in the aorta in AAA could be caused by increased macrophage infiltration, upregulation by increased MAC tissue levels, or some combination of these two mechanisms.

Our study strongly supports the hypothesis that MAC may accelerate the initiation and development of AAA through mediation of endothelial dysfunction, attraction and activation of macrophages, which lead to the secretion of MMP2 and MMP9 that destroy the wall of blood vessels and thereby form aneurysm (Fig. 1). Taken together, these results shed light on the important pathogenic role of MAC in aneurysms, point towards the molecular mechanism of MAC-activated signaling pathways in aneurysm, and suggest inhibition of MAC may provide a novel approach for the treatment/prevention of aneurysms.

6. Conclusion

In this review we summarized an increase in clinical and experimental evidence on the potential role of complement system in aortic aneurysms. The role of complement and MAC in artery aneurysms has only been suggested in human studies and has not been extensively studied in experimental models. Complement activation in the circulation has been identified in the course of the formation and rupture of artery aneurysms. Complement and MAC extensively deposit in aneurysm walls and more in rupture aneurysms than unruptured aneursyms. Complement also plays a critical role in the pathogenesis of reperfusion-ischemic injury after aneurysm repair. Experimental evidence indicates that C3a and C5a play a critical role in the development of elastase-induced AAA, CD59 plays a critical protective role, and MAC plays a critical pathogenic role in the development of AAA. Together, these finding lead us to postulate the following hypothesis that 1) after complement is activated by one or three complement activation pathways in the circulation, the MAC, a terminal complement activation product, mediates endothelial dysfunction in the artery wall. This process will lead to the migration of inflammatory cells such as macrophage, the promotion of the interaction with the damaged endothelial cells, and deposition of activated complement bioproducts such as C3a and C5a and MAC, and complement activators such as immunoglobins, CRP and OxLDL in the artery wall; 2) the deposition of immuneglobin and CRP, OxLDL locally activates the classical complement activation pathways; 3) complement activation byproducts such as C3a and C5a and MAC amplify the inflammatory process in the artery wall through the release of inflammatory mediators and the attraction of more inflammatory cells to the artery wall; 4) these inflammatory process mediate the release of MMP2 and MMP9, which will degrade the elastic lamellae and extracellular matrix and damage the smooth muscle cells, finally leading to artery wall weakening and the formation of aneurysm or even aneurysm rupture (Fig. 1).

Although the emerging evidence supports the role of complement in the pathogenesis of artery, there are still a number of questions that remain to be further studied. For example, the molecular and cellular mechanisms of C3a, C5a, and MAC, and the relative role of complement activation pathways in the pathogenesis of artery aneurysms still require further investigation with these different animal models. Whether the early complement components play a role in the pathogenesis of aneurysms has not been studied so far. Whether the restriction of complement activation and MAC formation serves as a novel approach for the treatment/prevention of aneurysm also warrants future studies.

7. Acknowledgment

This work was supported by R01 AI061174 (to X.Q.), by a Scientist Development Grant from the American Heart Association 0435483N (to X.Q.) and by Grant Aid In from the American Heart Association 10GRNT4370029 (to X.Q.).

8. References

International study group (1990). Criteria for diagnosis of Behcet's disease. International Study Group for Behcet's Disease. *Lancet* 335, 1078-1080.

Abe, K., Miyazaki, M., Koji, T., Furusu, A., Ozono, Y., Harada, T., Sakai, H., Nakane, P.K., & Kohno, S. (1998). Expression of decay accelerating factor mRNA and complement C3 mRNA in human diseased kidney. *Kidney international* 54, 120 130.

Acosta, J., Qin, X., & Halperin, J. (2004). Complement and complement regulatory proteins as potential molecular targets for vascular diseases. *Curr Pharm Des* 10, 203-211.

Acosta, J.A., Benzaquen, L.R., Goldstein, D.J., Tosteson, M.T., & Halperin, J.A. (1996). The transient pore formed by homologous terminal complement complexes functions as a bidirectional route for the transport of autocrine and paracrine signals across human cell membranes. *Mol Med* 2, 755-765.

Allaire, E., Forough, R., Clowes, M., Starcher, B., & Clowes, A.W. (1998). Local overexpression of TIMP-1 prevents aortic aneurysm degeneration and rupture in a rat model. *The Journal of clinical investigation* 102, 1413-1420.

An, G., Miwa, T., Song, W.L., Lawson, J.A., Rader, D.J., Zhang, Y., & Song, W.C. (2009). CD59 but not DAF deficiency accelerates atherosclerosis in female ApoE knockout mice. *Molecular immunology* 46, 1702-1709.

Baxter, B.T., Terrin, M.C., & Dalman, R.L. (2008). Medical management of small abdominal aortic aneurysms. *Circulation* 117, 1883-1889.

Benzaquen, L.R., Nicholson-Weller, A., & Halperin, J.A. (1994). Terminal complement proteins C5b-9 release basic fibroblast growth factor and platelet-derived growth factor from endothelial cells. *The Journal of experimental medicine* 179, 985-992.

Bradley, D.T., Badger, S.A., Bown, M.J., Sayers, R.D., & Hughes, A.E. (2010). Coding polymorphisms in the genes of the alternative complement pathway and abdominal aortic aneurysm. *International journal of immunogenetics.*

Breitner, S., Storkel, S., Reichel, W., & Loos, M. (1995). Complement components C1q, C1r/C1s, and C1INH in rheumatoid arthritis. Correlation of in situ hybridization and northern blot results with function and protein concentration in synovium and primary cell cultures. *Arthritis and rheumatism* 38, 492-498.

Brodbeck, W.G., Mold, C., Atkinson, J.P., & Medof, M.E. (2000). Cooperation between decay-accelerating factor and membrane cofactor protein in protecting cells from autologous complement attack. *J Immunol* 165, 3999-4006.

Caird, J., Napoli, C., Taggart, C., Farrell, M., & Bouchier-Hayes, D. (2006). Matrix metalloproteinases 2 and 9 in human atherosclerotic and non-atherosclerotic cerebral aneurysms. *Eur J Neurol* 13, 1098-1105.

Capella, J.F., Paik, D.C., Yin, N.X., Gervasoni, J.E., & Tilson, M.D. (1996). Complement activation and subclassification of tissue immunoglobulin G in the abdominal aortic aneurysm. *The Journal of surgical research* 65, 31-33.

Carney, D.F., Lang, T.J., & Shin, M.L. (1990). Multiple signal messengers generated by terminal complement complexes and their role in terminal complexes elimination. *J Immunol* 145, 621-629.

Chyatte, D., Bruno, G., Desai, S., & Todor, D.R. (1999). Inflammation and intracranial aneurysms. *Neurosurgery* 45, 1137-1146; discussion 1146-1137.

Collin, J., Araujo, L., Walton, J., & Lindsell, D. (1988). Oxford screening programme for abdominal aortic aneurysm in men aged 65 to 74 years. *Lancet* 2, 613-615.

Curci, J.A., Mao, D., Bohner, D.G., Allen, B.T., Rubin, B.G., Reilly, J.M., Sicard, G.A., & Thompson, R.W. (2000). Preoperative treatment with doxycycline reduces aortic wall expression and activation of matrix metalloproteinases in patients with abdominal aortic aneurysms. *J Vasc Surg* 31, 325-342.

Daugherty, A., & Cassis, L.A. (2004). Mouse models of abdominal aortic aneurysms. *Arteriosclerosis, thrombosis, and vascular biology* 24, 429-434.

Davitz, M.A., Low, M.G., & Nussenzweig, V. (1986). Release of decay-accelerating factor (DAF) from the cell membrane by phosphatidylinositol-specific phospholipase C (PIPLC). *J Exp Med* 163, 1150-1161.

de Waard, V., Bot, I., de Jager, S.C., Talib, S., Egashira, K., de Vries, M.R., Quax, P.H., Biessen, E.A., & van Berkel, T.J. (2010). Systemic MCP1/CCR2 blockade and leukocyte specific MCP1/CCR2 inhibition affect aortic aneurysm formation differently. *Atherosclerosis*.

Duftner, C., Seiler, R., Dejaco, C., Fraedrich, G., & Schirmer, M. (2006). Increasing evidence for immune-mediated processes and new therapeutic approaches in abdominal aortic aneurysms--a review. Annals of the New York Academy of *Sciences* 1085, 331-338.

Eliason, J.L., Hannawa, K.K., Ailawadi, G., Sinha, I., Ford, J.W., Deogracias, M.P., Roelofs, K.J., Woodrum, D.T., Ennis, T.L., Henke, P.K., *et al.* (2005). Neutrophil depletion inhibits experimental abdominal aortic aneurysm formation. *Circulation* 112, 232-240.

Fiane, A.E., Videm, V., Lingaas, P.S., Heggelund, L., Nielsen, E.W., Geiran, O.R., Fung, M., & Mollnes, T.E. (2003). Mechanism of complement activation and its role in the inflammatory response after thoracoabdominal aortic aneurysm repair. *Circulation* 108, 849-856.

Fisicaro, N., Aminian, A., Hinchliffe, S.J., Morgan, B.P., Pearse, M.J., D'Apice, A.J., & Cowan, P.J. (2000). The pig analogue of CD59 protects transgenic mouse hearts from injury by human complement. *Transplantation* 70, 963-968.

Fosbrink, M., Niculescu, F., Rus, V., Shin, M.L., & Rus, H. (2006). C5b-9-induced endothelial cell proliferation and migration are dependent on Akt inactivation of forkhead transcription factor FOXO1. *The Journal of biological chemistry* 281, 19009-19018.

Gao, C., Liu, X., Shi, H., Xu, S., Ji, Z., Wang, C., Wu, P., Liu, Z., & Zhao, S. (2009). Relationship between sympathetic nervous activity and inflammatory response after subarachnoid hemorrhage in a perforating canine model. *Auton Neurosci* 147, 70-74.

Gasque, P., Fontaine, M., & Morgan, B.P. (1995). Complement expression in human brain. Biosynthesis of terminal pathway components and regulators in human glial cells and cell lines. *J Immunol* 154, 4726-4733.

Gregory, A.K., Yin, N.X., Capella, J., Xia, S., Newman, K.M., & Tilson, M.D. (1996). Features of autoimmunity in the abdominal aortic aneurysm. *Arch Surg* 131, 85 88.

Gul, A. (2005). Behcet's disease as an autoinflammatory disorder. Curr Drug Targets *Inflamm Allergy* 4, 81-83.

Guo, R.F., & Ward, P.A. (2005). Role of C5a in inflammatory responses. *Annual review of immunology* 23, 821-852.

Haas, P.J., & van Strijp, J. (2007). Anaphylatoxins: their role in bacterial infection and inflammation. *Immunol Res* 37, 161-175.

Halas, Y.A., Rahal, E., Abdelnoor, A.M., Haddad, R., & Abchee, A. (2005). Serum C reactive protein and complement proteins in patients with acute myocardial infarction. *Immunopharmacol Immunotoxicol* 27, 405-416.

Halperin, J.A., Taratuska, A., & Nicholson-Weller, A. (1993). Terminal complement complex C5b-9 stimulates mitogenesis in 3T3 cells. *Journal of Clinical Investigation* 91, 1974-1978.

Hannawa, K.K., Eliason, J.L., & Upchurch, G.R., Jr. (2009). Gender differences in abdominal aortic aneurysms. *Vascular* 17 Suppl 1, S30-39.

Hansson, G.K., Holm, J., & Kral, J.G. (1984). Accumulation of IgG and complement factor C3 in human arterial endothelium and atherosclerotic lesions. *Acta Pathol Microbiol Immunol Scand [A]* 92, 429-435.

Harkin, D.W., Romaschin, A., Taylor, S.M., Rubin, B.B., & Lindsay, T.F. (2004). Complement C5a receptor antagonist attenuates multiple organ injury in a model of ruptured abdominal aortic aneurysm. *J Vasc Surg* 39, 196-206.

Haskard, D.O., Boyle, J.J., & Mason, J.C. (2008). The role of complement in atherosclerosis. *Curr Opin Lipidol* 19, 478-482.

Haug, E.S., Skomsvoll, J.F., Jacobsen, G., Halvorsen, T.B., Saether, O.D., & Myhre, H.O. (2003). Inflammatory aortic aneurysm is associated with increased incidence of autoimmune disease. *J Vasc Surg* 38, 492-497.

Hila, S., Soane, L., & Koski, C.L. (2001). Sublytic C5b-9-stimulated Schwann cell survival through PI 3-kinase-mediated phosphorylation of BAD. *Glia* 36, 58-67.

Holt, D.S., Botto, M., Bygrave, A.E., Hanna, S.M., Walport, M.J., & Morgan, B.P. (2001). Targeted deletion of the CD59 gene causes spontaneous intravascular hemolysis and hemoglobinuria. *Blood* 98, 442-449.

Jagadesham, V.P., Scott, D.J., & Carding, S.R. (2008). Abdominal aortic aneurysms: an autoimmune disease? *Trends in molecular medicine* 14, 522-529.

Kadoglou, N.P., & Liapis, C.D. (2004). Matrix metalloproteinases: contribution to pathogenesis, diagnosis, surveillance and treatment of abdominal aortic aneurysms. *Current medical research and opinion* 20, 419-432.

Kawano, T., & Yonekawa, Y. (1990). Serum complements as indicator for predictingvasospasm and its severity after aneurysmal subarachnoid hemorrhage. *Nippon geka hokan* 59, 189-197.

Kilgore, K.S., Flory, C.M., Miller, B.F., Evans, V.M., & Warren, J.S. (1996). The membrane attack complex of complement induces interleukin-8 and monocyte chemoattractant protein-1 secretion from human umbilical vein endothelial cells. *The American journal of pathology* 149, 953-961.

Kilgore, K.S., Schmid, E., Shanley, T.P., Flory, C.M., Maheswari, V., Tramontini, N.L., Cohen, H., Ward, P.A., Friedl, H.P., & Warren, J.S. (1997). Sublytic concentrations of the membrane attack complex of complement induce endothelial interleukin-8 and monocyte chemoattractant protein-1 through nuclear factor-kB activation. *Am J Pathol* 150, 2019-2031.

Krishna, S.M., Dear, A.E., Norman, P.E., & Golledge, J. (2010). Genetic and epigenetic mechanisms and their possible role in abdominal aortic aneurysm. *Atherosclerosis*.

Lewis, R.D., Jackson, C.L., Morgan, B.P., & Hughes, T.R. (2009). The membrane attack complex of complement drives the progression of atherosclerosis in apolipoprotein E knockout mice. *Molecular immunology*.

Lin, R.C., Herman, J., Henry, L., & Daniels, G.L. (1988). A family showing inheritance of the Inab phenotype. *Transfusion* 28, 427-429.

Longhi, M.P., Williams, A., Wise, M., Morgan, B.P., & Gallimore, A. (2007). CD59a deficiency exacerbates influenza-induced lung inflammation through complement-dependent and -independent mechanisms. *European journal of immunology* 37, 1266-1274.

Longo, G.M., Xiong, W., Greiner, T.C., Zhao, Y., Fiotti, N., & Baxter, B.T. (2002). Matrix metalloproteinases 2 and 9 work in concert to produce aortic aneurysms. The *Journal of clinical investigation* 110, 625-632.

Mayer, M.M. (1984). Complement. Historical perspectives and some current issues. *Complement (Basel, Switzerland) 1*, 2-26.

Medof, M.E., Lublin, D.M., Holers, V.M., Ayers, D.J., Getty, R.R., Leykam, J.F., Atkinson, J.P., & Tykocinski, M.L. (1987). Cloning and characterization of cDNAs encoding the complete sequence of decay-accelerating factor of human complement. *Proceedings of the National Academy of Sciences of the United States of America* 84, 2007-2011.

Meuwissen, M., van der Wal, A.C., Niessen, H.W., Koch, K.T., de Winter, R.J., van der Loos, C.M., Rittersma, S.Z., Chamuleau, S.A., Tijssen, J.G., Becker, A.E., *et al.* (2006). Colocalisation of intraplaque C reactive protein, complement, oxidised low density lipoprotein, and macrophages in stable and unstable angina and acute myocardial infarction. *J Clin Pathol* 59, 196-201.

Miller, F.J., Jr., Sharp, W.J., Fang, X., Oberley, L.W., Oberley, T.D., & Weintraub, N.L. (2002). Oxidative stress in human abdominal aortic aneurysms: a potential mediator of aneurysmal remodeling. *Arteriosclerosis, thrombosis, and vascular biology* 22, 560-565.

Miyata, K., Kawakami, K., Onimaru, T., Baba, Y., Ono, S., Hokonohara, M., Yoshinaga, M., & Terawaki, T. (1984). Circulating immune complexes and granulocytes chemotaxis in Kawasaki disease. *Japanese circulation journal* 48, 1350-1353.

Morgan, B.P. (1999). Regulation of the complement membrane attack pathway. *Crit Rev Immunol* 19, 173-198.

Morgan, B.P., & Gasque, P. (1997). Extrahepatic complement biosynthesis: where, when and why? *Clin Exp Immunol* 107, 1-7.

Mosorin, M., Juvonen, J., Biancari, F., Satta, J., Surcel, H.M., Leinonen, M., Saikku, P., & Juvonen, T. (2001). Use of doxycycline to decrease the growth rate of abdominal aortic aneurysms: a randomized, double-blind, placebo-controlled pilot study. *J Vasc Surg* 34, 606-610.

Newman, K.M., Ogata, Y., Malon, A.M., Irizarry, E., G&hi, R.H., Nagase, H., & Tilson, M.D. (1994). Identification of matrix metalloproteinases 3 (stromelysin-1) and 9 (gelatinase B) in abdominal aortic aneurysm. *Arterioscler Thromb* 14, 1315-1320.

Nicholson-Weller, A., & Halperin, J.A. (1993). Membrane signaling by complement C5b-9, the membrane attack complex. *Immunol Res* 12, 244-257.

Nicholson-Weller, A., Spicer, D.B., & Austen, K.F. (1985). Deficiency of the complement regulatory protein, "decay-accelerating factor," on membranes of granulocytes, monocytes, and platelets in paroxysmal nocturnal hemoglobinuria. *The New England journal of medicine* 312, 1091-1097.

Niculescu, F., Badea, T., & Rus, H. (1999a). Sublytic C5b-9 induces proliferation of human aortic smooth muscle cells: role of mitogen activated protein kinase and phosphatidylinositol 3-kinase. *Atherosclerosis* 142, 47-56.

Niculescu, F., & Rus, H. (1999). Complement activation and atherosclerosis. *Molecular immunology* 36, 949-955.

Niculescu, F., & Rus, H. (2004). The role of complement activation in atherosclerosis. *Immunol Res* 30, 73-80.

Niculescu, F., Rus, H., van Biesen, T., & Shin, M.L. (1997). Activation of Ras and mitogen-activated protein kinase pathway by terminal complement complexes is G protein dependent. *J Immunol* 158, 4405-4412.

Niculescu, F., Soane, L., Badea, T., Shin, M., & Rus, H. (1999b). Tyrosine phosphorylation and activation of Janus kinase 1 and STAT3 by sublytic C5b-9 complement complex in aortic endothelial cells. *Immunopharmacology* 42, 187 193.

Nijmeijer, R., Lagrand, W.K., Lubbers, Y.T., Visser, C.A., Meijer, C.J., Niessen, H.W., & Hack, C.E. (2003). C-reactive protein activates complement in infarcted human myocardium. *The American journal of pathology* 163, 269-275.

Nordon, I.M., Hinchliffe, R.J., Holt, P.J., Loftus, I.M., & Thompson, M.M. (2009). Review of current theories for abdominal aortic aneurysm pathogenesis. *Vascular* 17, 253-263.

Norwood, M.G., Sayers, R.D., Roscher, S., Lynch, N.J., Sutton, A.J., & Schwaeble, W.J. (2006). Consumption of mannan-binding lectin during abdominal aortic aneurysm repair. *Eur J Vasc Endovasc Surg* 31, 239-243.

Odegard, A., Aasland, J., Myhre, H.O., Mollnes, T.E., & Videm, V. (2007). The inflammatory response to stent grafting of the thoracic aorta. *Int Angiol* 26, 219 227.

Ostergaard, J.R. (1989). Risk factors in intracranial saccular aneurysms. Aspects on the formation and rupture of aneurysms, and development of cerebral vasospasm. *Acta neurologica Scandinavica* 80, 81-98.

Ostergaard, J.R., Kristensen, B.O., Svehag, S.E., Teisner, B., & Miletic, T. (1987). Immune complexes and complement activation following rupture of intracranial saccular aneurysms. *J Neurosurg* 66, 891-897.

Ozkan, S., Saritas, B., Aslim, E., Akay, T.H., & Aslamaci, S. (2007). Coronary bypass surgery in kawasaki disease in a four-year-old patient: case report. *Journal of cardiac surgery* 22, 511-513.

Pagano, M.B., Zhou, H.F., Ennis, T.L., Wu, X., Lambris, J.D., Atkinson, J.P., Thompson, R.W., Hourcade, D.E., & Pham, C.T. (2009). Complement-dependent neutrophil recruitment is critical for the development of elastase-induced abdominal aortic aneurysm. *Circulation* 119, 1805-1813.

Palombo, D., Maione, M., Cifiello, B.I., Udini, M., Maggio, D., & Lupo, M. (1999). Matrix metalloproteinases. Their role in degenerative chronic diseases of abdominal aorta. *The Journal of cardiovascular surgery* 40, 257-260.

Papadimitriou, J.C., Ramm, L.E., Drachenberg, C.B., Trump, B.F., & Shin, M.L. (1991). Quantitative analysis of adenine nucleotides during the prelytic phase of cell death mediated by C5b-9. *J Immunol* 147, 212-217.

Powell, J., & Greenhalgh, R.M. (1989). Cellular, enzymatic, and genetic factors in the pathogenesis of abdominal aortic aneurysms. *J Vasc Surg* 9, 297-304.

Pratt, J.R., Basheer, S.A., & Sacks, S.H. (2002). Local synthesis of complement component C3 regulates acute renal transplant rejection. *Nat Med* 8, 582-587.

Pyo, R., Lee, J.K., Shipley, J.M., Curci, J.A., Mao, D., Ziporin, S.J., Ennis, T.L., Shapiro, S.D., Senior, R.M., & Thompson, R.W. (2000). Targeted gene disruption of matrix metalloproteinase-9 (gelatinase B) suppresses development of experimental abdominal aortic aneurysms. *The Journal of clinical investigation* 105, 1641-1649.

Qin, X., & Gao, B. (2006). The complement system in liver diseases. *Cellular and molecular immunology* 3, 333-340.

Qin, X., Hu, W., Song, W., Grubissich, L., Hu, X., Wu, G., Ferris, S., Dobarro, M., & Halperin, J.A. (2009). Generation and phenotyping of mCd59a and mCd59b double-knockout mice. *American journal of hematology* 84, 65-70.

Qin, X., Krumrei, N., Grubissich, L., Dobarro, M., Aktas, H., Perez, G., & Halperin, J.A. (2003). Deficiency of the mouse complement regulatory protein mCd59b results in spontaneous hemolytic anemia with platelet activation and progressive male infertility. *Immunity* 18, 217-227.

Reid, M.E., Mallinson, G., Sim, R.B., Poole, J., Pausch, V., Merry, A.H., Liew, Y.W., & Tanner, M.J. (1991). Biochemical studies on red blood cells from a patient with the Inab phenotype (decay-accelerating factor deficiency). Blood *78*, 3291-3297.

Ross, R. (1999). Atherosclerosis--an inflammatory disease. *The New England journal of medicine* 340, 115-126.

Ryba, M., Jarzabek-Chorzelska, M., Chorzelski, T., & Pastuszko, M. (1992). Is vascular angiopathy following intracranial aneurysm rupture immunologically mediated? *Acta neurochirurgica* 117, 34-37.

Schmiedt, W., Kinscherf, R., Deigner, H.-P., Kamencic, H., Nauen, O., Kilo, J., Oelert, H., Metz, J., & Bhadki, S. (1998). Complement C6 deficiency protects against diet induced atherosclerosis in rabbits. *Arterioscler Thromb Vasc Biol* 18, 1790-1795.

Schneiderman, J., Bordin, G.M., Engelberg, I., Adar, R., Seiffert, D., Thinnes, T., Bernstein, E.F., Dilley, R.B., & Loskutoff, D.J. (1995). Expression of fibrinolytic genes in atherosclerotic abdominal aortic aneurysm wall. A possible mechanism for aneurysm expansion. *The Journal of clinical investigation* 96, 639-645.

Seifert, P.S., Hugo, F., Hansson, G.K., & Bhakdi, S. (1989). Prelesional complement activation in experimental atherosclerosis. Terminal C5b-9 complement deposition coincides with cholesterol accumulation in the aortic intima of hypercholesterolemic rabbits. *Laboratory investigation; a journal of technical methods and pathology* 60, 747-754.

Seifert, P.S., & Kazatchkine, M.D. (1988). The complement system in atherosclerosis. *Atherosclerosis* 73, 91-104.

Shankland, S.J., Pippin, J.W., & Couser, W.G. (1999). Complement (C5b-9) induces glomerular epithelial cell DNA synthesis but not proliferation in vitro. *Kidney international* 56, 538-548.

Shi, G.P., Sukhova, G.K., Grubb, A., Ducharme, A., Rhode, L.H., Lee, R.T., Ridker, P.M., Libby, P., & Chapman, H.A. (1999). Cystatin C deficiency in human atherosclerosis and aortic aneurysms. *The Journal of clinical investigation* 104, 1191-1197.

Shimizu, K., Mitchell, R.N., & Libby, P. (2006). Inflammation and cellular immune responses in abdominal aortic aneurysms. *Arteriosclerosis, thrombosis, and vascular biology* 26, 987-994.

Sivasankar, B., Donev, R.M., Longhi, M.P., Hughes, T.R., Davie, R., Cole, D.S., Morgan, B.P., & Marchbank, K.J. (2007). CD59a deficient mice display reduced B cell activity and antibody production in response to T-dependent antigens. *Molecular immunology* 44, 2978-2987.

Soane, L., Cho, H.J., Niculescu, F., Rus, H., & Shin, M.L. (2001). C5b-9 terminal complement complex protects oligodendrocytes from death by regulating Bad through phosphatidylinositol 3-kinase/Akt pathway. *J Immunol* 167, 2305-2311.

Stella, A., Gargiulo, M., Pasquinelli, G., Preda, P., Faggioli, G.L., Cenacchi, G., & D'Addato, M. (1991). The cellular component in the parietal infiltrate of inflammatory abdominal aortic aneurysms (IAAA). *European journal of vascular surgery* 5, 65-70.

Sugita, Y., Tobe, T., Oda, E., Tomita, M., Yasukawa, K., Yamaji, N., Takemoto, T., Furuichi, K., Takayama, M., & Yano, S. (1989). Molecular cloning and characterization of MACIF, an inhibitor of membrane channel formation of complement. *J Biochem (Tokyo)* 106, 555-557.

Sun, X., Funk, C.D., Deng, C., Sahu, A., Lambris, J.D., & Song, W.C. (1999). Role of decay-accelerating factor in regulating complement activation on the erythrocyte surface as revealed by gene targeting. *Proceedings of the National Academy of Sciences of the United States of America* 96, 628-633.

Tanaka, K., Iwamoto, Y., Ito, Y., Ishibashi, T., Nakabeppu, Y., Sekiguchi, M., & Sugioka, Y. (1995). Cyclic AMP-regulated synthesis of the tissue inhibitors of metalloproteinases suppresses the invasive potential of the human fibrosarcoma cell line HT1080. *Cancer Res* 55, 2927-2935.

Telen, M.J., & Green, A.M. (1989). The Inab phenotype: characterization of the membrane protein and complement regulatory defect. *Blood* 74, 437-441.

Thompson, R.W., Geraghty, P.J., & Lee, J.K. (2002). Abdominal aortic aneurysms: basic mechanisms and clinical implications. *Curr Probl Surg* 39, 110-230.

Thompson, R.W., Holmes, D.R., Mertens, R.A., Liao, S., Botney, M.D., Mecham, R.P., Welgus, H.G., & Parks, W.C. (1995). Production and localization of 92 kilodalton gelatinase in abdominal aortic aneurysms. An elastolytic metalloproteinase expressed by aneurysm-infiltrating macrophages. *The Journal of clinical investigation* 96, 318-326.

Torzewski, J., Oldroyd, R., Lachmann, P., Fitzsimmons, C., Proudfoot, D., & Bowyer, D. (1996). Complement-induced release of monocyte chemotactic protein-1 from human smooth muscle cells. A possible initiating event in the atherosclerotic lesion formation. *Arterioscler Thromb Vasc Biol* 16, 673-677.

Tulamo, R., Frosen, J., Junnikkala, S., Paetau, A., Kangasniemi, M., Pelaez, J., Hernesniemi, J., Niemela, M., & Meri, S. (2010a). Complement system becomes activated by the classical pathway in intracranial aneurysm walls. *Laboratory investigation; a journal of technical methods and pathology* 90, 168-179.

Tulamo, R., Frosen, J., Junnikkala, S., Paetau, A., Pitkaniemi, J., Kangasniemi, M., Niemela, M., Jaaskelainen, J., Jokitalo, E., Karatas, A., *et al.* (2006). Complement activation associates with saccular cerebral artery aneurysm wall degeneration and rupture. *Neurosurgery* 59, 1069-1076; discussion 1076-1067.

Tulamo, R., Frosen, J., Paetau, A., Seitsonen, S., Hernesniemi, J., Niemela, M., Jarvela, I., & Meri, S. (2010b). Lack of complement inhibitors in the outer intracranial artery aneurysm wall associates with complement terminal pathway activation. *The American journal of pathology* 177, 3224-3232.

Viedt, C., Hansch, G.M., Brandes, R.P., Kubler, W., & Kreuzer, J. (2000). The terminal complement complex C5b-9 stimulates interleukin-6 production in human smooth muscle cells through activation of transcription factors NF-kappaB and AP-1 [In Process Citation]. *Faseb J* 14, 2370-2372.

Vlaicu, R., Niculescu, F., Rus, H.G., & Cristea, A. (1985). Immunohistochemical localization of the terminal C5b-9 complement complex in human aortic fibrous plaque. *Atherosclerosis* 57, 163-177.

Wassef, M., Upchurch, G.R., Jr., Kuivaniemi, H., Thompson, R.W., & Tilson, M.D., 3rd (2007). Challenges and opportunities in abdominal aortic aneurysm research. *J Vasc Surg* 45, 192-198.

Weintraub, N.L. (2009). Understanding abdominal aortic aneurysm. *The New England journal of medicine* 361, 1114-1116.

Wu, G., Chen, T., Shahsafaei, A., Hu, W., Bronson, R.T., Shi, G.P., Halperin, J.A., Aktas, H., & Qin, X. (2010). Complement regulator CD59 protects against angiotensin II-induced abdominal aortic aneurysms in mice. *Circulation* 121, 1338-1346.

Wu, G., Hu, W., Shahsafaei, A., Song, W., Dobarro, M., Sukhova, G.K., Bronson, R.R., Shi, G.P., Rother, R.P., Halperin, J.A., *et al.* (2009). Complement regulator CD59 protects against atherosclerosis by restricting the formation of complement membrane attack complex. *Circulation research* 104, 550-558.

Yamana, K., Kosuga, K., Kinoshita, H., Uraguchi, K., Kinoshita, T., Hirata, Y., Akashi, H., Nakayama, T., & Ohishi, K. (1988). Vasculo-Behcet's disease: immunological study of the formation of aneurysm. *The Journal of cardiovascular surgery* 29, 751-755.

Yamashina, M., Ueda, E., Kinoshita, T., Takami, T., Ojima, A., Ono, H., Tanaka, H., Kondo, N., Orii, T., Okada, N., *et al.* (1990). Inherited complete deficiency of 20 kilodalton homologous restriction factor (CD59) as a cause of paroxysmal nocturnal hemoglobinuria. *The New England journal of medicine* 323, 1184-1189.

Yu, Q., Yu, R., & Qin, X. (2010). The good and evil of complement activation in HIV-1 infection. *Cellular & molecular immunology*, 7, 334-340

Yun, S., Leung, V.W., Botto, M., Boyle, J.J., & Haskard, D.O. (2008). Brief report: accelerated atherosclerosis in low-density lipoprotein receptor-deficient mice lacking the membrane-bound complement regulator CD59. *Arteriosclerosis, thrombosis, and vascular biology* 28, 1714-1716.

Zheng, X., Saunders, T.L., Camper, S.A., Samuelson, L.C., & Ginsburg, D. (1995). Vitronectin is not essential for normal mammalian development and fertility. *Proceedings of the National Academy of Sciences of the United States of America* 92, 12426-12430.

Zhou, X., Hu, W., & Qin, X. (2008). The role of complement in the mechanism of action of rituximab for B-cell lymphoma: implications for therapy. *Oncologist* 13, 954 966.

5

Immunoglobulin G4-Related Inflammatory Aortic Aneurysm

Mitsuaki Ishida and Hidetoshi Okabe
Shiga University of Medical Science
Japan

1. Introduction

1.1 The concept of immunoglobulin G4-related sclerosing disease

Immunoglobulin G4 (IgG4) is the rarest subclass of IgG, which is numbered 1 through 4 in the order of their discovery and serum concentration, and normally constitutes only 3 to 6% of the total IgG fraction (Oxelius, 2008). IgG4 antibody has unique structural and functional properties, and the production of IgG4 appears to be driven in part by T helper 2 (Th2) cytokines that mediate allergic responses and IgE production (Nirula et al., 2011). The presence of IgG4 autoantibody in bullous skin diseases and high serum IgG4 concentration in patients with atopic dermatitis, bronchial asthma and bullous skin diseases have indicated that IgG4 plays an important role in these diseases (Jones et al., 1988; Jarvis et al., 2007). However, little attention had been paid to IgG4, before Hamano et al. revealed that serum IgG4 concentration was markedly elevated in patients with sclerosing pancreatitis (also called autoimmune pancreatitis) in 2001 (Hamano et al., 2001). Moreover, the same group also reported that the lesions of sclerosing pancreatitis and retroperitoneal fibrosis had abundant infiltration of IgG4-positive plasma cells (Hamano et al., 2002). Since then, many extrapancreatic lesions that share the same histopathological and immunohistochemical features as autoimmune pancreatitis have been reported in various organs, and the distinct clinicopathological disease entity, termed "IgG4-related sclerosing disease", was established, because irrespective of origin of the organ, these lesions show common clinicopathological features (Kamisawa & Okamoto, 2008; Cheuk & Chan, 2010).

1.2 Clinicopathological features of IgG4-related sclerosing disease

The characteristic clinical features of IgG4-related sclerosing disease are as follows: mostly middle-aged and elderly are affected, male predominance, multiple synchronous or metachronous lesions can be seen in different organs, and the presentation of the patients depend on the involved site(s).

Laboratory tests show that high serum IgG, IgG4, and IgE concentrations, and usually low titers of autoantibodies, such as antinuclear antibodies and rheumatoid factor. In particular, high serum IgG4 concentration (>135mg/dL) is the most important diagnostic factor of IgG4-related sclerosing disease.

Dramatic response to steroid therapy is another characteristic clinical finding of IgG4-related sclerosing disease; a decline in the serum IgG4 level and a reduction of lymphocytes and IgG4-positive plasma cells in the involved tissues are frequently observed (Cheuk & Chan, 2010) (Table 1).

Age	Mostly middle-aged and elderly
Gender	Male predominance
Presentation	Symptom due to involved site(s) (usually mass formation)
Laboratory findings	Elevated IgG, IgG4 and IgE, especially IgG4 (>135mg/dL) Low titers of autoantibodies (e.g.: ANA, RF)
Treatment	Dramatic response to steroid therapy

Table 1. Clinical features of IgG4-related sclerosing disease

Pathologically, IgG4-related sclerosing disease is usually non-circumscribed and can extend into the surrounding tissues. The triad of pathological features of IgG4-related sclerosing disease is dense lymphoplasmacytic infiltration, sclerosis and obliterative phlebitis (Cheuk & Chan 2010) (Table 2). The variable proportion of the lymphoplasmacytic infiltrates and sclerosis in each case is responsible for the spectrum of histopathological patterns, such as pseudolymphomatous, mixed and sclerosing types (Cheuk & Chan, 2010).

In the pseudolymphomatous type, the presence of dense lymphocytes and plasma cells without atypia are the predominant features, and reactive lymphoid follicles are commonly observed. Eosinophil infiltration is also occasionally seen. The mixed pattern, which is the most common histological subtype of IgG4-related sclerosing disease, is characterized by the presence of patchy dense lymphoplasmacytic infiltration and sclerosis. Lastly, the sclerosing type is characterized by the predominance of sclerosis with patchy aggregates of lymphocytes and plasma cells.

The presence of obliterative phlebitis, which represents veins affected by segmental or circumferential transmural lymphoplasmacytic infiltrates, resulting in luminal occlusion, is also a characteristic finding of IgG4-related sclerosing disease.

Immunohistochemical studies revealed abundant IgG4-positive plasma cell infiltration, and the ratio of IgG4-/IgG-positive plasma cells is usually up to 40% (Cheuk & Chan 2010).

a) Lymphoplasmacytic infiltration with/without lymphoid follicles and frequent eosinophil infiltration
b) Sclerosis
c) Obliterative phlebitis
d) No myofibroblast proliferation
e) Abundant IgG4-positive plasma cell infiltration
f) The ratio of IgG4-/IgG-positive plasma cells >40%

Table 2. Pathological features of IgG4-related sclerosing disease

1.3 The spectrum of IgG4-related sclerosing disease

The concept of IgG4-related sclerosing disease has been expanded to include various organs since the first identification in the pancreas (autoimmune pancreatitis). Many extrapancreatic organs, such as bile duct (Zen et al., 2004), liver (Zen et al., 2004), salivary gland (Kitagawa et al., 2005), lacrymal gland (Sato et al., 2008), lung (Zen et al., 2005), breast (Zen et al., 2005), kidney and urinary tract (Watson et al., 2006; Cornell et al., 2007; Kim et al., 2011), prostate (Nishimori et al., 2007), retroperitonum (Hamano et al., 2002), central nervous system (Chan et al., 2009; Shimatsu et al., 2009), thyroid (Li et al., 2011), nasal cavity (Ishida et al., 2009; Moteki et al., 2010), skin (Cheuk et al., 2009) and lymph node (Cheuk et al., 2008; Sato et al., 2010) (Table 3), have been shown to have the same histopathological findings and abundant IgG4-positive plasma cell infiltration as autoimmune pancreatitis.

In addition, recently, a part of inflammatory aortic aneurysm has been regarded as a spectrum of IgG4-related sclerosing disease (Kasashima et al., 2008, 2009, 2010; Ishida et al., 2009).

Multiple synchronous or metachronous lesions can be seen in different organs in the patients with IgG4-related sclerosing disease.

Pancreas	Autoimmune pancreatitis
Bile duct	Sclerosing cholangitis
Gallbladder	Sclerosing cholecystitis
Liver	Inflammatory pseudotumor, hepatitis
Salivary gland	Sclerosing sialadenitis (Küttner's tumor)
Lacrimal gland	Sclerosing dacryoadenitis (Mickulicz's disease)
Nasal cavity	Inflammatory pseudotumor, rhinosinusitis
Lung	Inflammatory pseudotumor (plasma cell granuloma), interstitial pneumonia
Breast	Sclerosing mastitis
Kidney and urinary tract	Tubulointerstitial nephritis, inflammatory pseudotumor
Prostate	Prostatitis
Central nervous system	Hypophysitis, sclerosing pachmeningitis
Thyroid	Hashimoto's thyroiditis
Aorta	Inflammatory aortic aneurysm
Retroperitoneum	Retroperitoneal fibrosis
Skin	Cutaneous pseudolymphoma
Lymph node	Lymphadenopathy

Table 3. The spectrum of IgG4-related sclerosing disease

2. IgG4-related inflammatory aortic aneurysm

Inflammatory aortic aneurysm (IAA), first described by Walker et al. in 1972, is a distinct clinicopathological entity (Walker et al., 1972). They reported that approximately 10% of 187 patients undergoing resection of abdominal aortic aneurysm was IAA. The key distinguishing features of IAA from atherosclerotic aortic aneurysm are as follows: a) marked thickening of the aortic wall, b) fibrosis of the adjacent retroperitoneum, and c) rigid adherence of the adjacent structures to the anterior aneurysmal wall (Walker et al., 1972). Histopathologically, IAA of the abdominal aorta shows a striking fibrosclerotic change in the adventitia with dense lymphoplasmacytic infiltration (Hellmann et al., 2007).

Patients with IAA of the abdominal aorta are younger than patients with atherosclerotic abdominal aortic aneurysm (Paravastu et al., 2009). The clinical symptoms are usually non-specific, such as abdominal and back pain, fever, and general fatigue (Paravastu et al., 2009). Laboratory tests reveal that white blood counts and C-reactive protein levels are usually elevated (Walker et al. 1972). Elevated serum IgG concentration and the presence of autoantibodies are also frequently observed in the patients with IAA of the abdominal aorta (Vaglio A et al., 2003; Jagadesham et al., 2008)

IAA preferentially develops in the infrarenal abdominal aorta, and their presence in the ascending aorta and aortic arch is extremely rare (Ishida et al., 2009).

In 2008, Kasashima et al. proposed that IAA of the abdominal aorta can be divided into two subgroups: "IgG4-related" and "non-IgG4-related" (Kasashima et al., 2008). They reported that 4 of 10 patients with IAA of the abdominal aorta had high serum IgG4 concentration and abundant IgG4-positive plasma cell infiltrates in the aneurysmal wall, which are identical to the clinicopathological features of IgG4-related sclerosing disease. Henceforth, IgG4-related IAA of the thoracic aorta have also been reported (Ishida et al., 2009; Kasashima et al., 2010)

2.1.1 Abdominal aortic aneurysm

As shown Kasashima et al., there are clinicopathological differences between IgG4-related and non-IgG4-related IAA of the abdominal aorta (Kasashima, et al. 2008, 2009). With regard to incidence rate, IgG4-related IAA of the abdominal aorta accounts for 5% of all surgically resected abdominal aortic aneurysms, and 57% of IAA of the abdominal aorta (Kasashima et al. 2009).

Age/Gender	No difference
Aneurysmal diameter	No difference
Symptom	More frequency of abdominal or back pain in non-IgG4-related cases
History of autoimmune and allergic diseases	More frequent in IgG4-related cases (food or drug allergy, bronchial asthma and rheumatoid arthritis)
Serum IgG	No difference
Serum IgG4	Markedly higher in IgG4-related cases
Serum IgE	Higher in IgG4-related cases
Adventitial thickening	Thicker in IgG4-related cases
IgG-positive cells	Mildly superior in IgG4-related cases
IgG4-positive cells	More numerous in IgG4-related cases
IgG4/IgG cells ratio	More higher in IgG4-related cases
Neutrophils infiltration	Higher in non-IgG4-related cases
Eosinophils infiltration	Higher in IgG4-related cases
Lymphoid follicles	More frequent in IgG4-related cases
Obliterative phlebitis	More frequent in IgG4-related cases

Table 4. Clinicopathological differences between IgG4-related and non-IgG4-related inflammatory aortic aneurysms of the abdominal aorta.

Clinically, there are no differences in patient age, gender and aneurysmal diameter between IgG4-related and non-IgG4-related IAAs, however, IgG4-related cases are characterized by less frequent association with abdominal or back pain. The history of autoimmune diseases (such as rheumatoid arthritis and idiopathic thrombocytopenic purpura), bronchial asthma and food or drug allergy are more frequent in IgG4-related cases than non-IgG4-related cases. Characteristically, serum IgG4 concentration is significantly elevated in IgG4-related cases (>135 mg/dL), although serum IgG concentration is not different in both groups. In addition, IgE concentration is higher in IgG4-related cases. Aneurysmal rupture is more common in non-IgG4-related cases, because severe thickening of the aneurysmal wall and adhesion to the surrounding tissue may prevent rupture in IgG4-related cases (Kasashima et al., 2010) (Table 4).

Most reported cases of IgG4-related IAA of abdominal aorta have no association with other IgG4-related sclerosing diseases, however, some cases of IgG4-related IAA of the abdominal aorta with autoimmune pancreatitis have been reported (Ito et al., 2008; Tseng et al., 2009; Matsuki et al., 2010).

Pathologically, IgG4-related IAA fundamentally has the similar histopathological findings of IgG4-related sclerosing disease. IgG4-related IAA is characterized by significant thickening of the adventitia more so than non-IgG4-related cases (Figure 1), although all IAA cases generally have marked thickening of the adventitia (Figure 6). In IgG4-related cases, dense lymphoplasmacytic infiltrates with lymphoid follicles are observed in the adventitia (Figure 2). Eosinophil infiltration and perineural lymphoplasmacytic infiltration are common findings of IgG4-related cases (Figure 3), however, neutrophil infiltration is rarely seen. In contrast, neutrophil infiltration is occasionally seen in non-IgG4-related cases. In most IgG4-related cases, obliterative phlebitis, one of the characteristic findings of IgG4-related sclerosing disease, is present in the adventitia (Figure 4), although obliterative phlebitis is also observed in some non-IgG4-related cases, but at much lower frequency.

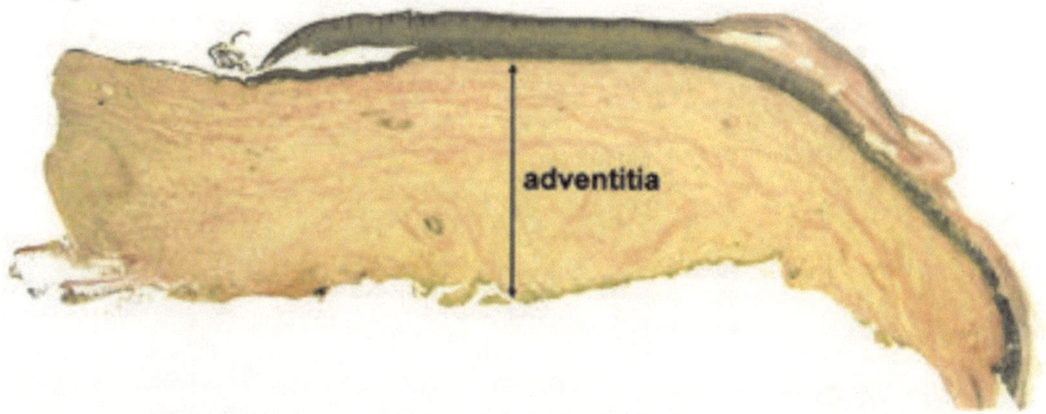

Fig. 1. Panoramic view of an IgG4-related inflammatory aortic aneurysm (Elastica van Gieson stain). Significant thickening of the adventitia is evident.

Atherosclerotic change is also observed in IgG4-related cases, because both IgG4-related and non-IgG4-related IAAs commonly affect middle-aged to elderly persons. However, atherosclerotic intimal thickening is more intense in non-IgG4-related cases (Kasashima et al., 2010).

Immunohistochemically, abundant IgG4-positive plasma cell infiltrate is observed in the adventitia of IgG4-related IAA (Figure 5), in contrast to non-IgG4-related IAA, which harbor only a few IgG4-positive plasma cells (Figure 7). The ratio of IgG4-/IgG-positive plasma cells is markedly higher in IgG4-related cases (usually >60%) as compared to non-IgG4-related cases (Kasashima et al., 2009).

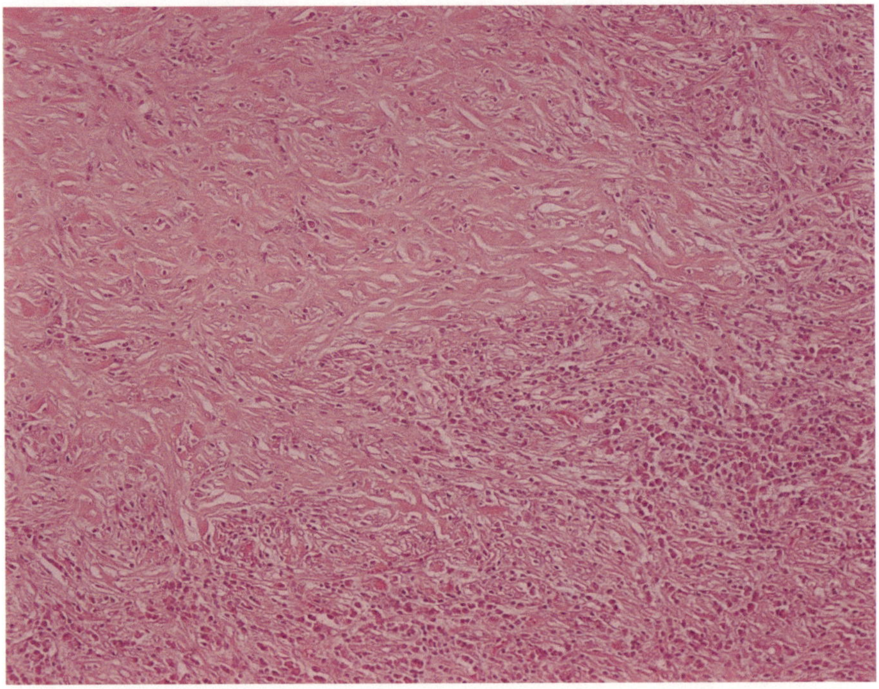

Fig. 2. Histopathological findings of IgG4-related inflammatory aortic aneurysm (H.E. stain). Lymphoplasmacytic infiltration and sclerosis in the adventitia.

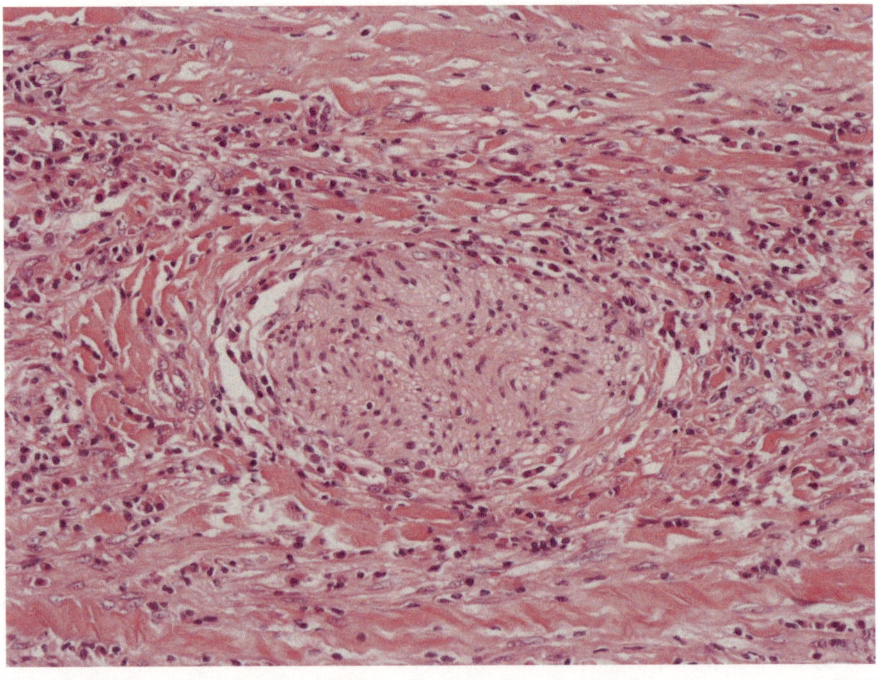

Fig. 3. Histopathological findings of IgG4-related inflammatory aortic aneurysm (H.E. stain). Perineural lymphoplasmacytic infiltration is occasionally observed.

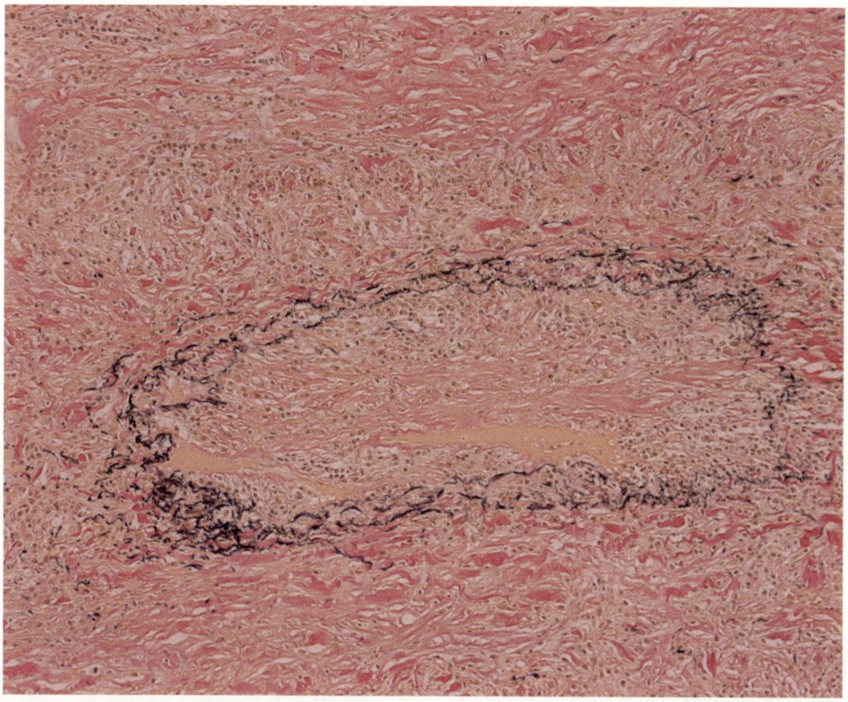

Fig. 4. Elastica van Gieson stain clearly showing obliterative phlebitis in the adventitia in IgG4-related inflammatory aortic aneurysm.

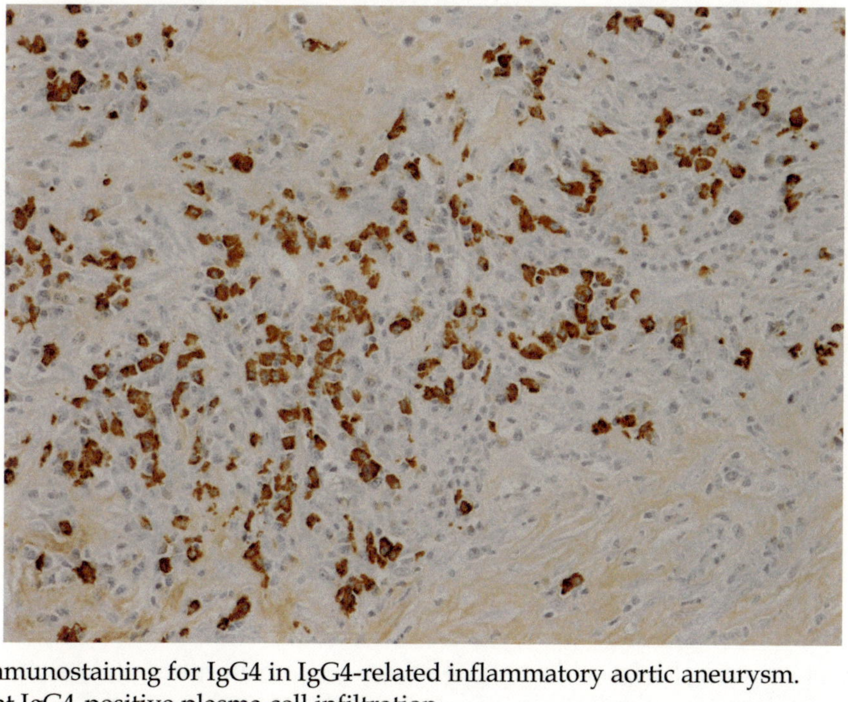

Fig. 5. Immunostaining for IgG4 in IgG4-related inflammatory aortic aneurysm. Abundant IgG4-positive plasma cell infiltration.

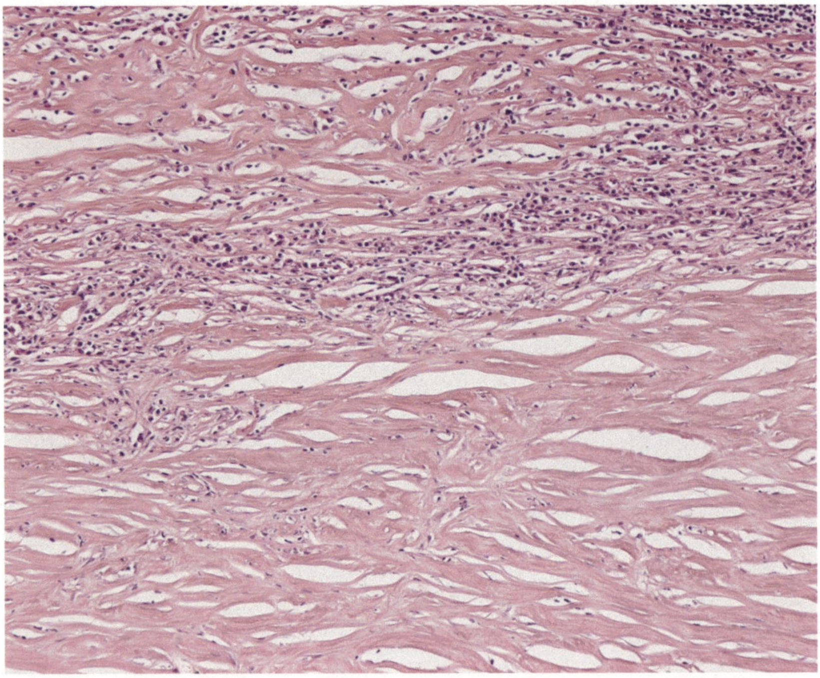

Fig. 6. Histopathological findings of non-IgG4-related inflammatory aortic aneurysm (H.E. stain). Lymphoplasmacytic infiltration and sclerosis are shown in the adventitia.

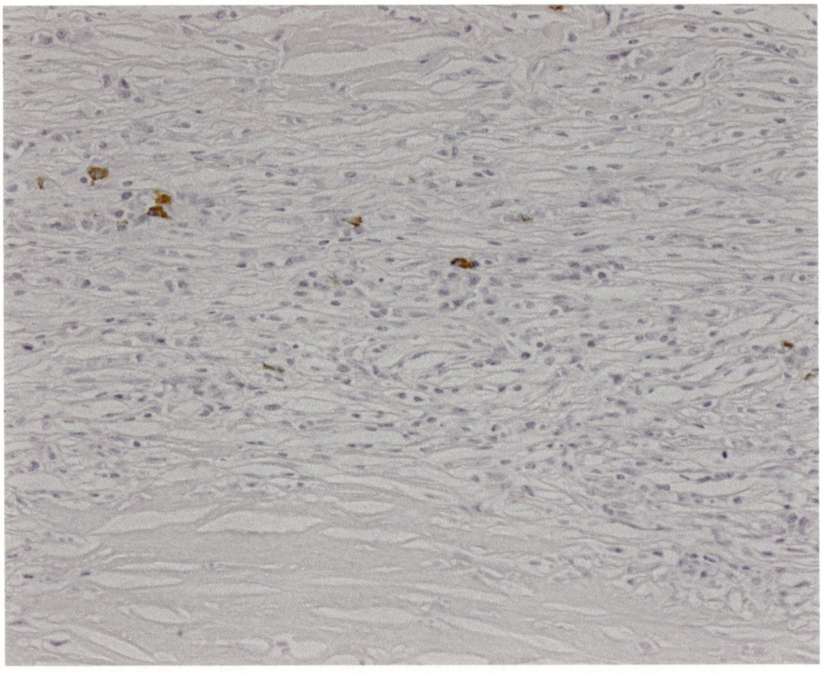

Fig. 7. Immunostaining for IgG4 in non-IgG4-related inflammatory aortic aneurysm. Only a few IgG4-positive plasma cells are detected in the adventitia.

2.1.2 Thoracic aortic aneurysm

In 2009, IgG4-related IAA of the aortic arch was first reported, and this report suggested that IgG4-related aortic lesion can occur in the thoracic aorta, as a counterpart of IgG4-related IAA of the abdominal aorta (Ishida et al., 2009). Since then, subsequent studies have revealed the clinicopathological features of IgG4-related lesions of the thoracic aorta. IgG4-related thoracic aortic lesions often represent aneurysmal cases, and several cases of lymphoplasmacytic aortitis without dilatation of the aorta are included in this entity, which may represent an early phase of IgG4-related aortic aneurysm (Kasashima et al., 2010; Stone et al., 2010).

Kasashima et al. reported that 4% of all surgically resected thoracic aortic lesions (which corresponded to 7% of thoracic aortic aneurysm) was IgG4-related. (Kasashima et al., 2010). These cases included inflammatory aneurysm, lymphoplasmacytic aortitis, and atherosclerotic aneurysms (Kasashima et al., 2010). Stone et al. reported that IgG4-related sclerosing lesions of thoracic aorta accounted for 9% of noninfectious thoracic aortitis and 75% of lymphoplasmacytic aortitis (Stone et al., 2010). These patients show similar clinical features to IgG4-related IAA of the abdominal aorta with a predilection for elderly males, medical history of bronchial asthma and allergy, and elevated white blood cell count and C-reactive protein levels. IgG4-related aortic aneurysm of the thoracic aorta develops frequently in the aortic arch and saccular form aneurysm (Kasashima et al., 2010). In addition, fibrous adherence to the surrounding tissue is more frequent as compared to non-IgG4-related cases (Kasashima et al., 2010).

Pathologically, IgG4-related IAA of the thoracic aorta also shows similar findings to IgG4-related IAA of the abdominal aorta including thickening of the adventitia, dense lymphoplasmacytic infiltration, obliterative phlebitis, frequent eosinophil infiltration, lymphoid follicle formation, and infrequent neutrophil infiltration. Immunohistochemically, abundant IgG4-positive plasma cell infiltration and high ratio of IgG4-/IgG-positive plasma cells (>60%) are observed (Ishida et al., 2009; Kasashima et al., 2010).

Interestingly, aortic dissection has been reported as one manifestation of IgG4-related lesions in the thoracic aorta (Stone et al., 2009, 2010). In such case, inflammation is denser in the media than in the adventitia, and medial laminar necrosis is also observed (Stone et al., 2009, 2010).

Some cases of IgG4-related lesions of the thoracic aorta associated with other IgG4-related sclerosing lesions, such as pancreas, submandibular gland and lymph node, have been reported (Stone et al., 2010).

2.2 Diagnostic criteria for IgG4-related IAA

The diagnostic criteria for IgG4-related IAA of the abdominal aorta have been previously outlined (Kasashima et al., 2009), and a recent study have found that these criteria may also be appropriate for IgG4-related thoracic aortic aneurysm (Kasashima et al., 2010).

a. Diffuse fibrous thickening of the adventitia (>4mm)
b. Abundant lymphoplasmacytic infiltrates
c. Numerous IgG4-positive plasma cells (60/ high-power fields)
d. Ratio of IgG4-/IgG-positive plasma cells >60%

2.3 Differential diagnosis of IgG4-related IAA

The chief differential diagnosis of IgG4-related IAA is non-IgG4-related IAA, which is not difficult due to the distinct features of each type. The clinicopathological differential diagnostic considerations are described in 2.1.2.

Takayasu arteritis must be taken into consideration during diagnosis of IgG4-related IAA of the thoracic aorta. Takayasu arteritis is well known as a "pulseless disease", which chiefly strikes young women, especially in Asian and South American countries, and mainly involves the ascending aorta, aortic arch, and their main branches, leading to the characteristic clinical findings of pulselessness and ophthalmic and/or cerebral disorders (Numano et al., 2000). Histopathologically, Takayasu arteritis is characterized by involvement of all three layers of the arterial wall, thickened adventitia with lymphocyte and histiocyte infiltrates, destruction of smooth muscles and elastic fiber network of the medina, occasional medial necrosis and intimal fibrosis and/or atherosclerotic changes (Numano, 2000). The inflammatory process appears to begin at the vaso vasorum in the adventitia and these inflammatory processes result in stenosis of vessel lumina and sometimes induce aneurysmal formation (Numano, 2000). IgG4-related IAA does not show vascular stricture and stenosis. Thus, the differential diagnostic features include patient's age, histopathological findings, especially involvement of all three arterial wall layers found only in Takayasu arteritis, and immunohistochemical findings for IgG4. In addition, epithelioid granuloma, giant cells, and fibrinoid necrosis are extremely rare in IgG4-related IAA (Kasashima et al. 2010).

Syphilitic aortitis is also included in the differential diagnosis, because it is also characterized by frequent aneurysmal formation and lymphoplasmacytic infiltration in the adventitia. Lymphoplasmacytic infiltration accompanying destruction of the medina and endarteritis obliterans of the vasa vasorum are usually observed in syphilitic aortitis (Heggtveit 1962), but not in IgG4-related IAA. The serological examination for *Treponema pallidum* agglutination is also useful.

a) Non-IgG4-related IAA
b) Takayasu areteritis
c) Syphilitic arteritis

Table 5. Chief differential diagnoses of IgG4-related IAA

3. The association with chronic periaortitis

Chronic periaortitis encompasses idiopathic retroperitoneal fibrosis, IAA and perianeurysmal retroperitoneal fibrosis (Jois et al., 2004). The histopathological characteristic are identical, which include periaortic fibrosis with extension to involve the adjacent structure, and lymphoplasmacytic infiltration in the aortic adventitia. These characteristic histopathological findings also correspond to IgG4-related sclerosing disease, and abundant IgG4-positive plasma cells infiltration is also observed in chronic periaortitis. Therefore, both retroperitoneal fibrosis and IgG4-related IAA of the abdominal aorta are recognized as a manifestation of "IgG4-related chronic periaortitis" (Kasashima et al., 2008, 2011), together with mediastinal fibrosis and IgG4-related IAA of the thoracic aorta (Ishida et al., 2009; Kasashima et al., 2011).

4. Treatment of IgG4-related IAA

Dramatic response to steroid therapy is the characteristic clinical finding of IgG4-related sclerosing disease. It is speculated that steroid therapy may be also effective in IgG4-related IAA, because adventitial thickening and fibrous adhesion to the surround organs may be reduced (Kasashima et al., 2009). However, most of the reported cases of IgG4-related IAA were surgically resected cases, therefore, steroid therapy was not administrated and no data is available.

Recently, some cases of IgG4-related IAA in whom steroid therapy could reduce the aneurysmal wall thickening and fibrous adhesion of IAA, have been reported (Kasashima et al., 2010; Yabe et al., 2010). However, it must be considered that the risk of aneurysmal rupture might be elevated by the thinning of the adventitia. Additional clinicopathological studies are required to establish the treatment strategy for IgG4-related IAA.

Finally, multiple metachronous or synchronous development is one of the characteristic findings of IgG4-related sclerosing disease, therefore, systemic surveillance and follow-up are required in cases of IgG4-related IAA.

5. Conclusion

IgG4-related sclerosing disease is a distinct clinicopathological entity and may manifest as IAA of the thoracic and abdominal aorta. IgG4-related IAA shows characteristic clinical features, and histopathological diagnostic criteria of IgG4-related IAA have been recently proposed. However, further studies are needed to clarify the spectrum of IgG4-related vascular lesions and treatment strategy of IgG4-related IAA.

6. References

Chan, SK.; Cheuk, W.; Chan, KT. & Chan, JK. (2009). IgG4-related sclerosing pachymeningitis: a previously unrecognized form of central nervous system involvement in IgG4-related sclerosing disease. *American Journal of Surgical Pathology*, Vol. 33, No. 8, (Aug), pp. 1249-1252, ISSN 0147-5185

Cheuk, W.; Yuen, HK.; Chu, SY.; Chiu, EK.; Lam, LK. & Chan JK. (2008). Lymphadenopathy of IgG4-related sclerosing disease. *American Journal of Surgical Pathology*, Vol. 32, No. 5, (May), pp. 671-681, ISSN 0147-5185

Cheuk, W.; Lee, KC.; Chong, LY.; Yuen, ST. & Chan, JK. (2009). IgG4-related sclerosing disease: a potential new etiology of cutaneous pseudolymphoma. *American Journal of Surgical Pathology*, Vol. 33, No. 11, (Nov), pp. 1713-1719, ISSN 0147-5185

Cheuk, W. & Chan, JK. (2010). IgG4-related sclerosing disease: a critical appraisal of an evolking clinicopathological entity. *Advances in Anatomic Pathology*, Vol. 17, No. 5, (Sep), pp. 303-332, ISSN 1072-4109

Cornell, LD. (2010). IgG4-related tubulointerstitial nephritis. *Kidney International*, Vol. 78, No. 10 (Nov), pp. 1016-1023, ISSN 0085-2538

Hamano, H.; Kawa, S.; Horiuchi, A.; Unno, H.; Furuya, N.; Akamatsu, T.; Fukushima, M.; Nikaido, T.; Nakayama, K.; Usuda, N. & Kiyosawa, K. (2001). High serum IgG4 concentration in patients with sclerosing pancreatitis. *New England Journal of Medicine*, Vol. 344, No. 10, (Mar), pp. 732-738, ISSN 0028-4793

Hamano, H.; Kawa, S.; Ochi, Y.; Unno, H.; Shiba, N.; Wajiki, M.; Nakazawa, K.; Shimojo, H. & Kiyosawa, K. (2002). Hydronephrosis associated with retroperitoneal fibrosis and sclerosing pancreatitis. *Lancet*, Vol. 359, No. 9315, (Apr), pp. 1403-1404, ISSN 0140-6736

Heggtveit, HA. (1964). Syphlitic aortitis. A clinicopathologic autopsy study of 100 cases, 1950 to 1960. *Circulation*, Vol. 29, (Mar), pp. 346-355, ISSN 0009-7322

Hellmann, DB.; Grand, DJ. & Freischlag, JA. (2007). Inflammatory abdominal aortic aneurysm. *JAMA-Journal of the American Medical Association*, Vol. 297. No. 4, (Jan), pp. 395-400, ISSN 0098-7384

Ishida, M.; Hotta, M.; Kushima, R.; Asai, T. & Okabe, H. (2009). IgG4-related inflammatory aortic aneurysm of the aortic arch. *Pathology International*, Vol. 59, No. 4, (Apr), pp. 269-273, ISSN 1320-5463

Ishida, M.; Hotta, M.; Kushima, R.; Shibayama, M.; Shimizu, T. & Okabe, H. (2009). Multiple IgG4-related sclerosing lesions in the maxillary sinus, parotid gland and nasal septum. *Pathology International*, Vol. 59, No. 9, (Sep), pp. 670-675, ISSN 1320-5463

Ito, H.; Kaizaki, Y.; Noda, Y.; Fujii, S. & Yamamoto, S. (2008). IgG4-related inflammatory abdominal aortic aneurysm associated with autoimmune pancreatitis. *Pathology International*, Vol. 58, No. 7, (Jul), pp. 421-426, ISSN 1320-5463

Jagadesham, VP.; Scott, DJ. & Carding, SR. (2008). Abdominal aortic aneurysms: an autoimmune disease? *Trends in Molecular Medicine*, Vol. 14, No. 12, (Dec), pp. 522-529, ISSN 1471-4914

Jarvis, D.; Zock, JP.; Heinrich, J.; Svanes, C.; Verlato, G.; Olivieri, M.; Villani, S.; Ponzio, M.; Leynaert, B.; Sunyer, J.; Dahlman-Hoglund, A.; Chinn, S.; Luczynska, C.; Norbäck, D. & Burney, P. (2007). Cat and dust mite allergen levels, specific IgG and IgG4, and respiratory symptoms in adults. *Journal of Allergy and Clinical Immunology*, Vol. 119, No. 3, (Mar), pp. 697-704, ISSN 0091-6749

Jois, RN.; Gaffney, K.; Marshall, T. & Scott, DG. (2004). Chronic periaortitis. *Rheumatology*, Vol. 43, No. 11, (Nov), pp. 1141-1146, ISSN 1462-0324

Jones, CC.; Hamilton, RG. & Jordon, RE. (1988). Subclass distribution of human IgG autoantibodies in pemphigus. *Journal of Clinical Immunology*, Vol. 8, No. 1, (Jan), pp. 43-49, ISSN 0271-9142

Kamisawa, T. & Okamoto, A. (2008). IgG4-related sclerosing disease. *World Journal of Gastroenterology*, Vol. 14, No. 25, (Jul), pp. 3948-3955, ISSN 1007-9327

Kasashima, S.; Zen, Y.; Kawashima, A.; Konishi, K.; Sasaki, H.; Endo, M.; Matsumoto, Y.; Kawakami, K.; Kasashima, F.; Moriya, M.; Kimura, K.; Ohtake, H. & Nakanuma, Y. (2008). Inflammatory abdominal aortic aneurysm: close relationship to IgG4-related periaortitis. *American Journal of Surgical Pathology*, Vol. 32, No. 2, (Feb), pp. 197-204, ISSN 0147-5185

Kasashima, S.; Zen, Y.; Kawashima, A.; Endo, M.; Matsumoto, Y. & Kasashima, F. (2009). A new clinicopathological entity of IgG4-related inflammatory abdominal aortic aneurysm. *Journal of Vascular Surgery*, Vol. 49,No. 5, (May), pp. 1264-1271, ISSN 0741-5214

Kasashima, S.; Zen, Y.; Kawashima, A.; Endo, M.; Matsumoto, Y.; Kasashima, F.; Ohtake, H. & Nakanuma, Y (2010). A clinicopathologic study of immunoglobulin G4-related sclerosing disease of the thoracic aorta. *Journal of Vascular Surgery*, Vol. 52,No. 6, (Dec), pp. 1587-1595, ISSN 0741-5214

Kasashima, S. & Zen, Y. (2011). IgG4-related inflammatory abdominal aortic aneurysm. *Current Opinion in Rheumatology*, Vol. 23, No. 1, (Jan), pp. 18-23, ISSN 1040-8711

Kim, SA.; Lee, SR.; Huh, J.; Shen, SS. & Ro, JY. (2011). IgG4-associated inflammatory pseudotumor of ureter: clinicopathologic and immunohistochemical study of 3 cases. *Human Pathology*, (in press), ISSN 0046-8177

Kitagawa, S.; Zen, Y.; Harada, K.; Sasaki, M.; Sato, Y.; Minato, H.; Watanabe, K.; Kurumaya, H.; Katayanagi, K.; Masuda, S.; Niwa, H.; Tsuneyama, K.; Saito, K.; Haratate, J.; Takagawa, K. & Nakanuma, Y. (2005). Abundant IgG4-positive plasma cell infiltration characterizes chronic sclerosing sialadenitis (Küttner's tumor). *American Journal of Surgical Pathology*, Vol. 29, No. 6, (Jun), pp. 783-791, ISSN 0147-5185

Li, Y.; Nishihara, E. & Kakudo, K. (2011). Hashimoto's thyroiditis: old concepts and new insights. *Current Opinion in Rheumatology*, Vol. 23, No. 1, (Jan), pp. 102-107, ISSN 1040-8711

Matsuki, Y.; Sato, K.; Fujikawa, A.; Kyoto, Y.; Hashimoto, H. & Hakozaki, Y. (2010). A case of incidentally detected IgG4-related sclerosing disease involving inflammatory abdominal aortic aneurysm and autoimmune pancreatitis. *Modern Rheumatology*, Vol. 20, No. 3, (Jun), pp. 306-310, ISSN 1439-7595

Moteki, H.; Yasuo, M.; Hamano, H.; Uehara, T. & Usami, SI. (2010). IgG4-related chronic rhinosinusitis: a new clinical entity of nasal disease. *Acta Oto-Laryngologica*, (in press), ISSN 0001-6489

Nirula, A.; Glaser, SM.; Kalled, SL. & Taylora, FR. (2011). What is IgG4? A review of the biology of a unique immunoglobulin subtype. *Current Opinion in Rheumatology*, Vol. 23, No. 1, (Jan), pp. 119-124, ISSN 1040-8711

Nishimori, I.; Kohsaki, T.; Onishi, S.; Shuin, T.; Kohsaki, S.; Ogawa, Y.; Matsumoto, M.; Hiroi, M.; Hamano, H. & Sawa, S. (2007). IgG4-related autoimmune prostatitis: two cases with or without autoimmune pancreatitis. *Internal Medicine*, Vol. 46, No. 24, pp. 1983-1989, ISSN 0918-2918

Numano, F.; Okawara, M.; Inomata, H. & Kobayashi, Y. (2000). Takayasu's arteritis. *Lancet*, Vol. 356, No. 9234, (Sep), pp. 1023-1025, ISSN 0140-6736

Numano, F. (2000). Vasa vasoritis, vasculitis and atherosclerosis. *International Journal of Cardiology*. Vol. 75, No. Suppl 1, (Aug), pp. S1-8, ISSN 0167-5273

Oxelius, VA. (2008). Immunoglobulin constant heavy G subclass chain genes in asthma and allergy. *Immunologic Research*, Vol. 40, No. 2, pp. 179-191, ISSN 0257-277X

Paravastu, SC.; Murray, D.; Ghosh, J.; Serracino-Inglott, F.; Smyth, JV. & Walker, MG. (2009). Inflammatory abdominal aortic aneurysms (IAAA): past and present. *Vascular and Endovascular Surgery*, Vol. 43, No. 4, (Aug-Sep), pp. 360-363, ISSN 1538-5744

Sato, Y.; Ohshima, K.; Ichimura, K.; Sato, M.; Yamadori, I.; Tanaka, T.; Takata, K.; Morito, T.; Kondo, E. & Yoshino, T. (2008). Ocular adnexal IgG4-related disease has uniform clinicopathology. *Pathology International*, Vol. 58, No. 8, (Aug), pp. 465-470, ISSN 1320-5463

Sato, Y.; Notohara, K.; Kojima, M.; Takata, K.; Masaki, Y. & Yoshino, T. (2010). IgG4-related disease: historical overview and pathology of hematological disorders. *Pathology International*, Vol. 60, No. 4, (Apr), pp. 247-258, ISSN 1320-5463

Shimatsu, A.; Oki, Y.; Fujisawa, I. & Sano, T. (2009). Pituitary and stalk lesions (infundibulo-hypophysitis) associated with immunoglobulin G4-related systemic disease: an emerging clinical entity. *Endocrine Journal*, Vol. 56, No. 9, pp. 1033-1041, ISSN 0918-8959

Stone, JH.; Khosroshahi, A.; Hilgenberg, A.; Spooner, A.; Isselbacher, EM. & Stone, JR. (2009). IgG4-related systemic disease and lymphoplasmacytic aortitis. *Arthritis & Rheumatism*, Vol. 60, No. 10, (Oct), pp. 3139-3145, ISSN 0004-3591

Stone, JH.; Khosroshahi, A.; Deshpande, V. & Stone, JR. (2010). IgG4-related systemic disease accounts for a significant proportion of thoracic lymphoplasmacytic aortitis cases. *Arthritis Care & Research*, Vol. 62, No. 3, (Mar), pp. 316-312, ISSN 2151-464X

Tseng, CW.; Tsai, JJ. & Chen, CC. (2009). Abdominal aortitis associated with autoimmune pancreatitis. *Clinical Gastroenterology and Hepatology*, Vol. 7, No. 1, (Jan), pp. e3-4, ISSN 1542-3565

Vaglio, A.; Corradi, D.; Manenti, L.; Ferretti, S.; Garini, G. & Buzio, C. (2003). Evidence of autoimmunity in chronic periaortitis: a prospective study. *American Journal of Medicine*, Vol. 114. No. 6, (Apr), pp. 454-462, ISSN 0002-9343

Walker, DI.; Bloor, K.; Williams, G. & Gillie, I. (1972). Inflammatory aneurysm of the abdominal aorta. *British Journal of Surgery*, Vol. 59, No. 8, (Aug), pp. 609-614, ISSN 0007-133

Watson, SJ.; Jenkins, DA. & Bellamy, CO. (2006). Nephropathy in IgG4-related systemic disease. *American Journal of Surgical Pathology*, Vol. 30, No. 11, (Nov), pp. 1472-1477, ISSN 0147-5185

Yabe, T.; Hamada, T.; Kubo, T.; Okawa, M.; Yamasaki, N.; Matsumura, Y.; Kitaoka, H. & Doi, Y. (2010). Inflammatory abdominal aortic aneurysm successfully treated with steroid therapy. *Journal of the American College of Cardiology*. Vol. 55, No. 25, (Jun), pp. 2877, ISSN 0735-1097

Zen, Y.; Harada, K.; Sasaki, M.; Sato, Y.; Tsuneyama, K.; Haratake, J.; Kurumaya, H.; Katayanagi, K.; Masuda, S.; Niwa, H.; Morimoto, H.; Miwa, A.; Uchiyama, A.; Portmann, BC. & Nakanuma, Y. (2004). IgG4-related sclerosing cholangitis with and without hepatic inflammatory pseudotumor, and sclerosing pancreatitis-associated sclerosing cholangitis: do they belong to a spectrum of sclerosing pancreatitis? *American Journal of Surgical Pathology*, Vol. 28, No. 9, (Sep), pp. 1193-1203, ISSN 0147-5185

Zen, Y.; Kasahara, Y.; Horita, K.; Miyayama, S.; Miura, S.; Kitagawa, S. & Nakanuma, Y. (2005). Inflammatory pseudotumor of the breast in a patient with a high serum IgG4 level: histologic similarity to sclerosing pancreatitis. *American Journal of Surgical Pathology*, Vol. 29, No. 2, (Feb), pp. 275-278, ISSN 0147-5185

Zen, Y.; Kitagawa, S.; Minato, H.; Kurumaya, H.; Katayanagi, K.; Masuda, S.; Niwa ,H.; Fujimura, M. & Nakanuma, Y. (2005). IgG4-positive plasma cells in inflammatory pseudotumor (plasma cell granuloma) of the lung. *Human Pathology*, Vol. 36, No. 7, (Jul), pp. 710-717, ISSN 0046-8177

6

Transcriptomic and Proteomic Profiles of Vascular Cells Involved in Human Abdominal Aortic Aneurysm

Florence Pinet[1,2,3,4] *et. al.* *
[1]*INSERM U744, Lille*
[2]*Institut Pasteur de Lille, Lille*
[3]*University of Nord de France, USDL, IFR 141, Lille*
[4]*Centre Hospitalier Régional et Universitaire de Lille*
France

1. Introduction

Abdominal aortic aneurysms (AAAs) are a potentially fatal disorder. Atherosclerotic changes followed by accelerated degradation of collagen and elastin, the main components of the extracellular matrix (ECM) in the vascular wall, cause the development of AAAs in deteriorating aortic walls that dilate progressively and may eventually rupture. Other alterations associated with AAAs include marked changes in the cellular composition of the aortic wall, especially the infiltration of macrophages and T-lymphocytes into the adventitia and a major reduction in the population of vascular smooth muscle cells (SMCs) (Lopez-Candales et al., 1997; Henderson et al., 1999).

AAA appear to be a consequence of complex mechanisms involving several potential factors: immunological, inflammatory, chemotactic, apoptotic, protease-related, angiogenic and fibrinolytic (Ailawadi et al., 2003). Recently, interleukin-8 and monocyte chemoattractant protein 1 expression were shown to be raised in the AAA biopsies compared to the abdominal aorta of controls, suggesting that pathways involving these proteins may be involved in AAA pathologies (Middleton et al., 2009). AAA is a disease associated with chronic inflammation in the aortic wall and leukotrienes are powerful lipid mediators released by inflammatory cells (Samuelsson, 1983). A recent study showed the increased expression of leukotriene C4 synthase together with the predominant formation of cysteinyl-leukotrienes in human AAA, linked with matrix metalloproteinases (MMP)

* Nicolas Lamblin[1,2,3,4], Philippe Ratajczak[1,2,3], David Hot[2,5,6], Emilie Dubois[1,2,3], Maggy Chwastyniak[1,2,3], Olivia Beseme[1,2,3], Hervé Drobecq[2,3,6], Yves Lemoine[2,5,6], Mohammad Koussa[4] and Philippe Amouyel[1,2,3,4]
1 *INSERM U744, Lille, France,*
2 *Institut Pasteur de Lille, Lille, France,*
3 *University of Nord de France, USDL, IFR 141, Lille, France,*
4 *Centre Hospitalier Régional et Universitaire de Lille, France,*
5 *Laboratoire d'Etudes Transcriptomiques et Génomiques Appliquées, Lille, France,*
6 *UMR CNRS 8161, France,*
7 *University of Nord de France, USTL, Villeneuve d'Ascq, France.*

production (Di Gennaro et al., 2010). This suggests a mechanism by which leukotrienes may promote matrix degradation in the AAA wall.

Despite reports that major atherosclerotic risk factors are related to AAA (Iribarren et al., 2007), we still lack the information about the process of aneurysmal degeneration (Wassef et al., 2007, Golledge et al., 2008) that we need to develop non-invasive approaches for its early detection. In aneurysm formation, collagen degradation exceeds its synthesis and together with excessive degradation of other ECM macromolecules, notably elastin, ultimately promotes rupture of these aneurysms. Increased local production of proteases, that is, enzymes capable of degrading collagen and elastin ECM proteins, have been identified in aneurysm sites (Dobrin & Mrkvicka, 1994; Knox et al., 1997; Thompson, 2006). The source of these proteases in humans is unclear, however, although many studies have measured their expression in cells from biopsies or tissues obtained after surgery (Wilson et al, 2006).

2. Purpose of the study

The aim of the study was to conduct a global comparison of the mRNA and protein expression profiles in the vascular cells to determine the genes involved in the pathological progression of aneurysmal disease by comparing the transcriptomic and proteomic profiles of SMCs and macrophages of patients with AAAs and those who have peripheral arterial occlusion (PAO) but no AAAs (verified by imaging). Using samples from two groups of patients in LILAS (the Lille Anevrysmal Study, described below), those with AAAs and others with PAO, we isolated SMCs from aortic tissue and monocytes (that were differentiated into macrophages) from blood. Although these diseases have common mechanisms, inflammatory cells essentially infiltrate the media and adventitia of the arterial wall in AAAs, whereas they are mostly in the intima in PAO. Because the factors that influence these distinctions are unknown, we designed a study that would allow us to distinguish "pro-aneurysmal" risk factors from those that are associated with atherogenesis and stenosis. We choose PAO disease as control diseases as Thompson *et al.,* (Thompson, 2002) described the separation of AAA disease from other atherosclerotic diseases like peripheral vascular disease and carotid disease.

Following recommendations for large-scale parallel quantitation of proteins (Kingsmore, 2006), we have constructed a protein microarray that contained on one slide 42 different antibodies representing proteins found by transcriptomic and proteomic analysis to be differentially modulated in macrophages and SMC from AAA and PAO patients. Finally, we performed the same analysis of plasma from the same patients to identify proteins involved in the aneurysmal process that are more easily detectable, as hypothesized that circulating biomarkers can reflect inflammation and degeneration in the AAA wall (Golledge et al., 2008).

3. Population study

The LILle Anevrysmal Study (LILAS) was a case-control study that enrolled 42 men, either AAA (case patients) or peripheral arterial occlusion (PAO) (control patients) who needed a vascular surgery or endovascular treatment at the Lille University Hospital Centre (Lille, France) (Lamblin et al., 2010). The ethics committee of the Lille University Hospital Center (France) approved the study (CCPPRB n° CP03/47 of 06 May 2003), and each patient provided written informed consent. The protocol required a blood sample (80 ml) to be taken at inclusion, before the surgery. All patients underwent the planned surgical

treatment and, when possible, surgeons removed the thrombus and took a sample of the aneurysm wall in the case patients (n=24) and a sample of the aortic wall during the bypass grafting for the control PAO patients (n=18).
The mean age of subjects was 65.6 ± 6.9 years but AAA patients were older (68.0 ± 6.1 years *versus* 62.3 ± 6.6 years). No other cardiovascular risk factors differed between the groups. In both groups, one third of the patients had hypertension and half dyslipidemia. Diabetes mellitus was found in 17% of the AAA group and 22% of the PAO group, an insignificant difference. Both groups also had similar percentages of family members with a history of heart disease (myocardial infarction and/or acute coronary syndrome): 29% in AAA patients and 35% in PAO patients. The AAA case patients (n=24) had a mean maximal external aortic diameter of 56.1 ± 11.3 [range: 46-95] mm. All the PAO patients had undergone recent vascular imaging of the aorta and lower limbs before surgery: none had AAAs or iliac, femoral or popliteal aneurysms. The groups did not differ concerning their cardiovascular treatment (Table 2, Lamblin et al, 2010). Before surgery, fewer than two thirds had antiplatelet treatment. Fewer AAA than PAO patients received ACE inhibitor treatment (21% *versus* 44%). Three of the 18 PAO patients took non-steroidal anti-inflammatory drugs and no AAA patients..
The difference of age between the two groups (AAA and PAO) of patients recruited in this study is consistent with literature on the mean age of onset of the disease in patients with similar risk factors. Also consistent with the literature is the finding that 30% of AAA patients and 50% of PAO patients have family members who have had a myocardial infarction or acute coronary syndrome.

4. Methods

4.1 Tissue biopsies from AAA and PAO patients

Aortic samples (Fig. 1) were obtained for 20 of the 24 AAA patients of the LILAS study. Because treatment procedures for PAO changed during the study period, from surgical to endovascular interventions, tissues were available for only the 4 of the 18 patients who had surgical treatment (Fig. 1).

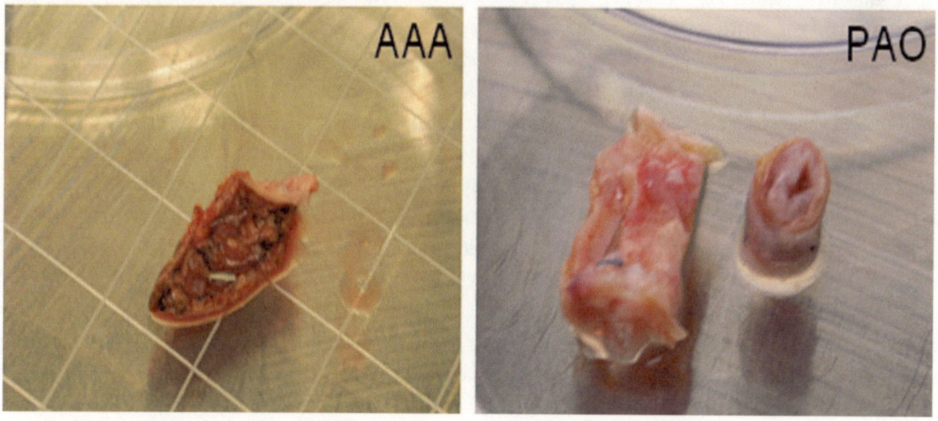

Fig. 1. Aneurysmal (AAA) and peripheral arterial occlusion (PAO) tissue used for culture of smooth muscle cells and macrophages. Example of biopsy tissue recovered for AAA (n=20) and PAO (n=4) patients.

4.2 Primary smooth muscle cells cultures

Human SMCs were obtained from all of the AAA tissue samples (n=20) and only one of the four samples from PAO patients. Individual cultures of human aortic SMCs were established for each patient by dissection of a residual segment of abdominal aorta and then cutting out the media into 1- to 2-mm^3 pieces and culturing them on dishes coated with collagen type 1. Cells began to migrate from the explant after 10 days and confluence was reached in one month.

4.3 Primary cultures of human monocytes-derived macrophages

Primary cultures of human macrophages are the cell models used most often *in vitro* for human macrophages, because only a simple venous blood sample is required to investigate qualitative or quantitative macrophage modifications in a case-control study. A highly-standardized primary culture had to be devised to take into account the individual genetic variability of each blood donor, as well as the behavioral and environmental influences, and hidden abnormalities (Korke et al., 2002). Primary cultures of human macrophages were prepared as previously described (Pinet et al., 2003), with a technique adapted from Boyum (Boyum, 1968).

4.4 Transcriptomic analysis of vascular cells from AAA and PAO patients

Specific oligonucleotides for 137 genes corresponding to 24 matrix metalloproteinases (MMP), 4 tissue inhibitors of metalloproteinases (TIMP), 20 ADAMs (a disintegrin and metalloproteinase), 20 ADAMTS (ADAMS with thrombospondin motifs), 65 other proteases and 4 control genes (hydroxymethylbilane synthase, beta-actin, NADPH oxidase 1, and Glyceraldehyde-3-phosphate dehydrogenase (GADPH)) were designed with OLIGOMER software (Mediagen, France) as previously described (Lamblin et al., 2010). Data were analyzed in comparison to a reference RNA, mixture from brain, colon, heart, placenta and testis, chosen for the expression of each protease and anti-protease in at least one of these tissues. We performed a self (Cy3)-self (Cy5) hybridization of the reference RNA and observed equivalent staining throughout the microarray, except for the renin gene which we excluded from the analysis (not shown). RNA samples were extracted from human SMCs and macrophages and only RNA with a RIN value >9 was analyzed. Each sample (5 µg) was analyzed with two slides according to a dye-swap strategy to account for labeling and detection differences between Cy5 and Cy3. Data analysis was performed with the statistical language R (v 2.0.1) (Ihaka & Gentelman, 1996), more specifically with the LIMMA library (Linear Models for MicroArray data) (Smyth et al, 2003). In accordance with the MIAME (Minimum Information About a Microarray Experiment) guidelines, we note the steps involved in data processing: 1) each microarray was scanned twice (at high and low intensity) for each wavelength of Cy3 and Cy5; 2) two separate normalization steps were conducted : first, pin-by-pin and second, a lowess fitness normalization. A moderated t-statistic with empirical Bayes shrinkage of the standard error was used to classify the statistically significant modulations (Lönnstedt & Speed, 2003). Because of multiple testing, p-values were corrected (Benjamini & Hochberg, 1995) to control for the false discovery rate. Genes with an adjusted p-value < 0.01 in at least three of five replications were considered further.

4.5 Proteomic analysis of vascular cells from AAA and PAO patients

Intracellular proteins from macrophages and SMCs of AAA and PAO patients were loaded (5 µg) on 2D gels. 2D-DIGE was performed as recently described (Dupont et al, 2008). Image analysis was performed with Progenesis SameSpots v2.0 software. The differences in protein spots were then analyzed. Spots were considered to have significantly different normalized spot volumes if the fold change was greater than 1.5 and the corresponding p value (one-way ANOVA analysis) was significant. The last step applied multivariate statistics to the selected spots by calculating q values (for the false discovery rate) and power. Spots corresponding to proteins differentially expressed between the different groups of samples were identified by MALDI-TOF following the protocol previously described (Acosta-Martin et al, 2009).

4.6 Protein microarray profiling of vascular cells and plasma from AAA and PAO patients

The protein arrays allowed us to monitor 42 protein-antibody pairs and detected the profile of differentially expressed proteins in aneurysmal disease. Four differentially expressed proteins were selected from 2D analysis of macrophages from the LILAS or an earlier study: HSP70, aconitase-1, GRP75 and beta-actin (Dupont et al, 2008). Four others were selected from microarray analysis, TIMP-3, ADAMTS10, fibronectin, and tenascin. Finally, four more were identified by the 2D-analysis of plasma from patients from LILAS (personal communications), apolipoprotein AII, vitronectin, transthyretin and factor H.

5. Results

Recently, laser microdissection was used to analyze mRNA expression from macrophages and SMCs from aneurysmal tissue of a rat model of AAA created using elastase infusion (Sho et al., 2005). They found that modulation of at least 5 mRNAs differed according to cell type and flow conditions and thus concluded that a global analysis of aneurysmal tissue could mask cellular responses specific to inflammation and flow. These recent data reinforce our strategy to quantify mRNA and protein expression in two types of vascular cells from patients with different pathologies: macrophages and SMCs from AAA and PAO patients, instead of analysing the whole AAA or PAO biopsies.

5.1 Primary smooth muscle cells cultures

All the cultured human SMCs had the same elongated, spindle-shaped morphology, and at confluence all cultures assumed a hill-and-valley pattern that was maintained throughout all subcultures (Fig. 2).

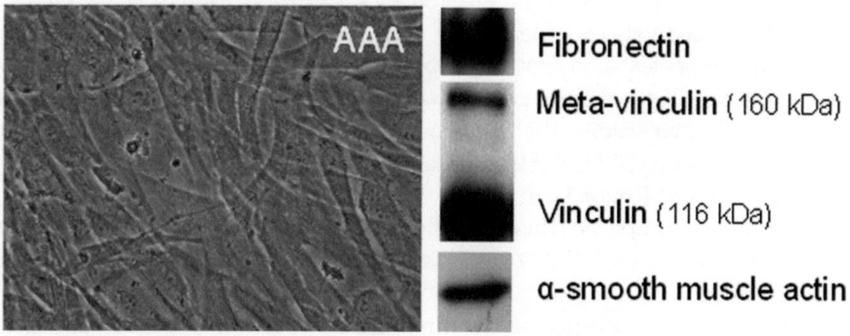

Fig. 2. Phase-contrast microscopy of smooth muscle cells obtained by explant from human AAA (n=20) and PAO (n=4) biopsies. Western blot analysis of SMC for fibronectin, meta-vinculin (160 kDa), vinculin (116 kDa) and α-smooth muscle actin.

Protein expression profiles determined by western blot analysis showed that all the cultures from both patient groups, expressed α-smooth muscle actin, vinculin and metavinculin. This finding indicates the presence of differentiated SMCs, as well as fibronectin, a component of basement membrane, that is indicative of a proliferative and secretory SMC phenotype (Fig. 2).

5.2 Primary cultures of human monocytes-derived macrophages

After, 12 days of culture, monocytes are differentiated into macrophages as shown by phase-contrast microscopy (Fig. 3).

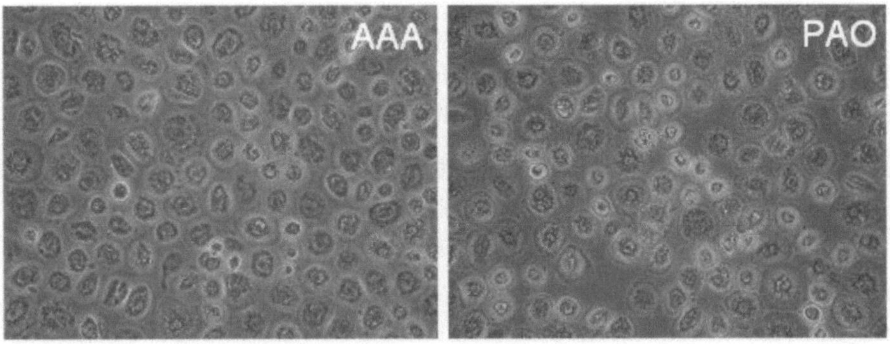

Fig. 3. Phase-contrast microscopy of macrophages prepared from blood samples obtained from human patients presenting AAA (n=16) and PAO (n=16).

The quality of macrophage cultures was evaluated by characterization of two markers, ECE-1 (Endothelin converting enzyme-1) mRNA and MMP-9 (Matrix metalloproteinase-9). ECE-1 mRNA was detected by RT-PCR on total RNA isolated from macrophages and MMP-9 activity was determined in culture medium by gelatin zymography (Pinet et al, 2003). Sixteen primary MDMs cultures, met these criteria and we observed no differences between macrophages obtained from AAA or PAO patients (Fig. 3).

5.3 Transcriptomic analysis of smooth muscle cells and macrophages from AAA and PAO patients

The importance of proteases as mediators of ECM degradation in vascular disease has been proved (Wight, 2005), as the role of other proteases and their inhibitors in AAA (Choke et al., 2005). Our global analysis on a dedicated array of proteases and anti-proteases was not limited by advance theories or hypotheses, precisely because it was intended to generate hypotheses. This technology enables more efficient selection of the possible genes involved in AAAs, as shown in two studies that used AAA specimens and a cDNA microarray (Tung et al., 2001) or quantitative RT-PCR (Higashikata et al., 2004).

We tested mRNA from SMCs of 12 different AAA patients and 2 mRNA samples from one PAO patient, and we compared them to the reference RNA. For human macrophages, mRNA expression ratio of AAA/PAO genes was tested from 4 different AAA patients and 5 different PAO patients.

The microarray analysis indicated that three mRNA sample species appeared to be significantly modulated with a q value (moderated p-value) <0.01 in SMCs from AAA compared with PAO patients: angiotensin converting enzyme (ACE), ADAMTS5 and ADAMTS8. In the AAA patients, ACE (AAA/PAO ratio: - 2.8 fold) was down-regulated, and ADAMTS5 (AAA/PAO ratio: 1.2 fold) and ADAMTS8 (AAA/PAO ratio: 1.3 fold) were very slightly but significantly up-regulated (Fig. 4A). The graphs of individual mRNA expression (AAA/PAO ratio) for these three genes show the variability between patients (Fig. 4B). Of the 137 genes analyzed first by microarrays and then by Q-PCR for selected genes, all showed significant and concordant up- or down-regulation of expression levels for CML samples. The down-regulation of ACE mRNA in AAA patients is not surprising as a recent meta-analysis showed that ACE I/D polymorphisms are associated with a significant risk of AAAs (Thompson et al., 2008), especially in patients with hypertension (Korcz et al., 2009). Similarly, we found that ADAMTS5 and ADAMTS8 were up-regulated in SMC of AAA compared with PAO patients. These two members of the ADAMTS family are involved in vascular lesion development and can degrade different proteoglycans present in blood vessels (Yao et al., 1994).

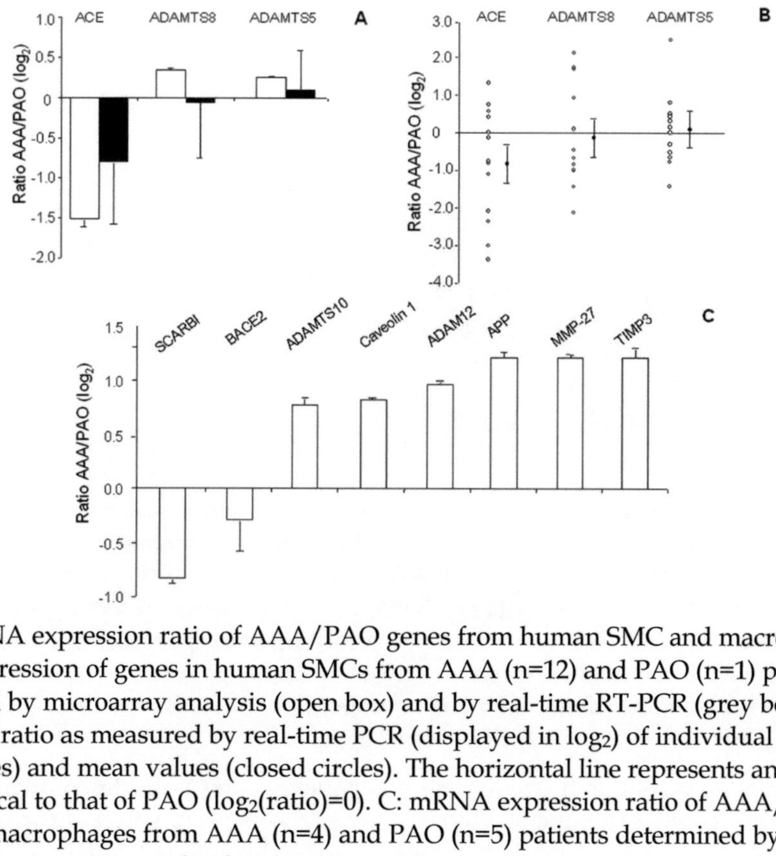

Fig. 4. mRNA expression ratio of AAA/PAO genes from human SMC and macrophages. A: mRNA expression of genes in human SMCs from AAA (n=12) and PAO (n=1) patients determined by microarray analysis (open box) and by real-time RT-PCR (grey box). B: Expression ratio as measured by real-time PCR (displayed in $\log_2$) of individual patients (open circles) and mean values (closed circles). The horizontal line represents an expression level identical to that of PAO ($\log_2$(ratio)=0). C: mRNA expression ratio of AAA/PAO genes in human macrophages from AAA (n=4) and PAO (n=5) patients determined by microarray analysis. Data are expressed in $\log_2$(ratio).

Figure 4C shows that the mRNA samples identified as differentially expressed in macrophages from AAA and PAO patients are different from those differentially modulated in SMCs. Differential modulation was observed in eight macrophage mRNA samples. Two were down-regulated in AAA compared with PAO patients: SCARB1 (scavenger receptor class B, member 1) AAA/PAO(ratio: 1.8) and BACE2 (beta-site APP-cleaving enzyme 2) (AAA/PAO ratio: 1.2). Six were up-regulated in AAA patients: caveolin 1 (AAA/PAO ratio:

1.8), ADAMTS10 (AAA/PAO ratio: 1.7), APP (amyloid precursor protein) (AAA/PAO ratio: 2.3), MMP-27 (AAA/PAO ratio: 2.3), ADAM12 (AAA/PAO ratio: 1.9) and TIMP3 (AAA/PAO ratio: 2.3). Microarray analysis of macrophages showed the modulation of other proteases and anti-proteases, but we were unable to validate these results by RT-PCR because of the limited amount of RNA obtained from cultures. Interestingly, TIMP-3, which we found to be up-regulated in macrophages from AAA patients, has been shown to be a potent inhibitor of ADAMTS5 (Kashiwagi et al., 2001). Nonetheless, our results are consistent with the data reported (Sho et al., 2005) and thus demonstrate the interest of analyzing cell-specific compared with tissue-specific responses.

5.4 Proteomic analysis of smooth muscle cells and macrophages from AAA and PAO patients

Proteins from macrophages and SMCs of AAA and PAO patients were analysed on 2D gels. An average image was established from the scanned gels for macrophages (Fig. 5A) and for SMC (Fig. 5B) from AAA and PAO patients.

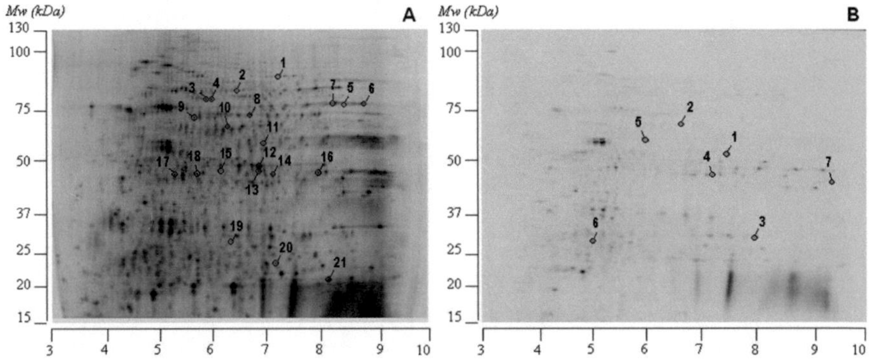

Fig. 5. Representative 2D-DIGE gel analysis of proteome of human macrophages (**A**) and smooth muscle cells (**B**) from LILAS patients. A : Macrophage proteins (5 µg) labeled with either Cy3 or Cy5 from patients presenting AAA (n=10) or PAO (n=12) were analyzed. B : SMC proteins (5 µg) labeled with either Cy3 or Cy5 from patients presenting AAA (n=10) or PAO (n=1) were analyzed. Gels were classified according to the presence of AAA or PAO. Polypeptidic spots differentially expressed between patients presenting AAA or PAO are indicated by a number and identified by this number in Table 1. The positions of *Mr* are indicated on the left and the *pI* on the bottom of the gels.

This differential analysis found twenty-one polypeptidic spots with differential abundance levels and a statistically reproducible difference over the series of gels. Four spots were up-regulated (spots 16, 17, 18 and 19) and 17 down-regulated (spots 1, 2, 3, 4, 5, 6, 7, 8, 9; 10, 11, 12, 13, 14, 15, 18 and 19) in macrophages from AAA compared with PAO patients (Fig. 5A). The intensity of each spot was calculated as the mean ± SD and expressed as a percentage of normalized volume. The same approach was used for the SMC proteins, although only two 2D gels were used for the PAO SMCs (Fig. 5B). This differential analysis found seven polypeptidic spots with differential abundance levels and a statistically reproducible difference over the series of gels. Two spots were up-regulated (spots 2 and 5) and 5 down-regulated (spots 1, 3, 4, 6, and 7) in SMC from AAA compared with PAO patients.

Table 1 summarizes the identity and factor of variation of proteins differentially expressed by macrophages and SMCs from AAA and PAO patients. Of the 21 polypeptidic spots differentially expressed for macrophages, 17 were identified by mass spectrometry and corresponded to 13 non-redundant proteins. Unfortunately, we were unable to identify proteins for SMC due to either the low intensity signal on the mass spectrometry or a low probability score.

Spot number	Accession number	Protein name	Protein function	Mean of normalized value of a spot* AAA	PAO	Fold-change ((AAA vs PAO)
Macrophages						
1		ND		0.005 ± 0.001	0.022 ± 0.008	0.23
2	P10636	Microtubule-associated protein tau	Promotes microtubule assembly and stability	0.008 ± 0.004	0.047 ± 0.018	0.18
3	P11142	Heat shock cognate 71 kDa protein	Chaperone	0.032 ± 0.011	0.078 ± 0.010	0.41
4		ND		0.012 ± 0.006	0.089 ± 0.025	0.13
5	P25705	ATP synthase subunit alpha	Produces ATP from ADP	0.005 ± 0.002	0.036 ± 0.010	0.14
6				0.029 ± 0.010	0.063 ± 0.023	0.47
7	P14618	Pyruvate kinase isozymes M1/M2	Glycolytic enzyme	0.019 ± 0.010	0.066 ± 0.024	0.29
8		ND		0.019 ± 0.005	0.090 ± 0.027	0.21
9	P30101	Protein disulfide-isomerase A3	Catalyzes the rearrangement of -S-S- bonds in proteins	0.080 ± 0.023	0.154 ± 0.055	0.52
10	P50395	Rab GDP dissociation inhibitor beta	Regulates the GDP/GTP exchange	0.072 ± 0.004	0.122 ± 0.016	0.59
11	P22695	Cytochrome b-c1 complex subunit 2	Part of the mitochondrial respiratory chain	0.036 ± 0.018	0.095 ± 0.022	0.38
12	P09467	Fructose-1,6-bisphosphatase 1	Carbohydrate biosynthesis	0.317 ± 0.077	0.771 ± 0.043	0.41
13				0.122 ± 0.023	0.284 ± 0.032	0.43
14				0.036 ± 0.013	0.073 ± 0.016	0.50
15	P40121	Macrophage-capping protein	locks the barbed ends of actin filaments	0.063 ± 0.009	0.109 ± 0.026	0.57
16	P04406	Glyceraldehyde-3-phosphate dehydrogenase	Carbohydrate degradation	0.22 ± 0.051	0.129 ± 0.025	1.71
17	P60709	Actin, cytoplasmic 1	Involved in various types of cell motility	0.266 ± 0.028	0.145 ± 0.037	1.83
18				0.266 ± 0.028	0.266 ± 0.028	0.26
18	P25774	Cathepsin S	Thiol protease	0.049 ± 0.011	0.031 ± 0.008	1.56
19	Q06830	Peroxiredoxin-1	Involved in redox regulation of the cell	0.260 ± 0.125	0.082 ± 0.011	3.18
20		ND		0.246 ± 0.05	0.386 ± 0.028	0.63

* spot number corresponds to spot indicated in Fig. 5.

Table 1. Detailed list of proteins differentially expressed between AAA and PAO samples.

Of the macrophage proteins identified, three are components of cytoskeleton: microtubule-associated protein tau (spot 2), beta-actin (spots 17 and 18) and macrophage-capping protein (spot 15) and cathepsin S (spot 18), has protease activity.
This dual transcriptomic and proteomic analysis of vascular cells from AAA and PAO patients revealed both the differences and the complementarity of microarray and 2D-electrophoresis technologies. Proteomic analysis identified only one protease, cathepsin S as differentially expressed in macrophages from AAA and PAO patients. This is consistent with previous reports showing an increase of cathepsin S activation in the wall of AAAs (Abisi et al., 2007; Abdul-Hussein et al., 2007). Still more recently, leukocyte cathepsin S was shown to be involved in macrophage apoptosis and increased SMC content and collagen deposition (De Nooijer et al., 2009). Interestingly, of the 13 proteins identified overall, three (microtubule-associated protein tau, beta-actin and macrophage-capping protein) are components of cytoskeleton, while the others are involved in protein metabolism and stress response. Unfortunately, we were unable to identify the SMC proteins corresponding to the polypeptidic spots differentially expressed.
Because of the different size of the proteome and transcriptome, we did not conduct a global correlation analysis of proteins and mRNA levels of SMCs and macrophages from these patients. Our strategy was to use specific and dedicated tools to identify the modulation of proteins and mRNAs in SMC and macrophages from AAA and PAO patients and to apply the same technology to their plasma samples.

5.5 Protein microarray profiling of SMCs, macrophages and plasma from AAA and PAO patients

Because of the limited amount of proteins available from macrophages and SMCs of our LILAS study, we used protein antibody array technology that has been shown to provide protein information in a systematic, reproducible and high-throughput fashion in several diseases (Sanchez-Carbayo et al., 2006; Weber et al., 2007).
The AAA/PAO ratio for each protein modulated is presented in detail in Table 2.
First, we analysed macrophages and SMCs proteins from LILAS patients. The microarray, revealed up-regulation in AAA patients of three macrophage proteins and down-regulation of six, as well as up-regulation of six SMC proteins and down-regulation of eight. All the proteins up-regulated in macrophages from AAA patients were also up-regulated in their SMCs: fibronectin, β-actin, tenascin. Five of six proteins down-regulated in AAA macrophages were also down-regulated in their SMCs: TIMP-3, ADAMTS5, HSP70, aconitase, GRP75.
Plasma analysis, of course, restricted the number of proteins available that could be detected as differentially modulated between the two groups. Interestingly, analysis of plasma from the LILAS patients showed only five proteins differentially expressed in plasma from AAA and PAO patients, three already selected from the macrophage and SMC samples, ADAMTS8 (AAA/PAO ratio: 0.9), ADAMTS5 (AAA/PAO ratio: 1.11) and TIMP-3 (AAA/PAO ratio: 1.15) and two only in plasma: ApoCIII (AAA/PAO ratio: 0.78) and alpha1-antitrypsin (AAA/PAO ratio: 0.88).
Of particular interest, however, is the finding that TIMP-3, ADAMTS5 and ADAMTS8 were differentially expressed in proteins from macrophages, SMCs and plasma. ADAMTS8 is known to degrade ECM proteoglycans and has the highest specific activity for cleaving aggrecan (Porter et al., 2005). Our data are in agreement with a report (Theocharis et al., 2001), which showed a decrease in the concentration of versican in human AAA. Unfortunately, tools to measure ADAMTS activity need to be developed (Wagstäter et al., 2008). Interestingly, TIMP-3 was shown to be modulated in the two cell types involved in

AAA, SMCs and macrophages and also in the plasma of the same patients, as shown with the overexpression of TIMP-3 in AAA tissue compared to aortic occlusive disease but they did not measure plasma TIMP-3 levels of the same patients as we did (Carell et al., 2002). The availability of TIMP assays allowed us to confirm the increased plasma levels of TIMP-3 in AAA patients (Lamblin et al., 2010).

Protein name	**AAA**	**PAO**	
	Mean value ± SD		**Ratio AAA/PAO**
Macrophages			
TIMP-3	521 ± 430	1409 ± 811	0.35
ADAMTS5	439 ± 501	1000 ± 633	0.43
ADAMTS10	611 ± 567	1190 ± 596	0.45
HSP70	3634 ± 1369	6971 ± 2559	0.55
GRP75	4909 ± 2331	8505 ± 1862	0.55
ACO-1	4171 ± 1315	7028 ± 2958	0.60
Tenascin	27566 ± 7751	16493 ± 3000	1.65
Fibronectin	29278 ± 6686	15586 ± 3607	1.75
Beta-actin	43479 ± 13524	23892 ± 6088	1.80
Smooth muscle cells*			
GRP75	6393 ± 1651	5126/8207	0.56/0.56
ADAMTS5	882 ± 403	1479/1431	0.59/0.59
TIMP-4	1247 ± 438	1977/2537	0.63/0.51
HSP70	7180 ± 1700	11358/8906	0.63/0.62
Transferrin	2895 ± 2153	4868/5076	0.67/0.59
ACO-1	6782 ± 2088	10076/8089	0.67/0.66
ApoAII	6009 ± 1392	8419/7622	0.71/0.63
Vitronectin	25237 ± 2568	31398/33481	0.80/0.71
Factor H	2339 ± 378	1733/1647	1.35/1.35
Tenascin	21849 ± 3847	14181/13722	1.54/1.49
Beta-actin	26599 ± 4899	16672/15917	1.59/1.56
Prealbumin	15339 ± 1272	16175/13780	1.60/1.57
ADAMTS8	962 ± 300	599/774	1.61/1.58
Fibronectin	23910 ± 4485	14154/15035	1.69/1.65
Plasma			
APOCIII	14867 ± 4892	18964 ± 6046	0.78
Alpha1-antitrypsin	60718 ± 6815	68871 ± 12632	0.88
ADAMTS8	2470 ± 523	2754 ± 594	0.90
ADAMTS5	2176 ± 720	1956 ± 754	1.11
TIMP-3	2448 ± 653	2132 ± 610	1.15

Macrophages and SMC analysis were performed respectively from 16 and 14 AAA and 16 and 11 PAO samples; Plasma analysis was performed from 24 AAA and 18 PAO samples.* Due to the limited number of SMC samples tested, we did not calculated SD for PAO patient and gave the value from 2 independent experiments performed.

Table 2. Expression ratio of proteins in macrophages. smooth muscle cells and plasma from AAA and PAO patients.

6. Conclusion

The limitations of this study are the relatively few tissue specimens allowing study of SMCs from PAO patients, because of changes in their treatment strategy (endovascular protheses rather than surgery). To our knowledge, this is the first study to combine several global analyses to assess the changes in the expression of genes and proteins of vascular cells involved in aneurysmal disease. Its strengths include the largest and most detailed view of changes in proteases and anti-proteases expression in patients presenting AAA. The protein array techniques confirmed that the differentially expressed proteins could also be detected in plasma. We found a restricted number of proteins differentially expressed between AAA and PAO patients: TIMP-3, ADAMTS5 and ADAMTS8that differ significantly in plasma of AAA patients compared to PAO approach. Combining transcriptomic and proteomic is a valid approach to a better understanding of the pathophysiology of AAA but strengthen the need to investigate multiple circulating biomarkers.

7. Acknowledgment

This work was supported by grants from "Fondation pour la Recherche Médicale", Région Nord Pas de Calais and a European FAD grant (Health-F2-2008-200647). All the authors declare that they have no conflicting financial interests.

8. References

Abisi, S., Burnand, K.G., Waltham, M., Humphries .J, Taylor, P.R. & Smith, A. (2007) Cysteine protease activity in the wall of abdominal aortic aneurysms. *Journal of Vascular Surgery* 46: 1260-1266.

Abdul-Hussein, H., Soekhoe, R.G., Weber, E., von der Thüsen, J.H., Kleemann, R., Mulder, A., van Bockel, J.H., Hanemaaijer, R. & Linderman, J.H. (2007) Collagen degradation in the abdominal aneurysm: a conspiracy of matrix metalloproteinase and cysteine collagenases. *American Journal of Pathology* 170: 809-817.

Acosta-Martin, A.E., Chwastyniak, M., Beseme, O., Drobecq, H., Amouyel, P. & Pinet, F. (2009) Impact of incomplete DNase I treatment on human macrophage proteome analysis. *Proteomics Clinical Applications* 3: 1236-1246.

Ailawadi, G., Eliason, J.L. & Upchurch Jr, G.R. (2003) Current concepts in the pathogenesis of abdominal aortic aneurysm. *Journal of Vascular Surgery* 38: 584-588.

Benjamini, Y. & Hochberg, Y. (1995) Controlling the false discovery rate: a practical and powerful approach to multiple testing. *Journal of Royal Statistical Society* 57: 289-300.

Boyum, A. (1968) Isolation of mononuclear cells and granulocytes from human blood. Isolation of mononuclear cells by one centrifugation, and of granulocytes by combining centrifugation and sedimentation at 1 g. *Scandinavian Journal of Clinical Laboratory Investigation Supplement* 68: 97:9-929.

Carrell, T.W.G., Burnand, K.G., Wells, G;M;A., Clements, J.M. & Smith, A. (2002) Stromelysin-1 (matrix metalloproteinase-3) and tissue inhibitor of metalloproteinase-3 are overexpressed in the wall of abdominal aortic aneurysms. *Circulation* 105: 477-482.

Choke, E., Cockerill, G., Wilson, W.R.W., Sayed, S., Dawson, J., Loftus, I. & Thompson, M.M. (2005) A review of biological factors implicated in abdominal aortic aneurysm rupture. *European Journal of Vascular Endovascular Surgery* 30 : 227-244.

De Nooijer, R., von der Thüssen, J.H., Leeuwenburgh, M.A., Overkleeft, H.S., Kraaijeveld, A.O., Dorland, R., van Santbrink, P.J., van Heiningen, S.H., Westra, M.M., Kovanen, P.T., Jukema, J.W., van der Wall, E.E., van Berkek , T.J., Shi, G.P. & Biessen, E.A. (2009) Leukocyte cathepsins S is a potent regulator of both cell and matrix turnover in advanced atherosclerosis. *Arteriosclerosis Thrombosis Vascular Biology* 29: 188-194.

Di Gennaro, A., Wagsäter, D., Mäyranpää, M.I., Gabrielsen, A., Swendenborg, J., Hamsten, A., Samuelsson, B., Eriksson, P & Haeggström, J.Z. (2010) Increased expression of leukotriene C_4 synthase and predominant formation of cysteinyl-leukotrienes in human abdominal aortic aneurysm. *Proceedings National Academy of Sciences USA* 107: 21093-21097.

Dobrin, P.B. & Mrkvicka, R. (1994) Failure of elastin or collagen as possible critical connective tissue alterations underlying aneurismal dilatation. *Cardiovascular Surgery* 2: 484-488.

Dupont, A., Chwastyniak, M., Beseme, O., Guihot, A.L., Drobecq, H., Amouyel, P. & Pinet, F. (2008) Application of saturation dye 2D-DIGE proteomics to characterize proteins modulated by oxidized low density lipoprotein treatment of human macrophages. *Journal of Proteome Research* 7: 3572-3582.

Golledge, J., Tsao, P.S., Dalman, R.L.& Norman, P.E. (2008) Circulating markers of abdominal aortic aneurysm presence and progression. *Circulation* 118; 2382-2392.

Henderson, E.L., Geng, Y.J., Sukhova, G.K., Whittemore, A.D., Knox, J. & Libby, P. (1999) Death of smooth muscle cells and expression of mediators of apoptosis by T lymphocytes in human abdominal aortic aneurysms. *Circulation* 99: 96-104.

Higashikata, T., Yamagishi, M., Saski, H., Minatoya, K., Ogino, H., Ishibashi-Ueda, H., Hao, H., Nagaya, N., Tomoike, H. & Sakamoto, A. (2004) Application of real-time RT-PCR to quantifying gene expression of matrix metalloproteinases and tissue inhibitors of metalloproteinases in human abdominal aortic aneurysm. *Atherosclerosis* 177: 353-360.

Ihaka, R. & Gentelman, R. (1996) R: a language for data analysis and graphics. *Journal of Computational Graphical Statistics* 5: 299-314.

Iribarren, C., Darbinian, J.A., Go, A.S., Fireman, B.H., Lee, C.D. & Grey, D.P. (2007) Traditional and novel risk factors for clinically diagnosed abdominal aortic aneurysm: The Kaiser multiphasic health checkup cohort study. *Annual Epidemiology* 17: 669-678.

Kashiwagi, M., Tortorella, M., Nagase, H. & Brew, K. (2001) TIMP-3 is a potent inhibitor of aggrecanase 1 (ADAM-TS4) and aggrecanase 2 (ADAM-TS5). *Journal of Biological Chemistry* 276: 12501-12504.

Kingsmore, S.F. (2006) Multiplexed protein measurement: technologies and applications of protein and antibody arrays. *Nature Review Drug Discovery* 5: 310-320.

Klein, T. & Bischoff, R. (2011) Active metalloproteases of the A disintegrin and metalloprotease (ADAM) family: biological function and structure. *Journal of Proteome Reearch* 10: 17-33.

Knox, J.B., Sukhova, G.K., Whittemore, A.D. & Libby, P. (1997) Evidence for altered balance between matrix metalloproteinases and their inhibitors in human aortic diseases. *Circulation* 95: 205-212.

Korcz, A., Mikolajczyk-Stecyna, J., Gabriel, M., Zowczak-Drabarczyk, M., Pawlaczyk, K., Kalafirov, M., Oszkinis, G. & Slomski, R. (2009) Angiotensin-converting enzyme (ACE, I/D) gene polymorphism and susceptibility to abdominal aortic aneurysm or aortoiliac occlusive disease. *Journal of Surgery Research* 153: 76-82.

Korke, R., Rink, A.., Seo, T.K., Chung, M.C., Beattle, C.W. & Hu, W.S. (2002) Genomic and proteomic perspectives in cell culture engineering. *Journal of Biotechnology* 94: 73-92.

Lamblin, N., Ratajczak, P., Hot, D., Dubois, E., Chwastyniak, M., Beseme, O., Drobecq, H., Lemoine, Y., Koussa, M., Amouyel, P. & Pinet, F. (2010) Profile of macrophages in human abdominal aortic aneurysms: a transcriptomic, proteomic and antibody protein array study. *Journal of Proteome Research* 9: 3720-3729.

Lönnstedt, I. & Speed, T.P. (2002) Replicated microarray data. *Statistica Sinica* 12: 31-46.

Lopez-Candales, A., Holmes, D.R., Liao, S., Scoot, M.J., Wickline, S.A. & Thompson, R.W. (1997) Decreased vascular smooth muscle cell density in medial degeneration of human abdominal aortic aneurysms. *American Journal of Pathology* 150: 993-1007.

Middleton, R.K., Bown, M.J., Lloyd, G.M., Jones, J.L., London, N.J. & Sayers, R.D. (2009) Characterisation of interleukin-8 and monocyte chemoattractant protein-1 expression within the abdominal aortic aneurysm and their association with mural inflammation. *European Journal of Vascular Endovascular Surgery* 37: 46-55.

Pinet, F., Dupont, A., Bencherif, N., Guihot, A.L., Quatannens, B & Amouyel P. (2003) Morphology, homogeneity and functionality of human monocytes-derived macrophages. *Cellular Molecular of Biology* 49: 899-905.

Porter, S., Clark, I.M., Kevorkian, L. & Edwards, D.R. (2005) The ADAMTS metalloproteinases. *Biochemical Journal* 386: 15-27.

Samuelsson, B. (1983) Leukotrienes: mediators of immediate hypersensitivity reactions and inflammation. *Science* 220: 568-575.

Sanchez-Carbayo, M., Socci, N.D., Lozano, J.J., Haab, B.B. & Cordon-Cardo, C. (2006) Profiling bladder cancer using targeted antibody arrays. *American Journal of Pathology* 168:93-103.

Sho, E., Sho, M., Najo, H., Kawamura, K., Masuda, H. & Dalman, R.L. (2005) Comparison of cell-type-specific vs transmural aortic gene expression in experimental aneurysms. *Journal of Vascular Surgery* 41: 844-852.

Smyth, G.K., Yang, Y.H. & Speed, T. (2003) Statistical issues in cDNA microarray data analysis. *Methods Molecular Biology* 224: 111-136.

Theocharis, A.D., Toslakis, I., Hjerpe, A. & Karamanos, N.K. (2001) Human abdominal aortic aneurysm is characterized by decreased versican concentration and specific downregulation of versican isoform V_0. *Atherosclerosis* 154: 367-376.

Thompson, R.W. (2002) Reflections on the pathogenesis of abdominal aortic aneurysms. *Cardiovasc Surg* 10 :389-394.

Thompson, R.W. (2006) Matrix metalloproteinase-8 and -9 are increased at the site of abdominal aortic aneurysm rupture. *Circulation* 113: 438-445.

Thompson, A.R., Drenos, F., Hafez, H. & Humphries, S.E. (2008) Candidate gene association studies in abdominal aortic aneurysm: a review and meta-analysis. *European Journal of Vascular Endovascular Surgery* 35: 19-30.

Tung, W.S., Lee, J.K. & Thompson, R.W. (2001) Simultaneous analysis of 1176 gene products in normal human aorta and abdominal aortic aneurysms using a membrane-based complementay DNA expression array. *Journal of Vascular Surgery* 34: 143-150.

Wagstäter, D., Björk, H., Zhu, C., Björkegren, J., Valen, G., Hamsten, A. & Eriksson, P. (2008) ADAMTS-4 and –8 are inflammatory regulated enzymes expressed in macrophage-rich areas of human atherosclerotic plaques. *Atherosclerosis* 196: 514-522.

Wassef, M., Upchurch, G.R., Kuivaniemi, H., Thompson, R.W. & Tilson III, M.D. (2007) Challenges and opportunities in abdominal aortic aneurysm research. *Journal of Vascular Surgery* 45: 192-198.

Weber, A., Hengge, U.R., Stricker, I., Tischoff, I., Markwart, A., Anhalt, K., Dietz, A., Wittekind, C. & Tannapfel, A. (2007) Protein microarrays for the detection of biomarkers in head and neck squamous cell carcinomas. *Journal of Pathology* 38:228-238.

Wight, T.N. (2005) The ADAMTS proteases, extracellular matrix, and vascular disease: waking the sleeping giant(s). *Arteriosclerosis Thrombosis Vascular Biology* 25: 12-14.

Wilson, W.R., Anderton, M., Schwalbe, E.C., Jones, J.L., Furness, P.N., Bell, P.R. & Thompson, M.M. (2006) Matrix metalloproteinase-8 and -9 are increased at the site of abdominal aortic aneurysm rupture. *Circulation* 113: 438-445.

Yao, L.Y., Moody, C., Schonherr, E., Wight, T.N. & Sandell, L.J. (1994) Identification of the proteoglycan versican in aorta and smooth muscle cells by DNA sequence anlaysis, in situ hybridisation and immunohistochemistry. *Matrix Biology* 14: 213-225.

7

Multifaceted Role of Angiotensin II in Vascular Inflammation and Aortic Aneurysmal Disease

Xiaoxi Ju, Ronald G. Tilton and Allan R. Brasier
University of Texas, Medical Branch, USA

1. Introduction

Aortic aneurysms and aortic dissections account for ~16,000 deaths in the United States annually (Kuivaniemi, et al., 2008). Recent evidence suggests that enhanced vascular inflammation underlies the progression of both abdominal aortic aneurysms and thoracic aortic aneurysms (Guo, et al., 2006a). Common pathologic features of vascular inflammation and aneurysmal disease include recruitment and activation of immune cells to the vessel wall, myofibroblast differentiation and extracellular matrix (ECM) remodeling. Recent preclinical work has implicated divergent signaling pathways downstream of the vasopressor angiotensin II (Ang II) peptide in controlling these activities. This work has elucidated two important paracrine signaling networks, one mediated by the NF-κB-IL-6 pathway controlling monocyte activation, and the second mediated by the TGF-β-Smad2 pathway controlling myofibroblast differentiation and T lymphocyte differentiation. Antagonism of Ang II signaling is being evaluated in the clinical management of patients with familial thoracic aneurysms. In this chapter, we will review the multifaceted role of Ang II in vascular inflammation in aortic aneurysmal disease.

1.1 Types of aortic aneurysms

Aortic aneurysms are primarily classified based on anatomic locations (Kuivaniemi, et al., 2008). Abdominal aortic aneurysms (AAA) primarily develop in the infrarenal segment of the abdominal aorta in humans or suprarenal aorta in rodent models. It predominantly affects elderly males, and is associated with hypertension, vascular inflammation and/or atherosclerosis (Guo, et al., 2006a). Initial pathological events in AAA involve recruitment and infiltration of leukocytes into the aortic adventitia and media, which are associated with the production of inflammatory cytokines, chemokine, and reactive oxygen species (ROS). Expression of macrophage activating cytokines is increased both systemically and locally in AAA. Importantly, as a major source of ECM-degrading matrix metalloproteinases (MMPs), recruited activated macrophages promote structural remodeling by degrading elastin and collagen in the vessel wall (Longo, et al., 2002). Moreover, in expanding aneurysmal tissues, increased infiltration of inflammatory cells may amplify MMP production by resident vascular cells (Pearce and Koch, 1996), facilitating aortic inflammation and structural remodeling.
In contrast, thoracic aortic aneurysms (TAA) are etiologically separable from AAA due to their strong genetic influence affecting areas including the ascending aorta, aortic arch,

and/or descending aorta. Common genetic disorders associated with TAAs include Marfan's Syndrome and Loeys-Dietz syndrome. Recent studies have also identified an inflammatory component in the etiology of TAA (Ejiri, et al., 2003). In TAA in patients undergoing surgical repair, enhanced expression of cytokines, such as interleukin-6 (IL-6) and interferon-γ (IFN-γ), as well as enhanced NADPH oxidase and reactive oxygen species (ROS) tone are found in aortic tissues. These events are spatially correlated with increased monocyte/macrophage accumulation and enhanced MMP production.

1.2 Cells and molecules implicated in inflammation in aortic aneurysms

The vascular inflammatory response involves complex interactions between recruited inflammatory cells (lymphocytes, monocytes, macrophages, neutrophils), vascular resident cells [endothelial cells (ECs), vascular smooth muscle cells (VSMCs) and adventitial fibroblasts] and the ECM. The ensuing inflammatory response increases expression of adhesion molecules, growth factors, cytokines and chemokines, that facilitates recruitment and local activation of inflammatory cells and matrix remodeling. Additionally, immune cells (macrophages, mast cells, B- and T- lymphocytes, neutrophils, along with VSMCs and adventitial fibroblasts) produce cytokines and enzymes, promoting an inflammatory reaction, extracellular matrix degradation, and neovascularization (Table 1).

Recruited CD68-expressing macrophages are found in both the adventitia and intima of aneurysms. They are attracted to the aortic wall by elastin degradation products, CC chemokines [e.g. monocyte chemotactic protein (MCP-1), RANTES, etc] and granulocyte-macrophage colony-stimulating factor (GM-CSF) (Rizas, et al., 2009). MCP-1 produced by VSMCs and fibroblasts (Tilson, et al., 2000) induces monocyte chemotaxis by binding to CC-chemokine receptor 2 (CCR2). MCP-1 is an important mediator in early pathogenesis of aortic aneurysms because CCR2 deficiency prevents aneurysm formation in various mouse models (Daugherty, et al., 2010; Tieu, et al., 2009). Additionally, macrophages express 5-lipooxygenase (5-LO), which produces macrophage inflammatory protein 1α (MIP-1α) to recruit T-cells in a paracrine fashion. Locally infiltrated T-cells then magnify the inflammatory cascade by secreting various CC and CXC chemokines, attracting other inflammatory cells to the aneurysmal tissue (Zhao, et al., 2004).

CD3+ T-cells are abundant immunomodulatory and pro-inflammatory cells recruited to aneurysmal tissues, accounting for ~50% of local hematopoietic cells (Kuivaniemi, et al., 2008). Most T-cell subtypes have been identified, including helper T-cells (Th cells), cytotoxic T-cells and natural killer T-cells (NKT) (Kuivaniemi, et al., 2008). Recent studies to identify Th cell subtypes, which are predominant in aneurysms, reported controversial results. Some suggested Th2 was predominant, while other studies suggested Th1 (Galle, et al., 2005; Schonbeck, et al., 2002).

Aortic resident cells also potentiate inflammation via interactions with recruited immune cells. Adventitial fibroblasts produce cytokines and chemokines such as IL-6, MCP-1, VEGF, and TNF (Tilson, et al., 2000), contributing to leukocytic chemotaxis and activation. Work from our laboratory has found that Ang II stimulates aortic adventitial fibroblasts to recruit monocytes via fibroblast-derived MCP-1, and that the recruited monocytes further promote fibroblast proliferation, adventitial thickening, and additional cytokine production. This fibroblast-monocyte amplification loop may critically mediate adventitial inflammation (Tieu, et al., 2010; Tieu, et al., 2009). Upon stimulation with TGF-β, fibroblasts differentiate into α-smooth muscle cell actin-expressing myofibroblasts (Desmouliere, et al., 1993). Myofibroblasts play a role in wound healing and fibrosis, and are associated with development of aneurysmal disease (Sakata, et al., 2007).

Cells	Molecules	Roles in Aortic Aneurysms
Fibroblasts	MMP-1	Collagen degradation
	MMP-2	Elastin and collagen degradation
	VEGF	Angiogenesis
	MCP-1	Monocyte chemotaxis
VSMCs	MMP-2	Elastin and collagen degradation
	MMP-13	Collagen degradation
	MT1-MMP	Elastin and collagen degradation; ProMMP-2 activation; facilitate macrophage migration
	MCP-1	Monocyte chemotaxis
	IL-6	Macrophage differentiation; MCP-1 induction; systemic acute-phase response
Macrophages	MMP-3	Elastin and collagen degradation; VEGF activation
	MMP-9	Elastin and collagen degradation; dominant gelatinase in late pathogenesis; TGF-β, VEGF activation; macrophage migration
	MMP-12	Elastin and collagen degradation
	MT1-MMP	Elastin and collagen degradation; ProMMP-2 activation; facilitate macrophage migration
	Cathepsins	ECM degradation; angiogenesis
	MIP-1α	T-cell chemotaxis
	IL-8	Neutrophil chemotaxis
	LTD4	MIP-1α induction
	TGF-β	Angiogenesis; MMP induction; Th17 differntiation; myofibroblast differntiation
	IL-6	Macrophage differentiation; MCP-1 induction; systemic inflammatory responses
Mast cells	Chymases	ProMMP activation; VSMC apoptosis; Ang II induction
	Tryptases	ProMMP activation
	LTD4	MIP-1α induction
Netrophils	MMP-8	Collagen degradation
	MMP-9	Elastin and collagen degradation; TGF-β, VEGF activation; macrophage migration
	Cathespins	ECM degradation; angiogenesis
	Netrophil elastase	Elastin degradation
NKT cells	IFN-γ	Th1 differentiation; macrophage activation
	IL-4	Th2 differentiation; humoral immunity
Th Cells	IFN-γ	Th1 differentiation; macrophage activation
	IL-4	Th2 differentiation; humoral immunity
	IL-17	Macrophage chemotaxis

Table 1. Major cell types and secreted molecules involved in vascular inflammatory response in aortic aneurysms.

Among the different enzymes secreted by immune and stromal cells, MMP-2, MMP-9, MMP-12, cathepsins, and neutrophil elastase cause ECM degeneration (Table 1). Chymase causes smooth muscle cell apoptosis, and MMP-3, MMP-8, and MMP-13 cause adventitial collagen degradation, promoting abdominal aortic aneurysm rupture.

Cytokines and chemokines such as IL-8, MIP-1α, and MCP-1 facilitate recruitment and proliferation of inflammatory cells (Table 1). Cytokines include TNF, interleukins, interferons, colony stimulating factors, and transforming growth factors, etc. They are produced by diverse cell types including macrophages, T-cells and monocytes, VSMCs and fibroblasts. Circulating cytokines interact with specific receptors on various cell types to activate JAK-STAT, NF-κB, and Smad signaling pathways, regulating expression of various genes controlling inflammatory response involving cell adhesion, permeability and apoptosis. Cytokine signaling is also known to increase mitochondrial ROS production, induce integrins to facilitate cellular adhesion and activate MMPs to modify ECM composition. Further, increased local cytokine expression is implicated in aortic aneurysms.

Vascular inflammation is an ordered process producing recruitment of activated leukocyte subtypes into the vessel wall, initiating complex interaction with vascular residential cells and ECM. This process is initiated and amplified by local secretion of adhesion molecules, chemotactic factors and cytokines, whose inducible expression are signaled by vascular injury and modulated by vasoactive peptides (Ang II), CD40 ligands, oxidized cholesterol, and advanced glycation end products. Of these, the effects of Ang II have been implicated in vascular inflammation and have emerged as an important clinical target for the treatment of human aneurysms associated with Marfan's disease.

2. Ang II-induced vascular inflammation

Angiotensin II (Ang II) is the major effector peptide of the renin-angiotensin system. In addition to its potent vasoconstrictor actions, Ang II exert pro-inflammatory activity in the vascular wall, inducing production of inflammatory cytokines, adhesion molecules, and formation of ROS, resulting in macrophage accumulation, myofibroblast differentiation, and localized aortic dilation followed by dissections (Ejiri, et al., 2003).

Ang II is a potent inducer of vascular inflammation producing acute thoracic and suprarenal aortic aneurysms and dissections in many mouse models (Daugherty, et al., 2010; Tieu, et al., 2009). Chronic subcutaneous infusion of Ang II peptide into atherosclerosis-prone hyperlipidemic apolipoprotein E-deficient (ApoE-/-) or LDL receptor (LDLR-/-) deficient mice produces thoracic and suprarenal aneurysms (Reiner, 2007) . Also in aged C57BL/6J mice, Ang II produces both suprarenal and ascending thoracic aneurysms and dissections, albeit at a lower frequency than in the presence of hyperlipidemia (Tieu, et al., 2009). Moreover, Ang II type I receptor and ACE polymorphisms are associated with AAA in humans (Jones, et al., 2008), suggesting that Ang II is tightly associated with aneurysmal diseases. The mouse models of acute Ang II infusion showed significant vascular inflammatory responses in aneurysmal tissues, including enhanced aortic cytokine/chemokine production, early macrophage recruitment, elastin degeneration, and intramural hematoma formation.

Ang II stimulates inflammatory chemokine expression and ROS production in EC and VSCMs, events implicated in the pathogenesis of aortic aneurysms (Ejiri, et al., 2003; Longo, et al., 2002). In ECs, Ang II up-regulates expression of the leukocyte adhesion molecules vascular cell adhesion molecule (VCAM-1), intercellular adhesion molecule (ICAM-1), and selectins (Pueyo, et al., 2000), facilitating monocyte adhesion and recruitment into the vascular wall. Once recruited, monocytes produce MMPs that mediate aortic wall remodeling in aneurysmal expansion, and migrate towards gradients of chemotactic cytokines (e.g. MCP-1, KC/Groβ, MIP-1α, etc). The actions of Ang II regulate many steps in these processes, inducing expression of chemokines MCP-1, KC/Groβ, and the cytokine IL-6 (Chen, et al., 2001; Han, et al., 1999). In VSMCs, Ang II is a potent inducer of cytokine and chemokine expression, including MCP-1 and IL-6. These molecules, in turn, cause more immune cell infiltration, further amplifying the inflammatory tone contributing to aneurysmal expansion.

The ability of Ang II to potently induce vascular inflammation involves the activation of two divergent signaling pathways important in the vascular stress response, the first being the nuclear factor-κB (NF-κB)-IL-6 signaling pathway, and the second, the transforming growth factor (TGF)-β-Smad pathway (Figure 1).

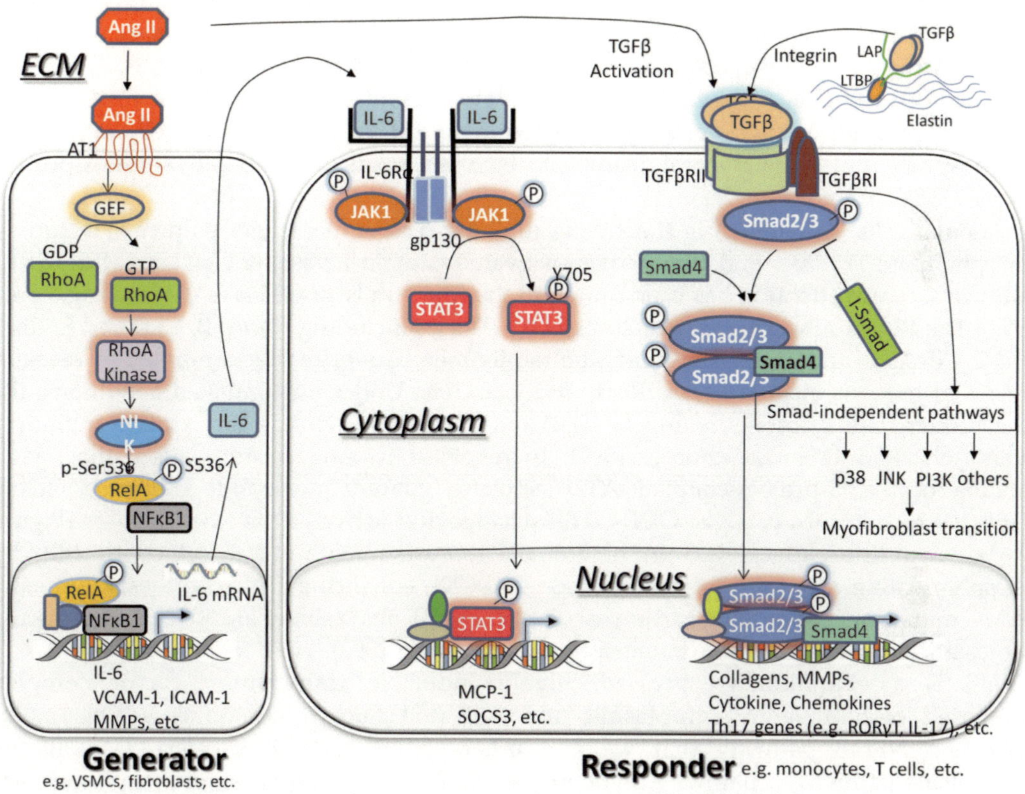

Fig. 1. Ang II-induced signaling pathways involved in vascular inflammatory events implicated in aortic aneurysms. The actions of Ang II involve cells directly responding to its actions schematically diagrammed as generators and downstream affected cells (responders) producing vascular inflammation and remodeling

3. The NF-κB-IL-6 pathway in Ang II-induced aortic aneurysms

A number of recent studies have demonstrated that NF-κB transcription factors play a central role in controlling the process of vascular inflammation. Responsive to vasoactive peptides such as Ang II, oxidized LDL, activated CD40 receptor, monocyte released cytokines, or advanced glycation end-products, activated NF-κB is known to control leucocyte adherence and chemotaxis, key steps in the process of vascular inflammation. Recently, an additional role for NF-κB in controlling monocyte activation via the IL-6 pathway has also been discovered. Here, locally secreted IL-6 activates vascular monocytes and induces cellular protection from ROS-induced stress via signaling through the downstream effector signal transducer and activator of transcription 3 (STAT3). In this way, the NF-κB –IL-6 signaling pathway plays multiple roles in initiating and sustaining vascular inflammation.

3.1 Mechanism of NF-κB activation by Ang II in VSMCs

Ang II initiates intracellular signaling by binding to two types of heterotrimeric guanosine (G) -protein coupled 7-transmembrane receptors, termed the type I (AT-1) and type II (AT-2) Ang II receptors (Griendling, et al., 1997). AT-1 is the major receptor normally expressed on ECs, VSMCs, cardiomyocytes and monocytes (Murphy, et al., 1991). These receptors are activated by Ang II ligand binding in a G protein-dependent manner. The activation of G protein-dependent signals activates phospholipase Cβ to increase intracellular inositol trisphosphate and diacylglycerol, leading to increase in calcium and activation of protein kinase C (PKC) isoforms.

In vascular cells, although Ang II activates multiple second messenger pathways including phospholipase D, PKC, and the mitogen activated protein kinase/erk kinase (MEK/ERK) pathways, recent attention has been drawn to the Rho family of GTPases (Griendling, et al., 1997). The Rho family is a group of 20-21 kDa GTPases including RhoA, B, C, D and E; Rac1 and 2; Cdc42Hs and TC10. The three Rho family members primarily expressed in vascular tissues in humans include RhoA, Rac1, and Cdc42Hs. Under unstimulated conditions, the Rho proteins are cytosolic, bound to GDP and guanine nucleotide dissociation inhibitors (Van Aelst and D'Souza-Schorey, 1997). In response to Ang II stimulation, the ligand binding of the G-protein-coupled AT-1 activates guanine nucleotide exchange factors (GEFs), which in turn catalyze GDP-GTP exchange and activates the Rho GTPases (Figure 1). Activated RhoA affects ROS production and controls smooth muscle cell contractility by phosphorylating myosin light chain kinase (MLCK), enhancing DNA synthesis, inducing VSMC migration, stimulating cardiovascular fibrosis (Kobayashi, et al., 2002), and inducing hemostatic and inflammatory proteins (Kobayashi, et al., 2002).

NF-κB is a ubiquitously-expressed, highly inducible transcription factor complex composed of both latent cytoplasmic and activated nuclear components. One major activation NF-κB pathway that we and others have defined is referred to as the "canonical" pathway, a pathway that controls nuclear targeting of latent cytoplasmic Rel A•NF-κB1 heterodimeric complexes. Rel A•NF-κB1 is retained in a cytoplasmic location by association with the IκBα inhibitor (Beg and Baldwin, 1993). Stimuli inducing the canonical NF-κB pathway activate the IKK kinase complex, resulting in IκBα phosphorylation at specific N-terminal serine residues, ultimately targeting it for proteosomal degradation (Ghosh and Baltimore, 1990). As a result, sequestered Rel A•NF-κB1 complexes are then released to enter the nucleus. Nuclear translocated Rel A•NF-κB1 then binds to specific regulatory sequences in cytokine and acute phase reactant promoters, activating their transcription.

Although initially the Ang II signaling pathway was thought to induce the canonical NF-κB activation pathway in VSMCs, detailed studies have shown that Ang II induces cell type-dependent activation of NF-κB pathways (Brasier, 2010). In non-vascular cells such as hepatocytes, PKC activation leads to cleavage of the IKK inhibitory TNFAIP3/A20 molecule and degradation of IkBα through the mechanisms as in canonical signaling induced by TNFα, resulting in activation of NF-κB translocation. In VSMCs, on the other hand, the Ang II-induced pathway is quite distinct from other cell types. A novel activation pathway independent of the well-recognized canonical pathway described above was identified by us and schematically diagrammed in Figure 1. In VSMCs, inactive NF-κB isoforms could be identified in unstimulated cells, and no significant changes in NF-κB abundance was observed in response to Ang II stimulation. Of importance, we found that Ang II stimulation rapidly induces phosphorylation of RelA at serine residue 536 in its COOH-terminal transactivating domain. Interestingly, we also found that phospho-Ser-536 RelA formation was blocked by RhoA inhibition, suggesting that Ser-536 phosphorylation was mediated upstream by RhoA. In addition, RhoA inhibition also blocked Ang II-induced IL-6 expression, indicating that Ang II-inducible phospho-Ser-536 RelA was required for IL-6 activation (Cui, et al., 2006).

Our studies in Ang II-stimulated VSMCs further showed that total RelA binding did not change on the native IL-6 promoter in response to Ang II, but fractional binding of phospho-Ser-536 RelA to the IL-6 promoter was increased (Choudhary, et al., 2007). These studies showed that Ang II induces NF-κB /RelA activation in VSMCs by increasing the relative abundance of phospho-Ser-536 RelA in the nucleoplasmic pool. We also confirmed Ang II-induced enhanced phospho-Ser-536 RelA formation in rat aortas treated with Ang II, establishing relevance to vascular signaling *in vivo* (Choudhary, et al., 2007; Cui, et al., 2006).

Our group further showed that Ang II-induced RelA Ser-536 phosphorylation is mediated by NF-κB-inducing kinase (NIK), the major regulated step controlling non-canonical NF-κB signaling. NIK inhibition prevented Ang II-induced Ser-536 phosphorylation and NF-κB-dependent transcription (Choudhary, et al., 2007), indicating that it is essential for RelA activation. We also found that NIK induced the activity of the RelA transactivation domain-1 and -2 in constitutively nuclear RelA proteins and that RelA formed an inducible nuclear complex with NIK in response to Ang II stimulation. The function and mechanism of this NIK·RelA complex in Ang II-induced vascular inflammation still requires further investigation.

Taken together, this data indicate that in VSMCs, where inactive NF-κB is constitutively nuclear, Ang II induces NF-κB -dependent transcription through an alternative pathway, being largely independent of IκB proteolysis, but mediated by the small GTPases Rac/RhoA, required for NIK·RelA complex formation and inducible phospho-Ser-536 RelA phosphorylation.

3.2 Vascular inflammatory actions of Ang II-induced NF-κB signaling

Ang II-induced NF-κB activation plays a central role in the development of aneurysms through regulation of gene expression of inflammatory molecules whose function broadly in the cascade of leukocyte recruitment and monocyte chemotaxis. These targets include pro-inflammatory cytokines (e.g. interleukins, etc.), chemokines (e.g. MCP-1, GM-CSF, etc.), adhesion molecules (e.g. E-selectin, ICAM-1, VCAM-1, etc.), and ECM-degrading MMPs.

A major target of Ang II-induced NF-κB activation is to activate expression of IL-6 by adventitial fibroblasts, recruited monocytes and VSMCs. Ang II induces rapid activation of

IL-6 transcription and translation (Han, et al., 1999). The transcriptional activation of IL-6 expression is mediated by NF-κB binding to its high affinity binding site in this proximal promoter of the IL-6 gene. This site is required for Ang II inducible expression since Ang II inducible activity is completely abolished by a promoter containing a point mutation that does not bind NF-κB (Han, et al., 1999). Together, these data suggest that NF-κB transcription factor is required for inducible expression of the IL-6 by Ang II.

IL-6 is a 26 kDa glycosylated cytokine that acts in a paracrine manner to signal through two distinct mechanisms, termed the classical initiated by membrane receptor binding, and the trans-signaling pathway mediated by soluble IL-6 Rα (Hou, et al., 2008). Classical IL-6 signaling is mediated via ligand binding to the IL-6Rα receptor on the cell membrane. The IL-6 trans-signaling pathway, on the other hand, involves circulating IL-6·IL-6Rα engagement with gp130 expressed on cells, enabling activation of the IL-6 signaling pathway in cells lacking IL-6Rα. In trans-signaling, proteolysis and/or alternative splicing lead to the generation of soluble IL-6 receptors (sIL-6R), which binds IL-6. The IL-6/sIL-6R complex can stimulate cells that only express gp130 but no IL-6R.

In IL-6-initiated classical signaling, the IL-6•IL-6Rα complex causes oligomerization with the ubiquitously expressed transmembrane gp130 β-subunit, inducing gp130 homodimerization, and subsequent formation of a hexameric IL-6•IL-Rα•gp130 complex (Boulanger, et al., 2003). This induces conformational changes of gp130, that trigger trans-autophosphorylation and activation of Janus tyrosine kinase JAK1, a specific Janus kinase mediating IL-6 signaling. JAK1 in turn induces tyrosine phosphorylation and activation of STAT isoforms STAT1 and STAT3 (Figure 1). As transcription factors, they then form homo- and heterodimers with each other, translocate to the nucleus, bind specific DNA sequences and enhance transcription of target genes via interactions with co-factors and co-activators such as p300/CREB-binding protein (CBP) and Positive Transcription Elongation Factor (PTEF-b) (Hou, et al., 2008).

IL-6 plays a major role in inducing systemic responses to the presence of vascular inflammation through the hepatic acute-phase response (Brasier, et al., 2002). IL-6 has diverse actions in multiple cell types of cardiovascular importance, including ECs, monocytes, platelets, hepatocytes and adipocytes. In the vessel, IL-6 promotes Ang II-induced ROS production because IL-6 deficiency protects against Ang II-induced endothelial dysfunction (Schrader, et al., 2007).

Importantly, a major action of IL-6 is to promote monocyte-to-macrophage differentiation, thus contributing to vascular inflammation. IL-6 stimulation increases esterase and phagocytic activities and enhances surface expression of Fc receptors, macrophage-colony stimulating factor (M-CSF) receptors, and the mature macrophage marker F4/80. Additionally, IL-6 induces expression of genes important for macrophage differentiation such as c-Jun, jun B, jun D, interferon-regulatory factor 1 (IRF1), JAK3, Egr-1 (Hou, et al., 2008). Moreover, IL-6 up-regulates MCP-1 expression (Biswas, et al., 1998; Tieu, et al., 2009) by vascular monocytic cells. MCP-1/CCR2 interactions are important in monocyte recruitment in the development of aneurysms (Boring, et al., 1998; Tieu, et al., 2009). Also, cell-cell interaction of monocytes and fibroblasts in cocultures induces IL-6 expression and macrophage activation, suggesting a role of IL-6 in monocyte-to-macrophage differentiation (Chomarat, et al., 2000; Tieu, et al., 2010). Recent studies demonstrated that IL-6-induced downstream gp130-JAK/STAT signaling pathway activation is also important for differentiation of monocytes (Hou, et al., 2008).

Recent studies indicate that enhanced IL-6 signaling is associated with vascular inflammation and aneurysm formation. IL-6 is elevated systemically and locally in patients and experimental models of aortic aneurysmal disease. IL-6 deficiency decreases aortic chemokine secretion and macrophage recruitment, and prevents aortic aneurysms and dissections in Ang II-infused mice (Tieu, et al., 2009). Conversely, in wild type mice, Ang II infusion potently induces IL-6 expression in the aorta, making IL-6 the most abundantly secreted cytokine that has yet been detected. IL-6 is predominantly expressed by fibroblasts and activated macrophages in the adventitia, with lesser amounts in the media and intimal layers (Recinos, et al., 2007). IL-6 signaling pathway was locally activated in Ang II-induced aortic aneurysms (Tieu, et al., 2009),where its action promotes monocytic activation and adventitial macrophage accumulation via a chemokine MCP-1-CCR2-based mechanism (Ishibashi, et al., 2004; Tieu, et al., 2009). These activated macrophages in the vessel wall produce pro-inflammatory cytokines, chemokines, ROS and MMPs, further facilitating local inflammation and remodeling.

4. The TGF-β-Smad pathway in Ang II signaling

The second pathway initiated by Ang II involves TGF-β receptor signaling pathway important in myofibroblast transition and vascular ECM remodeling, characteristic of aneurysmal disease. This cross-talk pathway is mediated by the effect of Ang II to upregulate TGF-β. TGF-β, in turn, induces the proliferation of adventitial fibroblasts and their phenotypic transition to myofibroblasts, that further promotes vascular remodeling with their enhanced mobility and secretory abilities. Additionally, Ang II-induced ECM decomposition and remodeling lead to monocytic chemotaxis and the release of latent TGF-β. TGF-β activation induces aortic Smad signaling, which further contributes to MMP production and macrophage recruitment. Finally, in conjunction with IL-6, TGF-β also modulates Th lymphocyte subsets by promoting Th17 cell differentiation via activation of Smad and STAT signaling.

4.1 TGF-β-Smad signaling mechanisms

TGF-β activates cells by binding to one of 7 type I TGF-β receptors (TGF-βRI) or 5 type II TGF-β receptors (TGF-βRII). In the cell, TGF-β signals through both Smad-dependent (Jones, et al., 2008) and Smad-independent (p38 MAP kinase-mediated) pathways (Funaba, et al., 2006). In the classic Smad-dependent pathway, ligand binding of TGF-β dimers leads to autophosphorylation and activation of a TGF-βRII homodimer, which in turn recruits and phosphorylates a TGF-βRI homodimer (Figure 1). TGF-βRI phosphorylates the appropriate receptor-activated Smad (R-Smad) (Jones, et al., 2008). Depending on the TGF-βRI that phosphorylates and activates them, there are 5 R-Smads in 2 groups (Smads 1, 5, 8; and Smads 2, 3). Once phosphorylated, R-Smad dissociates from TGF-βRI to form a complex with Smad4 (co-Smad), that translocates to the nucleus and regulates gene expression by binding to Smad binding elements. The signaling can also be regulated by inhibitory Smads (I-Smads), which attenuate the TGF-β response (Jones, et al., 2008).

4.2 Ang II and TGF-β interaction in TAAs

Recent studies have extensively focused on the role of TGF-β in the development of different forms of aortic aneurysms. Studies on TAAs caused by Marfan or Loeys-Dietz syndromes suggested a critical pathogenic role for increased TGF-β signaling in promoting abnormal vessel remodeling, dilatation, and aneurysmal expansion. Enhanced TGF-β signaling was implicated in aortic dilatation and aneurysm formation in Loeys-Dietz syndrome caused by mutations in the genes encoding TGF-βRI and TGF-βRII (Loeys, et al., 2005). In Marfan syndrome caused by mutations in the fibrillin-1 gene, bioavailability of TGF-β1is dysregulated (Chaudhry, et al., 2007), which contributes to the pathogenesis of TAAs (Dietz, et al., 2005; Neptune, et al., 2003). Normally, fibrillin-1 in the extracellular matrix regulates TGF-β activation by sequestering it in a complex with latent TGF-binding proteins (LTBPs). LTBPs associate matrix microfibrils with latency-associated peptide (LAP), regulating TGF-β matrix association and activation (Figure 1). Recent studies of fibrillin-1 deficient ($Fbn1^{-/-}$) mice have shown that several cardiovascular pathologies are caused by abnormal up-regulation of TGF-β signaling. Enhanced formation of activated TGF-β and phospho-Smad2, a downstream signaling protein activated by TGF-β, are detected in cardiovascular tissues. Importantly, neutralizing antibodies to TGF-β administered to $Fbn1^{-/-}$ mice reduce pathological abnormalities, suggesting a critical role of TGF-β signaling in the development and progression of TAA (Neptune, et al., 2003).

Interestingly, enhanced Ang II signaling, which is a potent inducer of cytokines and chemokines, has also been implicated in Marfan syndrome. Aortic Ang II concentration is increased in aortas of mice with fibrillin mutations (Nagashima, et al., 2001). Also, the Ang II type I receptor antagonist, Losartan, prevents aortic aneurysm formation in patients with Marfan syndrome (Habashi, et al., 2006). The ACE inhibitor perindopril reduced aortic diameter in Marfan syndrome patients and significantly reduced TGF-β levels and plasma levels of MMP-2 and MMP-3. In addition, Ang II enhances TGF-β actions by activating Smad pathway in a TGF-β-independent manner (Carvajal, et al., 2008). It also induces the production of a potent activator of TGF-β, thrombospondin-1 (Habashi, et al., 2006). These data suggest that Ang II activates TGF-β signaling, contributing to aneurysm formation. Ang II may activate TGF-β signaling by regulating its transcription and/or its activation from the latent form (Habashi, et al., 2006). Previous studies have shown that in renal disease, Ang II regulates TGF-β signaling activation by activating tumor necrosis factor TNF-α-converting enzyme (TACE), which through the cleavage of vasorin, controls TGF-β-mediated epithelial-to-mesenchymal transition (Shah and Catt, 2006).

In a mouse model with fibrillin deficiency (mgR), an inflammatory-fibroproliferative response has been described in aneurysm formation. Homozygous mgR mice die between 3 and 6 months of age of dissecting TAAs, and adventitial inflammation may accelerate pathogenesis by stimulating unregulated degradation of elastic matrix. In this mouse model, enhanced monocyte/macrophage infiltration is also pronounced at late stages of disease progression (Pereira, et al., 1999). Additionally, aortas from these mice secrete a GxxPG-containing fibrillin-1 fragment that is able to induce macrophage chemotaxis (Guo, et al., 2006b). Together, these findings suggest that inflammation is important in extracellular matrix degradation associated with fibrillin deficiency-induced TAAs. Two recent reports by the Dietz's group of Johns Hopkins University suggested that the effects of Ang II on aneurysm progression in MFS was mediated through a noncanonical TGF-beta signaling pathway involving extracellular signal-regulated kinase (ERK). It was reported that ERK activation contributed to aortic aneurysm progression in MFS (Holm, et al., 20111). Using a mouse model haplo-insufficient for Fbn-1 ($Fbn1^{C1039G/+}$), this group found that ERK1/2 was activated and that ERK inhibition, but not Smad4 deficiency, eliminated aneurysm development in MFS. It also was reported that AT1 receptor blocker losartan abrogated aneurysm progression by inhibiting TGF-beta-mediated ERK activation through AT2 (Habashi, et al., 2011).

Increased expression and activation of TGF-β are found in Ang II-induced AAAs. Preliminary studies from our group also demonstrated that Ang II induced Smad2/3 phosphorylation in mouse aortas. However, the precise role of TGF-β activity in inflammation in aneurysms remains contradictory. One study reported that TGF-β neutralizing antibodies afforded significant protection from Ang II-induced inflammatory aneurysms after Cxcl10 targeting (King, et al., 2009), while other studies showed that TGF-β played a protective role in AAA formation and TGF-β neutralization increased Ang II-induced aneurysm and monocyte invasiveness in C57BL/6 mice (Dai, et al., 2005; Wang, et al., 2010). Controversial results indicating the protective role of TGF-β in AAA formation may be explained by the concentration-dependent bipolar actions of TGF-β. With a higher dose of Ang II infusion in aged C57BL/6 mice (Tieu, et al., 2009), our preliminary studies showed that TGF-β neutralization decreased incidence of Ang II-induced aneurysm and adventitial thickening. Emerging evidence highlights the complex and context-dependent biphasic effects of TGF-β in the pathogenesis of aneurysm (Jones, et al., 2008), that can be partially explained by interaction with different receptors when TGF-β concentration changes (Goumans, et al., 2002). It may also be important to consider the variable roles of TGF-β during the dynamic transition from predisposition to terminal events. Thus, the detailed role of TGF-β in inflammatory aneurysms may be very complex and merits further exploration.

Also, we have recently demonstrated that co-culture of monocytes with adventitial fibroblasts resulted in enhanced expression of IL-6, MCP-1 and IL-6-dependent macrophage differentiation (Tieu, et al., 2009). It is interesting to speculate that TGF-β may play a role in this process as a paracrine factor (Dietz, 2010). TGF-β is known to induce IL-6 and MCP-1 expression (Seong, et al., 2009; Zhang, et al., 2009), monocyte recruitment and differentiation and myofibroblast formation, which in turn may amplify the process through secretion of TGF-β, MMPs, or even MCP-1 (Dagouassat, et al., 2010).

4.3 Effects of TGF-β-Smad signaling activation in aneurysms

TGF-β has both angiogenic and antiangiogenic effects (Goumans, et al., 2002), diametric actions thought to be controlled by the ratio of TGF-β signals via different receptors. Also, TGF-β produces opposing effects on mast cells to inhibit maturation or induce apoptosis, depending on their developmental stage and the TGF-β concentration (Rizas, et al., 2009).

Additionally, TGF-β controls both ECM synthesis and degradation (Jones, et al., 2008). TGF-β promotes ECM degradation by inducing MMP-2 and MMP-9 production (Kim, et al., 2007). On the other hand, TGF-β stimulates both fibroblasts (Varga and Jimenez, 1986) and myofibroblasts (Mishra, et al., 2007) to synthesize collagen I, that provides load-bearing characteristics, and collagen III, that provides tensile properties to the aortic wall (van Keulen, et al., 2000). TGF-β also induces α-smooth muscle actin expression in fibroblasts and promotes myofibroblast transdifferentiation (Vaughan, et al., 2000). The expression of α-smooth muscle actin was found to be significantly increased in adventitial fibroblasts of inflammatory aortic aneurysms, suggesting inflammatory remodeling in aneurysmal disease may be partly mediated by the proliferation of adventitial myofibroblasts (Sakata, et al., 2007).

It is also noteworthy that TGF-β engages in adaptive immunity by promoting the differentiation of naïve CD4+ T helper cells (Th0) to T helper 17 (Th17) cells via activation of Smad and STAT signaling, depending on the coinstantaneous presence of IL-6 or IL-21 (Reiner, 2007). TGF-β activation is critical and required for differentiation of Th17 cells (Melton, et al., 2010). It activates signature transcription factor RORγT (retinoic-acid receptor related orphan receptor gt) and cytokine IL-17 expression (Oukka, 2008). IL-17 mediates the production of inflammatory cytokines by stromal cells, which results in recruitment of leukocytes, thus creating a link between innate and adaptive immunity. Th17 cells and IL-17A have been implicated in the pathogenesis of autoimmune and inflammatory diseases (Tesmer, et al., 2008), and only recently in cardiovascular disease (Cheng, et al., 2008). Increased circulating Th17 cells and Th17 cell infiltration into the aorta are found in Ang II-induced hypertension, and IL-17 deficiency blunts these responses and prevents hypertension (Madhur, et al., 2010). Further, Th17 cells as well as IL-17 expression in atherosclerosis are increased, and blockade of IL-17A reduced aortic macrophage infiltration, cytokine secretion, and atherosclerotic plaque formation. Interestingly, IL-6 expression is induced by IL-17 and reduced by blockade of IL-17A signaling (Smith, et al., 2010), suggesting the proinflammatory effects of IL-6 could also be mediated by Th17 cells. Importantly, IL-17 and, by extension, Th17 cells, may contribute to inflammatory processes by promoting monocyte chemotaxis, adhersion and migration. It has recently been found that IL-17 mediated monocyte migration partially through MCP-1 induction (Shahrara, et al., 2010). IL-17A treatment of aortas from atherosclerotic mice promoted aortic CXCL1 expression and monocyte adhesion (Smith, et al., 2010). These studies highlight an important proinflammatory role for T cells, especially the Th17 subset, in vascular inflammation.

5. Conclusion

Recent preclinical research has indicated that Ang II influences development and progression of aortic aneurysmal disease in two important ways. First, Ang II affects the process of vascular inflammation by promoting macrophage accumulation, activation, local ROS production and aortic aneurysms in the suprarenal and thoracic aorta, followed by dissections through the NF-κB-IL-6 signaling pathway. Second, Ang II promotes myofibroblast transition and ECM remodeling - both characteristic of aneurysmal disease - by a TGF-β1-Smad pathway. Currently, there are still many important unresolved questions. For example, 1) the role of NF-κB RelA activation in the development of aneurysms; 2) the mechanism through which Ang II activates TGF-β in the vessel wall; 3) the precise role of TGF-β signaling in Ang II-induced aortic aneurysms; 4) the role of myofibroblast formation in the development of aortic remodeling and aneurysms; 5) the role of TGF-β signaling on Th17 cell differentiation and recruitment in the development of Ang II-induced aneurysms; and 6) clinical relevance of TGF-β neutralization in aneurysmal disease. Further elucidation of these issues will identify new targets for therapeutic intervention and biomarker development.

6. Acknowledgment

We thank Adrian Recinos and Hong Sun for discussions and advice. Work in our laboratories is supported by NIH grants R01HL70925 (ARB), R01DK079053 (RGT), P50 HL083794 (D. Milewicz), and support from the Ted Nash Long Life Foundation.

7. References

Beg, A. A. & Baldwin, A. S., Jr. (1993) The I kappa B proteins: multifunctional regulators of Rel/NF-kappa B transcription factors. Genes Dev, Vol. 7, No. 11, pp. 2064-2070, ISSN 0890-9369

Biswas, P., Delfanti, F., Bernasconi, S., Mengozzi, M., Cota, M., Polentarutti, N., Mantovani, A., Lazzarin, A., Sozzani, S. & Poli, G. (1998) Interleukin-6 induces monocyte chemotactic protein-1 in peripheral blood mononuclear cells and in the U937 cell line. Blood, Vol. 91, No. 1, pp. 258-265, ISSN 0006-4971

Boulanger, M. J., Chow, D. C., Brevnova, E. E. & Garcia, K. C. (2003) Hexameric structure and assembly of the interleukin-6/IL-6 alpha-receptor/gp130 complex. Science, Vol. 300, No. 5628, pp. 2101-2104, ISSN 1095-9203

Brasier, A. R. (2010) The nuclear factor-kappaB-interleukin-6 signalling pathway mediating vascular inflammation. Cardiovasc Res, Vol. 86, No. 2, pp. 211-218, ISSN 1755-3245

Brasier, A. R., Recinos, A., 3rd & Eledrisi, M. S. (2002) Vascular inflammation and the renin-angiotensin system. Arterioscler Thromb Vasc Biol, Vol. 22, No. 8, pp. 1257-1266, ISSN 1524-4636

Carvajal, G., Rodriguez-Vita, J., Rodrigues-Diez, R., Sanchez-Lopez, E., Ruperez, M., Cartier, C., Esteban, V., Ortiz, A., Egido, J., Mezzano, S. A. & Ruiz-Ortega, M. (2008) Angiotensin II activates the Smad pathway during epithelial mesenchymal transdifferentiation. Kidney Int, Vol. 74, No. 5, pp. 585-595, ISSN 1523-1755

Chaudhry, S. S., Cain, S. A., Morgan, A., Dallas, S. L., Shuttleworth, C. A. & Kielty, C. M. (2007) Fibrillin-1 regulates the bioavailability of TGFbeta1. J Cell Biol, Vol. 176, No. 3, pp. 355-367, ISSN 0021-9525

Chen, H. J., Li, D. Y., Saldeen, T., Phillips, M. I. & Mehta, J. L. (2001) Attenuation of tissue P-selectin and MCP-1 expression and intimal proliferation by AT(1) receptor blockade in hyperlipidemic rabbits. Biochem Biophys Res Commun, Vol. 282, No. 2, pp. 474-479, ISSN 0006-291X

Cheng, X., Yu, X., Ding, Y. J., Fu, Q. Q., Xie, J. J., Tang, T. T., Yao, R., Chen, Y. & Liao, Y. H. (2008) The Th17/Treg imbalance in patients with acute coronary syndrome. Clin Immunol, Vol. 127, No. 1, pp. 89-97, ISSN 1521-6616

Chomarat, P., Banchereau, J., Davoust, J. & Palucka, A. K. (2000) IL-6 switches the differentiation of monocytes from dendritic cells to macrophages. Nat Immunol, Vol. 1, No. 6, pp. 510-514, ISSN 1529-2908

Choudhary, S., Lu, M., Cui, R. & Brasier, A. R. (2007) Involvement of a novel Rac/RhoA guanosine triphosphatase-nuclear factor-kappaB inducing kinase signaling pathway mediating angiotensin II-induced RelA transactivation. Mol Endocrinol, Vol. 21, No. 9, pp. 2203-2217, ISSN 0888-8809

Cui, R., Tieu, B., Recinos, A., Tilton, R. G. & Brasier, A. R. (2006) RhoA mediates angiotensin II-induced phospho-Ser536 nuclear factor kappaB/RelA subunit exchange on the interleukin-6 promoter in VSMCs. Circ Res, Vol. 99, No. 7, pp. 723-730, ISSN 1524-4571

Dagouassat, M., Suffee, N., Hlawaty, H., Haddad, O., Charni, F., Laguillier, C., Vassy, R., Martin, L., Schischmanoff, P. O., Gattegno, L., Oudar, O., Sutton, A. & Charnaux, N. (2010) Monocyte chemoattractant protein-1 (MCP-1)/CCL2 secreted by hepatic myofibroblasts promotes migration and invasion of human hepatoma cells. Int J Cancer, Vol. 126, No. 5, pp. 1095-1108, ISSN 1097-0215

Dai, J., Losy, F., Guinault, A. M., Pages, C., Anegon, I., Desgranges, P., Becquemin, J. P. & Allaire, E. (2005) Overexpression of transforming growth factor-beta1 stabilizes already-formed aortic aneurysms: a first approach to induction of functional healing by endovascular gene therapy. Circulation, Vol. 112, No. 7, pp. 1008-1015, ISSN 1524-4539

Daugherty, A., Rateri, D. L., Charo, I. F., Owens, A. P., Howatt, D. A. & Cassis, L. A. (2010) Angiotensin II infusion promotes ascending aortic aneurysms: attenuation by CCR2 deficiency in apoE-/- mice. Clin Sci (Lond), Vol. 118, No. 11, pp. 681-689, ISSN 1470-8736

Desmouliere, A., Geinoz, A., Gabbiani, F. & Gabbiani, G. (1993) Transforming growth factor-beta 1 induces alpha-smooth muscle actin expression in granulation tissue myofibroblasts and in quiescent and growing cultured fibroblasts. J Cell Biol, Vol. 122, No. 1, pp. 103-111, ISSN 0021-9525

Dietz, H. C. (2010) TGF-beta in the pathogenesis and prevention of disease: a matter of aneurysmic proportions. J Clin Invest, Vol. 120, No. 2, pp. 403-407, ISSN 1558-8238

Dietz, H. C., Loeys, B., Carta, L. & Ramirez, F. (2005) Recent progress towards a molecular understanding of Marfan syndrome. Am J Med Genet C Semin Med Genet, Vol. 139C, No. 1, pp. 4-9, ISSN 1552-4868

Ejiri, J., Inoue, N., Tsukube, T., Munezane, T., Hino, Y., Kobayashi, S., Hirata, K., Kawashima, S., Imajoh-Ohmi, S., Hayashi, Y., Yokozaki, H., Okita, Y. & Yokoyama, M. (2003) Oxidative stress in the pathogenesis of thoracic aortic aneurysm: protective role of statin and angiotensin II type 1 receptor blocker. Cardiovasc Res, Vol. 59, No. 4, pp. 988-996, ISSN 0008-6363

Funaba, M., Ikeda, T., Murakami, M., Ogawa, K., Nishino, Y., Tsuchida, K., Sugino, H. & Abe, M. (2006) Involvement of p38 MAP kinase and Smad3 in TGF-beta-mediated mast cell functions. Cell Signal, Vol. 18, No. 12, pp. 2154-2161, ISSN 0898-6568

Galle, C., Schandene, L., Stordeur, P., Peignois, Y., Ferreira, J., Wautrecht, J. C., Dereume, J. P. & Goldman, M. (2005) Predominance of type 1 CD4+ T cells in human abdominal aortic aneurysm. Clin Exp Immunol, Vol. 142, No. 3, pp. 519-527, ISSN 0009-9104

Ghosh, S. & Baltimore, D. (1990) Activation in vitro of NF-kappa B by phosphorylation of its inhibitor I kappa B. Nature, Vol. 344, No. 6267, pp. 678-682, ISSN 0028-0836

Goumans, M. J., Valdimarsdottir, G., Itoh, S., Rosendahl, A., Sideras, P. & ten Dijke, P. (2002) Balancing the activation state of the endothelium via two distinct TGF-beta type I receptors. EMBO J, Vol. 21, No. 7, pp. 1743-1753, ISSN 0261-4189

Griendling, K. K., Ushio-Fukai, M., Lassegue, B. & Alexander, R. W. (1997) Angiotensin II signaling in vascular smooth muscle. New concepts. Hypertension, Vol. 29, No. 1 Pt 2, pp. 366-373, ISSN 0194-911X

Guo, D. C., Papke, C. L., He, R. & Milewicz, D. M. (2006a) Pathogenesis of thoracic and abdominal aortic aneurysms. Ann N Y Acad Sci, Vol. 1085, pp. 339-352, ISSN 0077-8923

Guo, G., Booms, P., Halushka, M., Dietz, H. C., Ney, A., Stricker, S., Hecht, J., Mundlos, S. & Robinson, P. N. (2006b) Induction of macrophage chemotaxis by aortic extracts of the mgR Marfan mouse model and a GxxPG-containing fibrillin-1 fragment. Circulation, Vol. 114, No. 17, pp. 1855-1862, ISSN 1524-4539

Habashi, J.P., Doyle, J.J., Holm, T.M., Aziz, H., Schoenhoff, F., Bedja, D., Chen, Y., Modiri, A.N., Judge, D.P. & Dietz, H.C. (2011) Angiotensin II type 2 receptor signaling attenuates aortic aneurysm in mice through ERK antagonism. *Science*. Vol. 332, No. 6027, pp. 361-365, ISSN 0036-8075

Habashi, J. P., Judge, D. P., Holm, T. M., Cohn, R. D., Loeys, B. L., Cooper, T. K., Myers, L., Klein, E. C., Liu, G., Calvi, C., Podowski, M., Neptune, E. R., Halushka, M. K., Bedja, D., Gabrielson, K., Rifkin, D. B., Carta, L., Ramirez, F., Huso, D. L. & Dietz, H. C. (2006) Losartan, an AT1 antagonist, prevents aortic aneurysm in a mouse model of Marfan syndrome. Science, Vol. 312, No. 5770, pp. 117-121, ISSN 1095-9203

Han, Y., Runge, M. S. & Brasier, A. R. (1999) Angiotensin II induces interleukin-6 transcription in vascular smooth muscle cells through pleiotropic activation of nuclear factor-kappa B transcription factors. Circ Res, Vol. 84, No. 6, pp. 695-703, ISSN 0009-7330

Holm, T.M., Habashi, J.P., Doyle, J.J., Bedja, D., Chen, Y., van Erp, C., Lindsay, M.E., Kim, D., Schoenhoff, F., Cohn, R.D., Loeys, B.L., Thomas, C.J., Patnaik, S., Marugan, J.J., Judge, D.P. & Dietz, H.C. (2011) Noncanonical TGFβ signaling contributes to aortic aneurysm progression in Marfan syndrome mice. *Science*. Vol. 332, No. 6027, pp. 358-361, ISSN 0036-8075

Hou, T., Tieu, B. C., Ray, S., Recinos Iii, A., Cui, R., Tilton, R. G. & Brasier, A. R. (2008) Roles of IL-6-gp130 Signaling in Vascular Inflammation. Curr Cardiol Rev, Vol. 4, No. 3, pp. 179-192, ISSN 1875-6557

Ishibashi, M., Egashira, K., Zhao, Q., Hiasa, K., Ohtani, K., Ihara, Y., Charo, I. F., Kura, S., Tsuzuki, T., Takeshita, A. & Sunagawa, K. (2004) Bone marrow-derived monocyte chemoattractant protein-1 receptor CCR2 is critical in angiotensin II-induced acceleration of atherosclerosis and aneurysm formation in hypercholesterolemic mice. Arterioscler Thromb Vasc Biol, Vol. 24, No. 11, pp. e174-178, ISSN 1524-4636

Jones, G. T., Thompson, A. R., van Bockxmeer, F. M., Hafez, H., Cooper, J. A., Golledge, J., Humphries, S. E., Norman, P. E. & van Rij, A. M. (2008) Angiotensin II type 1 receptor 1166C polymorphism is associated with abdominal aortic aneurysm in three independent cohorts. Arterioscler Thromb Vasc Biol, Vol. 28, No. 4, pp. 764-770, ISSN 1524-4636

Kim, E. S., Sohn, Y. W. & Moon, A. (2007) TGF-beta-induced transcriptional activation of MMP-2 is mediated by activating transcription factor (ATF)2 in human breast epithelial cells. Cancer Lett, Vol. 252, No. 1, pp. 147-156, ISSN 0304-3835

King, V. L., Lin, A. Y., Kristo, F., Anderson, T. J., Ahluwalia, N., Hardy, G. J., Owens, A. P., 3rd, Howatt, D. A., Shen, D., Tager, A. M., Luster, A. D., Daugherty, A. & Gerszten, R. E. (2009) Interferon-gamma and the interferon-inducible chemokine CXCL10 protect against aneurysm formation and rupture. Circulation, Vol. 119, No. 3, pp. 426-435, ISSN 1524-4539

Kobayashi, N., Nakano, S., Mita, S., Kobayashi, T., Honda, T., Tsubokou, Y. & Matsuoka, H. (2002) Involvement of Rho-kinase pathway for angiotensin II-induced plasminogen activator inhibitor-1 gene expression and cardiovascular remodeling in hypertensive rats. J Pharmacol Exp Ther, Vol. 301, No. 2, pp. 459-466, ISSN 0022-3565

Kuivaniemi, H., Platsoucas, C. D. & Tilson, M. D., 3rd (2008) Aortic aneurysms: an immune disease with a strong genetic component. Circulation, Vol. 117, No. 2, pp. 242-252, ISSN 1524-4539

Loeys, B. L., Chen, J., Neptune, E. R., Judge, D. P., Podowski, M., Holm, T., Meyers, J., Leitch, C. C., Katsanis, N., Sharifi, N., Xu, F. L., Myers, L. A., Spevak, P. J.,

Cameron, D. E., De Backer, J., Hellemans, J., Chen, Y., Davis, E. C., Webb, C. L., Kress, W., Coucke, P., Rifkin, D. B., De Paepe, A. M. & Dietz, H. C. (2005) A syndrome of altered cardiovascular, craniofacial, neurocognitive and skeletal development caused by mutations in TGFBR1 or TGFBR2. Nat Genet, Vol. 37, No. 3, pp. 275-281, ISSN 1061-4036

Longo, G. M., Xiong, W., Greiner, T. C., Zhao, Y., Fiotti, N. & Baxter, B. T. (2002) Matrix metalloproteinases 2 and 9 work in concert to produce aortic aneurysms. J Clin Invest, Vol. 110, No. 5, pp. 625-632, ISSN 0021-9738

Madhur, M. S., Lob, H. E., McCann, L. A., Iwakura, Y., Blinder, Y., Guzik, T. J. & Harrison, D. G. (2010) Interleukin 17 promotes angiotensin II-induced hypertension and vascular dysfunction. Hypertension, Vol. 55, No. 2, pp. 500-507, ISSN 1524-4563

Massague, J. (1998) TGF-beta signal transduction. Annu Rev Biochem, Vol. 67, pp. 753-791, ISSN 0066-4154

McAllister-Lucas, L. M. & Lucas, P. C. (2008) Finally, MALT1 is a protease! Nat Immunol, Vol. 9, No. 3, pp. 231-233, ISSN 1529-2916

Melton, A. C., Bailey-Bucktrout, S. L., Travis, M. A., Fife, B. T., Bluestone, J. A. & Sheppard, D. (2010) Expression of alphavbeta8 integrin on dendritic cells regulates Th17 cell development and experimental autoimmune encephalomyelitis in mice. J Clin Invest, Vol. 120, No. 12, pp. 4436-4444, ISSN 1558-8238

Mishra, R., Zhu, L., Eckert, R. L. & Simonson, M. S. (2007) TGF-beta-regulated collagen type I accumulation: role of Src-based signals. Am J Physiol Cell Physiol, Vol. 292, No. 4, pp. C1361-1369, ISSN 0363-6143

Murphy, T. J., Alexander, R. W., Griendling, K. K., Runge, M. S. & Bernstein, K. E. (1991) Isolation of a cDNA encoding the vascular type-1 angiotensin II receptor. Nature, Vol. 351, No. 6323, pp. 233-236, ISSN 0028-0836

Nagashima, H., Sakomura, Y., Aoka, Y., Uto, K., Kameyama, K., Ogawa, M., Aomi, S., Koyanagi, H., Ishizuka, N., Naruse, M., Kawana, M. & Kasanuki, H. (2001) Angiotensin II type 2 receptor mediates vascular smooth muscle cell apoptosis in cystic medial degeneration associated with Marfan's syndrome. Circulation, Vol. 104, No. 12 Suppl 1, pp. I282-287, ISSN 1524-4539

Neptune, E. R., Frischmeyer, P. A., Arking, D. E., Myers, L., Bunton, T. E., Gayraud, B., Ramirez, F., Sakai, L. Y. & Dietz, H. C. (2003) Dysregulation of TGF-beta activation contributes to pathogenesis in Marfan syndrome. Nat Genet, Vol. 33, No. 3, pp. 407-411, ISSN 1061-4036

Oukka, M. (2008) Th17 cells in immunity and autoimmunity. Ann Rheum Dis, Vol. 67 Suppl 3, pp. iii26-29, ISSN 1468-2060

Pearce, W. H. & Koch, A. E. (1996) Cellular components and features of immune response in abdominal aortic aneurysms. Ann N Y Acad Sci, Vol. 800, pp. 175-185, ISSN 0077-8923

Pereira, L., Lee, S. Y., Gayraud, B., Andrikopoulos, K., Shapiro, S. D., Bunton, T., Biery, N. J., Dietz, H. C., Sakai, L. Y. & Ramirez, F. (1999) Pathogenetic sequence for aneurysm revealed in mice underexpressing fibrillin-1. Proc Natl Acad Sci U S A, Vol. 96, No. 7, pp. 3819-3823, ISSN 0027-8424

Pueyo, M. E., Gonzalez, W., Nicoletti, A., Savoie, F., Arnal, J. F. & Michel, J. B. (2000) Angiotensin II stimulates endothelial vascular cell adhesion molecule-1 via nuclear factor-kappaB activation induced by intracellular oxidative stress. Arterioscler Thromb Vasc Biol, Vol. 20, No. 3, pp. 645-651, ISSN 1079-5642

Recinos, A., 3rd, LeJeune, W. S., Sun, H., Lee, C. Y., Tieu, B. C., Lu, M., Hou, T., Boldogh, I., Tilton, R. G. & Brasier, A. R. (2007) Angiotensin II induces IL-6 expression and the Jak-STAT3 pathway in aortic adventitia of LDL receptor-deficient mice. Atherosclerosis, Vol. 194, No. 1, pp. 125-133, ISSN 1879-1484

Reiner, S. L. (2007) Development in motion: helper T cells at work. Cell, Vol. 129, No. 1, pp. 33-36, ISSN 0092-8674

Rizas, K. D., Ippagunta, N. & Tilson, M. D., 3rd (2009) Immune cells and molecular mediators in the pathogenesis of the abdominal aortic aneurysm. Cardiol Rev, Vol. 17, No. 5, pp. 201-210, ISSN 1538-4683

Sakata, N., Nabeshima, K., Iwasaki, H., Tashiro, T., Uesugi, N., Nakashima, O., Ito, H., Kawanami, T., Furuya, K. & Kojima, M. (2007) Possible involvement of myofibroblast in the development of inflammatory aortic aneurysm. Pathol Res Pract, Vol. 203, No. 1, pp. 21-29, ISSN 0344-0338

Schonbeck, U., Sukhova, G. K., Gerdes, N. & Libby, P. (2002) T(H)2 predominant immune responses prevail in human abdominal aortic aneurysm. Am J Pathol, Vol. 161, No. 2, pp. 499-506, ISSN 0002-9440

Schrader, L. I., Kinzenbaw, D. A., Johnson, A. W., Faraci, F. M. & Didion, S. P. (2007) IL-6 deficiency protects against angiotensin II induced endothelial dysfunction and hypertrophy. Arterioscler Thromb Vasc Biol, Vol. 27, No. 12, pp. 2576-2581, ISSN 1524-4636

Seong, G. J., Hong, S., Jung, S. A., Lee, J. J., Lim, E., Kim, S. J. & Lee, J. H. (2009) TGF-beta-induced interleukin-6 participates in transdifferentiation of human Tenon's fibroblasts to myofibroblasts. Mol Vis, Vol. 15, pp. 2123-2128, ISSN 1090-0535

Shah, B. H. & Catt, K. J. (2006) TACE-dependent EGF receptor activation in angiotensin-II-induced kidney disease. Trends Pharmacol Sci, Vol. 27, No. 5, pp. 235-237, ISSN 0165-6147

Shahrara, S., Pickens, S. R., Mandelin, A. M., 2nd, Karpus, W. J., Huang, Q., Kolls, J. K. & Pope, R. M. (2010) IL-17-mediated monocyte migration occurs partially through CC chemokine ligand 2/monocyte chemoattractant protein-1 induction. J Immunol, Vol. 184, No. 8, pp. 4479-4487, ISSN 1550-6606

Smith, E., Prasad, K. M., Butcher, M., Dobrian, A., Kolls, J. K., Ley, K. & Galkina, E. (2010) Blockade of interleukin-17A results in reduced atherosclerosis in apolipoprotein E-deficient mice. Circulation, Vol. 121, No. 15, pp. 1746-1755, ISSN 1524-4539

Tesmer, L. A., Lundy, S. K., Sarkar, S. & Fox, D. A. (2008) Th17 cells in human disease. Immunol Rev, Vol. 223, pp. 87-113, ISSN 1600-065X

Tieu, B. C., Ju, X., Lee, C., Sun, H., Lejeune, W., Recinos, A., 3rd, Brasier, A. R. & Tilton, R. G. (2010) Aortic Adventitial Fibroblasts Participate in Angiotensin-Induced Vascular Wall Inflammation and Remodeling. J Vasc Res, Vol. 48, No. 3, pp. 261-272, ISSN 1423-0135

Tieu, B. C., Lee, C., Sun, H., Lejeune, W., Recinos, A., 3rd, Ju, X., Spratt, H., Guo, D. C., Milewicz, D., Tilton, R. G. & Brasier, A. R. (2009) An adventitial IL-6/MCP1 amplification loop accelerates macrophage-mediated vascular inflammation leading to aortic dissection in mice. J Clin Invest, Vol. 119, No. 12, pp. 3637-3651, ISSN 1558-8238

Tilson, M. D., Fu, C., Xia, S. X., Syn, D., Yoon, Y. & McCaffrey, T. (2000) Expression of molecular messages for angiogenesis by fibroblasts from aneurysmal abdominal aorta versus dermal fibroblasts. Int J Surg Investig, Vol. 1, No. 5, pp. 453-457, ISSN 1028-5229

Van Aelst, L. & D'Souza-Schorey, C. (1997) Rho GTPases and signaling networks. Genes Dev, Vol. 11, No. 18, pp. 2295-2322, ISSN 0890-9369

van Keulen, C. J., van den Akker, E., van den Berg, F. G., Pals, G. & Rauwerda, J. A. (2000) The role of type III collagen in family members of patients with abdominal aortic aneurysms. Eur J Vasc Endovasc Surg, Vol. 20, No. 4, pp. 379-385, ISSN 1078-5884

Varga, J. & Jimenez, S. A. (1986) Stimulation of normal human fibroblast collagen production and processing by transforming growth factor-beta. Biochem Biophys Res Commun, Vol. 138, No. 2, pp. 974-980, ISSN 0006-291X

Vaughan, M. B., Howard, E. W. & Tomasek, J. J. (2000) Transforming growth factor-beta1 promotes the morphological and functional differentiation of the myofibroblast. Exp Cell Res, Vol. 257, No. 1, pp. 180-189, ISSN 0014-4827

Wang, Y., Ait-Oufella, H., Herbin, O., Bonnin, P., Ramkhelawon, B., Taleb, S., Huang, J., Offenstadt, G., Combadiere, C., Renia, L., Johnson, J. L., Tharaux, P. L., Tedgui, A. & Mallat, Z. (2010) TGF-beta activity protects against inflammatory aortic aneurysm progression and complications in angiotensin II-infused mice. J Clin Invest, Vol. 120, No. 2, pp. 422-432, ISSN 1558-8238

Zhang, F., Tsai, S., Kato, K., Yamanouchi, D., Wang, C., Rafii, S., Liu, B. & Kent, K. C. (2009) Transforming growth factor-beta promotes recruitment of bone marrow cells and bone marrow-derived mesenchymal stem cells through stimulation of MCP-1 production in vascular smooth muscle cells. J Biol Chem, Vol. 284, No. 26, pp. 17564-17574, ISSN 0021-9258

Zhao, L., Moos, M. P., Grabner, R., Pedrono, F., Fan, J., Kaiser, B., John, N., Schmidt, S., Spanbroek, R., Lotzer, K., Huang, L., Cui, J., Rader, D. J., Evans, J. F., Habenicht, A. J. & Funk, C. D. (2004) The 5-lipoxygenase pathway promotes pathogenesis of hyperlipidemia-dependent aortic aneurysm. Nat Med, Vol. 10, No. 9, pp. 966-973, ISSN 1078-8956

8

Aortitis and Aortic Aneurysm in Systemic Vasculitis

Ana García-Martínez, Sergio Prieto-González, Pedro Arguis, Georgina Espígol, José Hernández-Rodríguez and Maria C Cid
Vasculitis Research Unit, Departments of Emergency Medicine and Systemic Autoimmune Diseases, Hospital Clínic, University of Barcelona, Institut d'Investigacions Biomèdiques August Pi i Sunyer, Barcelona
Spain

1. Introduction

Vasculitis encompasses a heterogeneous group of disorders characterized by inflammation of blood vessels. Inflammation affects vessels of any type and size, and causes a wide range of clinical manifestations, depending on the vascular bed involved. The preferential size of involved vessels and the targeted tissues determine the clinical presentation and serve as key elements for classification (Watts & Scott, 2009). Vasculitis may occur as a primary process or may be secondary to an underlying disease such as infection, malignancy or other systemic autoimmune or chronic inflammatory diseases. Blood vessel inflammation results in abnormal vascular remodelling with the potential of severe clinical consequences. In some instances, inflammation leads to intimal hyperplasia resulting in vascular stenoses and ischemia of the tributary tissues. In other settings, inflammation causes disruption of the vessel wall architecture leading to aneurysm formation and eventual dissection or rupture.

Aortitis is the term used to define inflammation of one or more layers of the aortic wall and may have an infectious or non-infectious origin (Gornik & Creager, 2008). Non-infectious aortitis is usually part of the spectrum of vascular involvement occurring in primary large-vessel vasculitis including giant-cell arteritis (GCA) of the elderly and Takayasu's arteritis (TAK). Aortitis is a major component of these diseases and may lead to severe complications including aortic aneurysm, dissection or stenosis.

Aortitis may also present as a circumscribed condition named isolated aortitis. This term refers to aortitis incidentally found at the time of histopathological examination of aortas obtained from necropsy studies or from patients who have undergone surgical repair of aortic aneurysm or aortic valve replacement. Existing studies are retrospective and most patients have not been prospectively and systematically evaluated in search for a systemic vasculitis or other chronic inflammatory diseases. There is some controversy about whether isolated aortitis is a specific condition or represents an incomplete view of a systemic disease.

Occasionally, aortitis may occur in the setting of other primary systemic vasculitis, particularly antineutrophil cytoplasmic antibody (ANCA)-associated vasculitis (Chirinos et al., 2004; Lee et al., 2008), and other autoimmune disorders or chronic inflammatory diseases (i.e. sarcoidosis, Crohn's disease, ankylosing spondylitis, Behçet's disease, Cogan's disease, and IgG4-related disease) (Domenech et al., 2005; Gluth et al., 2006; Palazzi et al.,

2010; Stone, 2011; Weiler et al., 2000; Okada et al., 1997). The main causes of primary and secondary aortitis are summarized in table 1.
Chronic periaortitis is an additional form of aortic inflammation that encompasses a variety of conditions and is characterized by inflammatory involvement of the outer layer of the aorta and surrounding tissues. Chronic periaortitis may occasionally occur in patients with small-medium sized vessel vasculitis.
This chapter will particularly focus on aortic inflammation and its consequences in the context of the primary large-vessel vasculitis.

NON INFECTIOUS AORTITIS	
Primary vasculitis	
Large-vessel vasculitis	Giant-cell arteritis Takayasu's arteritis
Other vasculitis	Granulomatosis with polyangiitis (Wegener's) Microscopic polyangiitis
Vasculitis associated with chronic inflammatory or autoimmune conditions	Rheumatoid arthritis Sarcoidosis Systemic lupus erythematosus Behçet disease Cogan syndrome HLA-B27 associated spondyloarthropaties Crohn's disease Relapsing polychondritis IgG4-related disease
Isolated aortitis	
Chronic periaortitis	Retroperitoneal fibrosis Inflammatory abdominal aortic aneurysm Perianeurysmal aortitis
INFECTIOUS AORTITIS	
Bacterial	*Salmonella spp* *Staphylococcus spp* *Streptococcus pneumoniae* *Treponema pallidum spp*
Mycobacterial	*Mycobacterium tuberculosis*

Table 1. Causes of aortic inflammation

2. Aortic inflammation in primary systemic vasculitis

2.1 Vasculitis leading to aortic inflammation

Primary large-vessel vasculitis encompasses GCA and TAK which represent the most common disorders associated with non-infectious aortitis. Although histologically similar, GCA and TAK are considered distinct disease entities based on demographic and clinical features. While GCA affects aged people and is usually associated with cranial symptoms, TAK predominantly affects patients younger than 40 years, primarily involves the aorta and its major branches but generally spares the cranial arteries. These features usually allow a clear clinical differentiation between these two vasculitides. However the increasing recognition of large-artery involvement in GCA during the past decade widens the overlap features between both entities and some authors suggest that they may be part of the spectrum of a single disorder (Maksimowicz-McKinnon & Hoffman, 2009).

2.1.1 Giant-cell arteritis

GCA is a systemic vasculitis involving large and medium sized vessels in patients older than 50 years. The preferential involvement of the cranial arteries determines the classical symptoms of GCA (headache, jaw claudication, scalp tenderness) and its more frequent vaso-occlusive complication (visual loss usually due to anterior ischemic optic neuritis). About half of the patients have polymyalgia rheumatica and the majority have prominent systemic symptoms (fever, anemia of chronic disease type, and weight loss) and elevation of acute phase reactants.

Although early descriptions of GCA identified the cranial arteries as the main target of the disease, subsequent reports indicated more widespread vascular involvement (Hunder, 2006). First report of aortic involvement was in 1937 (Sproul & Hawthorne, 1937) and described post-mortem chronic diffuse inflammation with giant cells in the aorta and iliac arteries of two men without apparent premortem symptoms of vasculitis. Over the following years, additional cases were reported (Bonnin & Lander, 1956; Cardell & Hanley, 1951; Cooke & Cloake, 1946; Heptinstall et al., 1954) confirming the potential of GCA to involve large-vessels.

In 1972 Ostberg (Ostberg, 1972) systematically investigated the aorta and its major branches in necropsies from 13 patients with GCA. Inflammatory involvement of the aorta was present in 12 out of the 13 patients (90%). Although the necropsy nature of this survey may be biased towards the inclusion of more severe cases, these findings suggest that aortic involvement might be frequent in GCA.

More recently, other authors have investigated the prevalence of aortitis in specimens obtained from patients who underwent aortic reconstructive surgery because of aortic aneurysm, aortic dissection or aortic valve insufficiency. Table 2 summarizes the main findings of these studies (Burke et al., 2008; Gelsomino et al., 2005; Homme et al., 2006; Kerr et al., 2000; Liang et al., 2009; Miller et al., 2006; Nesi et al., 2009; Pacini et al., 2008; Rojo-Leyva et al., 2000). Histopathologic analysis of removed aortic fragments revealed chronic inflammation in about 1,7 to 8,7% of patients subjected to aortic surgery. Patients with aortic inflammation were predominantly women and the age average was 65 years. Among these patients, 5-20% had an underlying chronic inflammatory disease, mainly GCA. The design of these retrospective studies is not aimed to estimate the frequency of aortic involvement in GCA but underlines the fact that GCA accounts for a significant proportion of complicated inflammatory aortitis.

In the past decade, the vast development of imaging techniques has facilitated the non-invasive detection of signs suggestive of aortic inflammation in living individuals in early phases, before the development of clinically relevant aortic complications (Pipitone et al., 2008) (Figures 1 and 2). In this setting, three prospective studies have been conducted to determine the prevalence of aortitis in patients with recent-onset GCA. Blockmans et al. performed a systematic 18F-Fluorodeoxyglucose (FDG) Positron Emission Tomography (FDG-PET) to 35 newly diagnosed GCA patients and found FDG uptake suggestive of active inflammation in both the abdominal and the thoracic aorta in approximatelly half of the patients (Blockmans et al., 2006). Agard et al. studied 22 patients with computed tomography angiography (CTA) during the first month after GCA diagnosis. Although some of these patients had received treatment at the time of the CTA, the authors demonstrated radiological signs of aortitis in 45% of patients in the thoracic aorta and in 23% in the abdominal aorta. Finally, in a prospective study performed by the authors in 40 newly diagnosed GCA patients using CTA, radiologic findings suggesting aortitis were detected in 65% of patients, which represents the higher prevalence of aortitis found by means of imaging techniques (Cid et al., 2009; Prieto-Gonzalez et al., 2009).

Reference	Specimen	NIA (%)	Gender (M/F)	Age (mean)	LVV	Other diagnosis	Isolated aortitis (%)	Treatment	Follow-up (mo)	New aneurysms
Kerr, 2000	1069 TA and AA	19 (1,7)	7/12	73	19 GCA	-	-	0	12-48	-
Rojo-Leyva, 2000	383 TA 681 AA	52 (4,3)	17/35	63	4 GCA 1 TAK	1 SLE 1 SS, 1 IBD 1 RPF 1 RF 1 GPA 1 PAN	36 (69,2)	11 GC	1-144	6 (untreated)
Gelsomino, 2005	386 TA and aortic valve	NA	1/9	74	10 GCA	-	-	2 GC	-	1 AAA (untreated)
Homme & Miller, 2006	513 TA and aortic valve	45 (8,7)	8/37	64	14 GCA 6 TAK	2 RA 1 rective arthritis	21 (46,6)	19 GC	35-196	7 (3 untreated)
Burke, 2008	NA	52	16/36	58	5 GCA	1 Crohn 1 SLE 1 SNA	44 (84,6)	-	-	-
Pacini, 2008	788 TA	38 (4,8)	14/24	73	30 GCA 1 TAK	1 Behçet 1 SLE	5 (0.6)	0	26-125	1 (AAA)
Nesi, 2009	338 TA	7 (2)	2/5	>65	7 GCA	-	-	-	-	-
Pacini, 2008	788 TA	38 (4,8)	14/24	73	30 GCA 1 TAK	1 Behçet 1 SLE	-	0	26-125	1 (AAA)

AA: abdominal aorta; AAA: abdominal aortic aneurysm; GC: glucocorticoids; GCA: giant-cell arteritis; NIA:non- infectious aortitis; IBD: inflammatory bowel disease; IS: inmunosupressive agents; LVV: large-vessel vasculitis; M/F: male/female; mo: months; PAN: polyarteritis nodosa; SLE: systemic lupus erythematosus; SNA: seronegative arthritis; SS: systemic sclerosis; RA: rheumatoid arthritis; RPF: retroperitoneal fibrosis; RF: rheumatic fever; TA: thoracic aorta;TAK: Takayasu's arteritis; GPA: granulomatosis with polyangiits (Wegener's), NA: no available information.

Table 2. Prevalence of aortitis and associated diseases in surgical specimens.

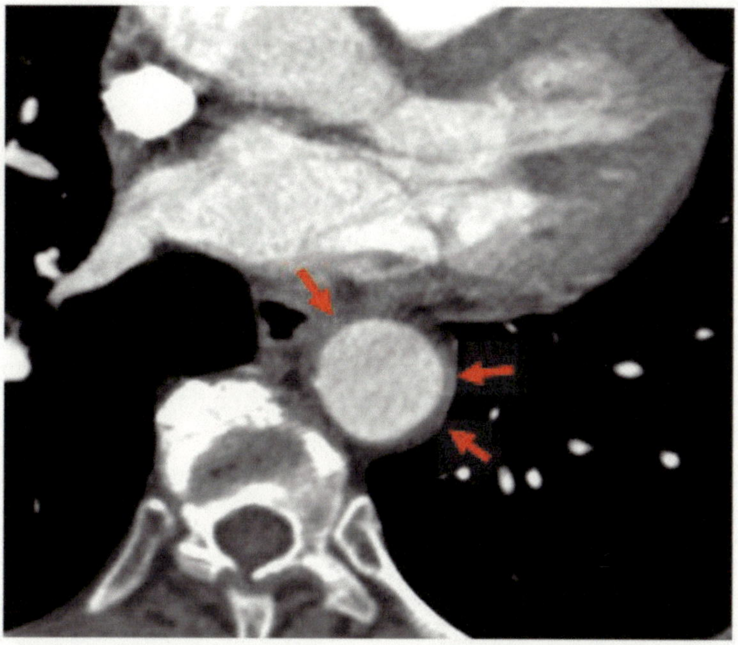

Fig. 1. Cross-sectional view of a CT angiography of a patient with newly diagnosed GCA displaying a marked circumferential thickening of the aortic wall.

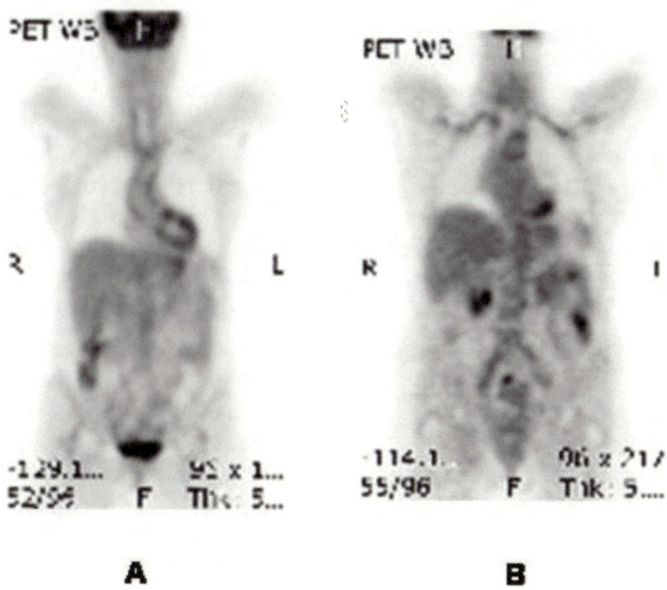

Fig. 2. ^{18}F-FDG-PET scan of a patient with GCA prior to corticosteroid treatment.
(A) Markedly abnormal uptake of ^{18}F-FDG in the ascending thoracic aorta and carotid arteries. (B) Increased ^{18}F-FDG uptake in the aortic arch, abdominal aorta, iliac, subclavian and axillary arteries.

2.1.2 Takayasu's arteritis

TAK is a rare chronic inflammatory granulomatous disease of unknown aetiology that affects predominantly young women. It has a worldwide distribution but higher prevalence has been reported among Asian populations. TAK primarily affects the aorta and its major branches. Pulmonary arteries can also be involved (Kerr et al., 1994; Mwipatayi et al., 2005). Aortitis may affect either an aortic segment or involve the entire aorta. Although there is considerable variability in disease expression between different geographical areas, the initial vascular lesion frequently occurs in the middle or proximal segment of the left subclavian artery close to the aorta. In Japanese patients, aortitis has been described mostly in the ascending aorta and the aortic arch whereas in Indian patients inflammation apparently occurs firstly in the abdominal aorta, subsequently extending towards the thoracic segments. (Hata et al., 1996). Aortic involvement is very common in TAK. In different series of patients with TAK who underwent imaging studies, aortic involvement had been detected in more than 70% of cases.

2.1.3 Isolated aortitis

Vasculitis limited to the aorta has been found in post-mortem studies or has been incidentally diagnosed in specimens obtained from surgical repair of aortic aneurysms. The prevalence of isolated aortitis in the general population is unknown due to the subclinical course of this entity.

In a retrospective review of 1204 aortic surgical specimens obtained over a 20-year period at the Cleveland Clinic, idiopathic aortitis was found in 52 patients (4.3%) (Rojo-Leyva et al., 2000). Sixty-nine percent of these patients had no previous history of systemic vasculitis and only 31% of patients had prior history of systemic illnesses known to be associated with aortitis. Indications for surgery in patients with isolated aortitis consisted of manifestations related to aortic aneurysm (large aneurysm size or progressive enlargement, aortic dissection, or aortic valve dysfunction), or coronary artery disease and only in 1 patient aortitis was detected at the time of thymoma ressection. In 96% of patients with aneurysm formation and idiopathic aortitis, the disease was only identified within the thoracic aorta whereas aortic aneurysms not associated with idiopathic aortitis occurred predominantly in the abdominal aorta (67%).

In another recent retrospective study, noninfectious aortitis was detected in 64 patients of a series of 766 patients with ascending thoracic aneurysm who underwent surgical repair, representing 8.4% of the series. The majority of patients were asymptomatic or had aneurysm-related symptoms only, being aneurysm incidentally discovered in a chest x-ray or echocardiography. The majority of aortitis (81.3%) were of the isolated variant, with no history of chronic inflammatory diseases. Among the remaining, GCA was the entity more frequently associated with aortitis. Eighty-nine percent of patients with noninfectious aortitis (57/64) underwent vascular imaging, and additional vascular abnormalities were present in 72% of them. Additional imaging findings included stenoses and/or ectasia of the major aortic branches (42.1%), descending thoracic aneurysm (31.6%), descending thoracic and abdominal aneurysms (21.1%), and abdominal aneurysms (7%). The median follow up in this study was 15.4 months, which was insufficient to determine the outcome of these additional vascular abnormalities (Liang et al., 2009). Data from these and other surgical series are summarized in table 2.

Therefore, in the majority but not all patients with apparently isolated aortitis, a more widespread involvement indicating systemic large-vessel vasculitis or an associated condition can be detected. Existing studies assessing potentially associated diseases in these patients are retrospective and almost certainly underestimate the prevalence of pre-existing conditions because many patients with incidentally discovered aortitis had not been systematically subjected to an extensive clinical evaluation or imaging study.

2.1.4 ANCA-associated vasculitis

Large-vessel involvement and associated complications such as aortic stenoses, aneurysm, or dissection have been occasionally reported in patients with small-medium sized vessels such as ANCA- associated vasculitis, particularly granulomatosis with polyangiitis (Wegener's) (GPA). Reported cases, have well-sustained diagnosis and have no epidemiologic, clinical or histopathologic features of GCA or TAK that might suggest misclassification (Chirinos et al., 2004). These findings suggest that aortitis may be part of the spectrum of vascular involvement in ANCA-associated vasculitis.

2.1.5 Chronic periaortitis

Chronic periaortitis includes several modalities of aortic inflammatory involvement including retroperitoneal fibrosis, inflammatory aortic aneurysm and perianeurysmal retroperitoneal fibrosis. The last two conditions convey aortic dilatation. The abdominal aorta is most frequently involved. Retroperitoneal fibrosis is idiopathic in most cases but may occur in the context of small and medium sized vessel vasculitis, particularly GPA. It has also been described in association with microscopic poliangiitis and its renal limited variant, and hepatitis C virus-associated cryoglobulinemia. Idiopathic retroperitoneal fibrosis may accompany other autoimmune diseases such as rheumatoid arthritis, systemic lupus erythematosus, autoimmune thyroiditis) or may be part of other fibrosing disorders including orbital pseudotumor, mediastinal fibrosis, sclerosing cholangitis, and Riedel's thyroiditis. Histopathologically there is a marked aortic adventitial inflammation with inflammatory involvement of vasa vasorum extending towards the retroperitoneal small vessels and retroperitoneum itself. Inflammatory changes are thought to trigger a fibrotic response of variable intensity (Vaglio et al., 2003; Levine et al., 2006).

2.2 Clinical manifestations derived from aortitis

Aortic inflammation is usually asymptomatic until complications derived from inflammation -induced vascular remodelling occur. Clinical manifestations are dominated by other components of the associated disease. In patients with GCA cranial, systemic and polymyalgic symptoms dominate the clinical picture. TAK disease is usually more silent and indolent and initial manifestations are frequently derived from involvement of the aortic branches (vascular bruits, weak or absent pulses, limb claudication, hypertension, dizziness or light-headedness) (Kerr GS et al., 1994; Macsimowicz-Mckinnon et al., 2007). Aortitis may contribute to the inflammation-associated non-specific signs and symptoms such as fever, anemia, weigh loss or malaise highly frequent in GCA and also present in a substantial proportion of TAK patients. Complications derived from aortitis are usually manifest and patients may present with severe symptoms related to aortic aneurysm enlargement or rupture (i.e. chest pain, abdominal pain, back pain) or aortic valve insufficiency (i.e. dyspnea and heart failure,) (Garcia-Martinez et al., 2008; Nuenninghoff et al., 2003a; Nuenninghoff et al., 2003b).

2.3 Histopathological features

Aortitis is characterized by patchy areas of medial necrosis and focal loss of medial smooth muscle cells, along with adjacent infiltration of lymphocytes, plasma cells, and histiocytes. Multinucleated giant cells, if present, are generally found at the borders of necrotic zones. The aorta of TAK patients may show thickening of the aortic wall with fibrotic rindlike adventitia, and intense medial and adventitial inflammation with granulomas. It can be indistinghishable from aortitis found in GCA. In general, histological features of non-infectious aortitis are similar and there are no specific features helpful in distinguishing isolated aortitis from GCA or TAK (Kerr et al., 2000; Miller et al., 2006; Gravanis, 2000; Hall et al., 1985; miller et al., 2006).

2.4 Diagnosis and assessment of aortic inflammation

In GCA, diagnosis is usually obtained by temporal artery biopsy. The detection of aortitis may have diagnostic usefulness in patients with suspected GCA when temporal artery biopsy is not informative or is unavailable. In TAK, the diagnosis is largely based on the combination of clinical information, laboratory evaluation, and diagnostic imaging (Mukhtyar et al., 2009). Imaging is an essential tool for the diagnosis of TAK because the involved vessels are not routinely available for histopathologic examination and in both conditions imaging techniques play a critical role in evidencing aortitis. Among imaging modalities, percutaneous intravascular angiography has been traditionally the gold standard investigation for the diagnosis of TAK, providing high-quality images of the arterial lumen frequently altered in involved vessels. Typical lesions appear as long, smooth, tapered stenoses or sometimes complete occlusions intermingled with areas of dilatation. Collateral circulation is often prominent because of the slow progression of the disease. Modern non-invasive diagnostic modalities including ultrasonography, PET-scan, computed tomography scanning and magnetic resonance angiography have progressively replaced conventional angiography for diagnosis of large vessel involvement because of their reduced risks and the ability to provide information not only about the lumen but also about the vessel wall. Specific MRI sequences such as delayed contrast-enhanced MRI may allow the detection of edema and arterial wall thickening at a reversible stage, prior to the development of luminal stenosis. MRI/MRA may provide useful information avoiding the risks associated with arterial puncture, iodinated contrast load and radiation exposure. Currently, conventional angiography is basically used to guide endovascular intervention procedures or to combine imaging with the detection of central blood pressure in patients with significant limb artery stenoses.

Systematic evaluation of patients with large-vessel vasculitis with imaging studies such as color duplex ultrasonography (US), CTA, FDG-PET, angiography, and magnetic resonance imaging (MRI) or MR angiography (MRA) has been performed by several investigators (Agard et al., 2008; Andrews et al., 2004; Andrews & Mason, 2007; Blockmans et al., 2008; Blockmans et al., 2009; Both et al., 2008; Hautzel et al., 2008; Henes et al., 2008; Narvaez et al., 2005; Pipitone et al., 2008; Prieto-Gonzalez et al., 2009; Walter et al., 2005; Webb & Al-Nahhas 2006). These techniques offer different but complementary information to assess large vessel involvement with relative advantages and disadvantages which are summarized in Table 3 (Tso E et al., 2002; Blockmans et al., 2009; Cid et al., 2009;).

Technique	Findings	Advantages	Disadvantges
Color Dupplex US	Wall thickening Hipoechoic halo Reduced pulsation Stenoses/occlusions /dilatations Lumen patency assessment	Inexpensive Repeatable No radiation No IV contrast needed Communication with the patient during the procedure Good resolution for small arteries	Not suitable for structures below air or bone
MRI/MRA	Wall thickening Contrast enhancement Stenosis/occlusions /dilatations Lumen patency assessment	No radiation Repeatable	Expensive Not suitable for patients with claustrophhobia No feasible with metal devices Limited resolution for small vessels Gadolinium contrast contraindicated if impaired renal function
CTA	Wall thickening Contrast enhancement Stenosis/occlusions /dilatations Lumen patency assessment	Rapid and available Inexpensive Repeatable	Contraindicated if renal insufficiency or iodine allergy Radiation exposure
FDG-PET	FDG uptake by metabolically active cells such as inflammatory infiltrate	Repeatable Whole body assessment	Expensive Not widely available No lumen patency assessment No resolution for vessels < 4 mm Setting and results not standardized Requires normal blood glucose concentration Not suitable for cranial arteries due to strong cerebral uptake
Angiography	Lumen patency assessment (smooth, long and tapered stenoses or occlusions)	Therapeutic procedures (angioplasty and/or stent placement) High resolution for small vessels Central blood pressure detection	Invasive Radiation Contraindicated if renal insufficiency or iodine allergy No information about the vessel wall

Table 3. Imaging techniques applied to assess large-vessel vasculitis

3. Aortic complications in patients with large-vessel vasculitis

Aortitis may eventually lead to aortic complications in patients with large-vessel vasculitis. After the initial inflammatory injury, abnormal vascular remodelling may eventually cause aortic structural damage and clinical complications such as aortic aneurysm, dissection, or aortic valve insufficiency secondary to aortic root dilatation (Salvarani et al., 2008). Patients with GCA tend to develop complications derived from aortic dilatation or dissection whereas patients with TAK more commonly develop aortic stenosis but may also develop dilatation of the ascending aorta and aortic valve insufficiency.

3.1 Aortic complications in patients with GCA

GCA patients are at an increased risk of developing aortic complications. In a retrospective population-based study, GCA patients were 17.3 times more likely to develop thoracic aortic aneurysms and 2.4 times more likely to develop abdominal aortic aneurysms during follow-up than individuals of the same age from the general population (Evans et al., 1995). The prevalence of aortic complications during follow-up ranged from 9.5 to 18% in three series of patients with GCA (Evans et al., 1995; González-Gay et al., 2004; Nuenninghoff et al., 2003a). Table 4 summarizes the main results of these studies.

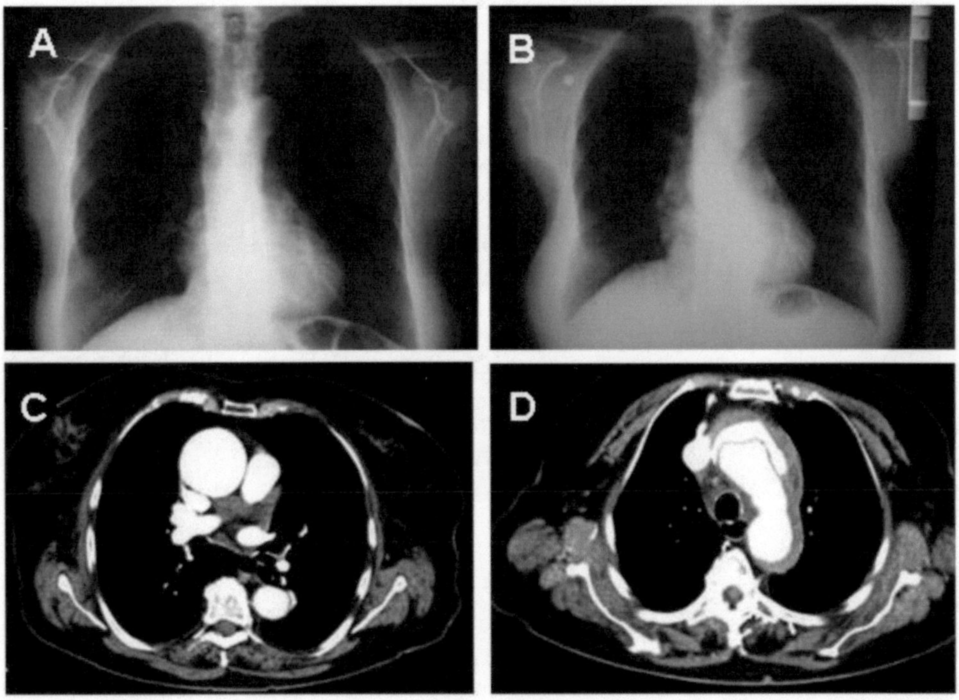

Fig. 3. (A) Chest x-ray of a 68 -years old woman at the time of GCA diagnosis. (B) Four years later the chest radiograph of the same patient showed mediastinum broadening and aortic aneurysm was confirmed by CT-scan. (C) CT scan of another patient wit GCA demonstrating an aneurysm with a maximum diameter of 5 cm at the ascending thoracic aorta. (D) Aortic dissection at the ascending aortic segment in a patient with GCA presenting with chest pain.

	Evans (n=96)	Nuenninghoff (n=168)	González-Gay (n=210)	García-Martínez (n=54)
Design of the study	Retrospective	Retrospective	Retrospective	Prospective cross-sectional evaluation
GCA diagnosis	1950-1985	1950-1999	1981-2001	1995-2001
Follow-up	8.6 yr (1 mo – 28 yr)	7.6 yr (3.9 – 13.5)	Not recorded	5.4 yr (4-10.5)
Aortic complications	16 (16.6%)	30 (18%)	20 (9.5%)	12 (22.2%)
Type of aortic complication	2 TAD at GCA diagnosis 9 TAA 5 AAA	18 TAA 16 AAA	16 TAA 6 AAA	11 thoracic dilatation/aneurysm 1 AAA
Time of complication discovery after GCA diagnosis	TAA: 5.75 yr (2.5 mo-20 yr) AAA: 2.5 yr (1.3-7.6)	TAA: 10.9 yr (4.5-13.3) TAD: 1.1 yr (0.2-2.1) AAA: 6.3 yr (1.1-13.3) AAD: 7.6 yr	3.2 yr (0-13.5)	5.4 yr (4-10.5)
Histophatologic aortitis	4 / 6	5 / 7 in TA 0 / 1 in AA	Not recorded	0/2 (*)
CS treatment	1 yr (< 1 mo-4.2 yr)	Not recorded	Not recorded	Patients were treated uniformly and those with ASD were able to withdraw CS in a shorter period of time

TAA: thoracic aortic aneurysm; TAD: thoracic aortic dissection; AAA: abdominal aortic aneurysm; AAD: abdominal aortic dissection; CAD: coronary artery disease; yr: years; mo: months;.
ASD: aortic structural damage (aneurysm or dilatation)
(*) Only scattered small infiltrates were observed.

Table 4. Studies evaluating aortic complications in patients with GCA

Overall, these studies suggest that aortic aneurysms are late complications, usually detected several years after the diagnosis of GCA, even in patients that have achieved sustained remission and have been able to withdraw corticosteroid therapy. Only 10% of patients with GCA evaluated by CT angiography imaging exhibit slight dilatation of the aortic wall at the time of diagnosis (Prieto-Gonzalez et al., 2009). Apparently, aortic dissection may occur in earlier phases even in the absence of aortic aneurysmal disease and sometimes represents the initial event leading to the diagnosis of GCA. In this setting, aortic dissection may occur in patients with active inflammation which is demonstrated by histopathologic examination of the aortic specimen obtained after surgical repair or necropsy (Lie, 1995; Nuenninghoff et al., 2003a). Although the entire aorta may be involved, aneurysms and dissections preferentially develop in the thoracic segments, mainly the ascending aorta. Although survival rates are not decreased in patients with GCA, the development of aortic rupture is a catastrophic event that carries high morbidity and mortality (Evans et al., 1995; Nuenninghoff et al., 2003a).

In a prospective cross-sectional analysis of 54 GCA patients who were screened with a defined protocol after a median follow-up of 5.4 years (range 4-10.5 years), García-Martínez A et al found significant aortic structural damage (aneurysm or dilatation) in 22% of patients which was higher than the prevalence observed in previous retrospective studies (García-Martínez et al., 2008). Almost half of the patients in this cohort were candidates to surgical repair because of the size of the aneurysm. The ascending aorta was the segment involved in three quarters of patients. Aortic structural damage was significantly more frequent in men and was not associated with the presence of traditional cardiovascular risk factors. When these patients were re-screened after longer follow-up (median 8.8 years, range 8-10.5) additional aortic aneurysms appeared in few additional patients who had non-dilated aortas in the initial study and one of them developed aortic dissection. Histopathological study of the aorta of this patient did not evidence persistence of active aortic inflammation but there was marked loss and disruption of elastic lamelae.

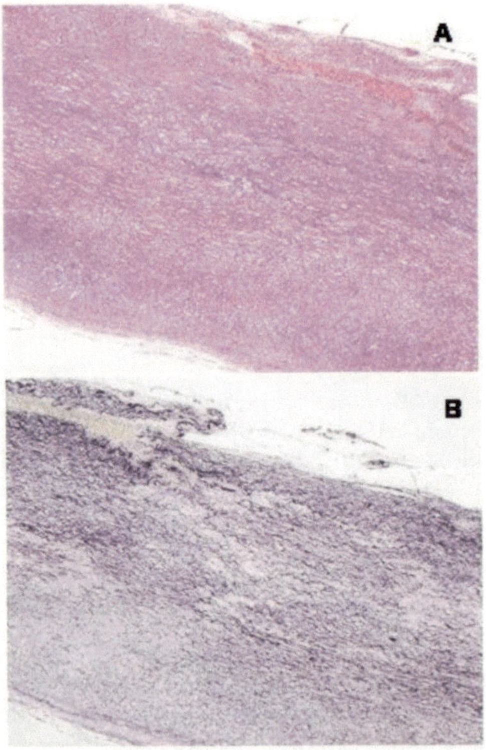

Fig. 4. Post-mortem aortic specimen obtained from a patient who died from aortic dissection 9 years after the diagnosis of GCA. A) Hematoxylin-eosin staining showing absence of inflammation. B) Orcein staining of a serial section disclosing extensive disruption of the elastic fibres, probably due to the initial injury.

Persistence of inflammatory infiltrates has been described in some aortic specimens obtained from necropsies or from patients with aortic aneurysm that have undergone surgery years after the diagnosis of GCA (Evans et al., 1995; Lie, 1995; Nuenninghoff et al., 2003a; Zehr et al., 2005). As a result of these findings, aortic complications are considered to be the result of persistent aortic inflammation and the ensuing weakening of the aortic wall. However, in a prospective cross-sectional evaluation, persistence of clinically or analytically detectable disease activity was not found to be associated with increased risk of aortic structural damage (García-Martínez A et al 2008). Patients with aortic dilatation experienced less relapses during follow-up, had lower corticosteroid requirements and exhibited lower acute-phase reactants than patients without aortic aneurysm or dilatation. Histopathological review of the aortic wall in patients who underwent surgery for aneurysm repair evidenced only minimal inflammatory infiltrates but important loss and disruption of elastic lamellae even in areas devoid of inflammation, probably as a consequence of the initial injury (Figure 4). The aneurysmal aortic wall exhibited increased expression of matrix metalloproteinase (MMP)-2 but not MMP-9 which suggests ongoing remodelling process more than persistent aortic inflammation (García-Martínez et al., 2008). Thus, aortic dilatation develops as a consequence of complex and probably multifactorial mechanisms. On the basis of these studies it is likely that aortic inflammation and subsequent maladaptative remodelling determine the weakening of the aortic wall, which subjected to mechanical stress, may eventually undergo dilatation and aneurysm formation over time.

The life-threatening nature of the potential complications derived from aortic structural damage makes mandatory to subject GCA patients to a continuous surveillance by clinical examination and imaging, even patients in long-term sustained remission. The best cost-benefit screening procedure has not been established but a reasonable approach would include performance of a chest X-ray and abdominal US examination every one or two years and echocardiogram if aortic bruits are detected.

3.2 Aortic complications in patients with Takayasu's arteritis

As the disease progresses abnormal vascular remodelling leads to the combination of arterial stenosis/occlusion with arterial aneurysms. However, while stenotic lesions appear in almost all patients with TA only 27% of patients develop arterial aneurysms (Kerr GS et al., 1994). Symptoms derived from involvement of the aortic branches, usually dominate the clinical picture and may combine with symptoms derived form aortic involvement. Patients may experience symptoms due to vertebrobasilar insufficiency (vertigo, syncope), upper- and lower-extremity claudication, transient ischemic attacks or stroke, coronary heart disease, or mesenteric ischemia, among others.

In the aorta stenoses/occlusions are mainly located at the aortic arch, the descending aorta and the abdominal aorta, and aortic aneurysms preferentially develop at the ascending thoracic aorta (Kerr et al., 1994; Mwipatayi, 2005). More than 70% of patients develop hypertension, mainly of renovascular origin but aortic stenosis leading to atypical aortic coarctation may also contribute. Blood pressure treatment and control may be a serious problem in these patients since arm blood pressure measurement may not be accurate. TAK patients may also develop aortic dilatation or aneurysm with risk of rupture. Aortic valve incompetence has been reported in up to one quarter of patients and is generally due to annular or ascending aortic dilatation but also as a result of secondary aortic valve changes such as fibrous thickening, retraction, and calcification. Congestive heart failure is present in up to one fourth of patients who have TAK and usually occurs as a consequence of uncontrolled hypertension or aortic regurgitation (Kerr et al. 1994; Macksimowicz-Mckinnon et al. 2007).

4. Treatment of aortitis and aortic complications

Treatment of primary large vessel vasculitis is addressed to eliminate clinical symptoms and suppress inflammatory activity wherever it is present, including the aorta and its branches. However current therapies are not able to completely abrogate inflammation in most cases and are not able to prevent complications derived from inflammation-induced vascular remodelling which may need to be addressed with surgery or revascularization procedures. High dose glucocorticoids are the mainstay of initial therapy to induce remission in large-vessel vasculitis which must be combined with immunosuppressive agents in the majority of patients with TAK.

4.1 Giant-cell arteritis

Prednisone or equivalent is usually given to patients with GCA at 1 mg/Kg/day, up to 60 mg/day for 1 month with subsequent tapering. Low-dose prednisone is maintained for 2-3 years until complete discontinuation which is achieved by approximately half of the patients. Between 40-60% of patients experience a relapsing course. Methotrexate and azathioprine have shown modest corticosteroid sparing effects in clinical trials (Mahr et al. 2007; Hoffman et al. 2002; Cid et al., 2007) and can be used to reduce glucocorticoid exposure in patients with relapsing outcome or with glucocorticoid-related side effects (Mukhtyar et al., 2009). A randomized clinical trial did not show benefit of infliximab over placebo in maintaining remission in patients with newly-diagnosed GCA (Hoffman et al.,2007). Glucocorticoid treatment is usually adjusted according to remission of cranial, systemic or polymyalgic symptoms and normalization of acute phase reactants. Response of aortic inflammation has not been taken into account because the substantial prevalence of aortitis and its potential delayed complications has not been appreciated until very recently. Imaging techniques may have promise in assessing the effect of treatment on large-vessel inflammation but their sensitivity and specificity are not fully established and, at present, it is premature to adapt therapeutic adjustments to the persistence or resolution of imaging abnormalities.

Since the discovery that aortitis and aortic complications are frequent in GCA is relatively recent, there is no evidence supporting whether the discovery of aortic dilatation may have therapeutic implications. It is not clear whether aortic dilatation results from persistent subclinical inflammation, previous injury, abnormal remodelling, hemodynamic factors or a combination of these. Surgical aortic repair in GCA patients should be performed according to standard current guidelines for the general population with aortic disease and preferably in patients in remission (Zehr et al. 2005). Since GCA targets aged people, advanced age or co-morbidities may unacceptably increase the risk of elective surgery and convenience of surgical repair must be carefully weighted in an individual basis. Endovascular repair of aortic aneurysm may be an interesting option but the experience is limited. Moreover, most of the existing evidence regarding endovascular repair of aortic aneurysm has been obtained from abdominal and thoracic descending aneurysms. Endovascular repair of ascending aortic dilatation, common in GCA, is technically more difficult (The United Kingdom EVAR trial investigators, 2010a; The United Kingdom EVAR trial investigators, 2010b; Kolvenbach et al., 2011).

4.2 Takayasu arteritis

For TAK patients, an initial prednisone dose of 1 mg/Kg/day (max 60 mg/day) maintained for 1 month and gradually tapered is recommended. With this treatment, 93% of patients achieve disease remission. However, remission is sustained in only 20% of patients. More than 70% of patients need adjuvant therapy and long-term low-dose glucocorticoid is frequently required by most patients. Recommendations about immunosuppressive agents are based on open-label studies. Methotrexate, azathioprine and mycophenolate are the most frequently used. Open-label studies support the potential usefulness of infliximab for refractory patients (Mukhtyar et al., 2009; Molloy et al., 2008)

TAK is a chronic relapsing disease and flares and anatomic progression of vascular lesions occur in the majority of patients during follow-up.

One of the challenges in TAK is to find better surrogate markers of disease activity and ongoing inflammation. Clinical data are often non-specific and acute-phase reactants may be unreliable indicators. Previous studies of patients undergoing periodic imaging surveillance showed inconsistencies in the relationship between acute-phase reactants and the development of new vascular lesions during follow-up. In a review of patients with clinically inactive disease, new angiographic changes appeared in 60% of them and surgical aortic biopsy specimens revealed histological evidence of persistent inflammatory infiltrates in 44% of the samples (Kerr et al., 1994).

Serial imaging has been used for long in the follow-up of patients with TAK since symptoms usually occur when severe disruption of the normal vascular architecture has occurred. Serial imaging is very useful in detecting new lesions or changes in the existing ones and allows an objective assessment of disease stability or progression. MRI angiography may reveal early signs of vascular inflammation in patients with TAK and is currently being evaluated as a potential tool to assess disease activity and response to treatment in prospective clinical studies (Andrews & Mason 2007). However, qualitative changes suggestive of active disease versus fibrotic scarring do not always accurately predict response to therapy. (Tso et al., 2002) .

Vascular remodelling and scarring may lead to fixed vascular lesions that will not be reversed by pharmacologic therapy. Revascularization or surgical repair should be considered if stenotic or occlusive lesions lead to significant haemodynamic effects with ischemic symptoms, or if aneurysmal enlargement results in increased risk of rupture, dissection or in case of aortic valve regurgitation (Mukhtyar et al., 2009).

For correction of stenoses and occlusions of the aorta and its branches the largest body of experience comes from bypass graft procedures where good long-term outcomes have been achieved. On average, a 20 to 30% rate of restenosis or occlusion is reported on long-term follow-up. Revascularization can also be achieved by percutaneous transluminal angioplasty (PTA). PTA is less invasive than vascular surgery and is currently the revascularization procedure of choice. Angioplasty is usually successful but the rate of restenosis during follow-up is higher than with vascular surgery. Endovascular angioplasty has shown better outcomes for lesions that are short and not already occluded. To prevent restenosis, stents are currently used although conventional stents have been associated with high rates of failure in long-term follow-up studies. The long-term impact of angioplasty in patients with TAK is still uncertain because there have been no reports describing the outcome of angioplasty with or without stenting after periods longer than 10 years. Encouraging results have been reported with the use of drug-eluting stents in atheromatous vascular disease. Their benefit in the treatment of patients with TAK needs to be determined (Liang et al., 2009).

In patients with hypertension, anatomical correction of lesions such as renal artery or aortic stenosis should also be performed. When needed, the most common procedure to repair aortic stenosis has been an aortoaortic bypass with the use of a prosthetic graft. Angioplasty with or without stenting may also be of use to treat discrete stenosis of the aorta. Aortic aneurysm should be repaired according to the current guidelines for general population. Aortic valve incompetence with aortic ring expansion may necessitate root and aortic valve replacement or valvuloplasty. Complex vascular reconstructions (i.e. complete aortic arch replacement) may be need by patients with multiple stenosis.

Patients with TAK have lower rates of sustained vessel patency for angioplasty and arterial bypass procedures than patients undergoing intervention for atherosclerosis or other vascular diseases. Failure has been associated with the presence of active disease at the time of surgery. Thus, in order to improve the life-span of the revascularized vessel and minimize the risk of surgical dehiscence, interventions should ideally be performed during inactive disease. However, when an earlier surgical intervention is mandatory it can also be successfully accomplished during the acute stage. In this scenario, treatment with steroids and/or immunosuppressive agents should be continued after surgery. Some authors recommend to carefully select the anastomotic site excluding inflamed vascular areas in order to avoid occlusion of the reconstructed vessel, anastomotic disruption or aneurysm development at the site of anastomosis (Ogino et al., 2008).

Recent advances in immunosuppressive and surgical therapies, including endovascular interventions, have improved the outcome of patients with TAK. However, longer follow-up studies are still necessary to get statistically valid conclusions about the impact of these therapies on the natural history of TAK. In addition, patients with TAK may develop accelerated atherosclerosis as a consequence of systemic chronic inflammation and long-term hypertension. Therefore, in order to improve the long-term outcome of these patients, a careful control of traditional vascular risk factors is crucial to prevent the potential vascular complications associated with atherosclerosis.

4.3 Isolated aortitis

Patients with incidentally discovered noninfectious aortitis should be evaluated for additional areas of arterial disease and for signs and symptoms of systemic inflammatory conditions potentially associated with aortitis. The evaluation should include a full patient interview, a complete physical examination with particular focus on the vascular system, and appropriate laboratory testing including acute phase reactants. Imaging of the entire aorta and its main branches with MRI or CTA to exclude abnormalities in other vascular beds should be considered.

It is not clear at present whether patients with incidentally discovered aortitis in whom a systemic vasculitis or systemic disease has been reasonably ruled out should receive therapy with glucocorticoids and/or immunosuppressants following resection of the affected aortic segment. Data from retrospective studies indicate that the longterm outcome of patients with isolated aortitis is generally good. However, in a retrospective study performed at the Cleveland Clinic in which 36 out of the 52 patients with idiopathic aortitis were followed for a mean of 3.25 years, 6 out of the 25 patients not receiving therapy after the initial surgery developed new aortic aneurysm during follow-up. Conversely, recurrent aneurysms were not identified among 11 corticosteroid-treated patients, in spite that treatment schedule was not standardized and some patients received very short courses of corticosteroids (Rojo-Leyva F., et al 2008).

Therefore, the decision to treat with glucocorticoids or immunosuppressive agents should be individually considered, depending on the clinical presentation and the location and extent of inflammation. Patients with idiopathic aortitis require careful and periodic surveillance during follow-up because small case series have identified a propensity toward aneurysm formation in other vascular beds over time. Prospective follow-up studies of patients with isolated aortitis are required to further clarify this point.

5. Conclusions

Over the past decade, the improvement and wider use of imaging techniques has motivated an increasing appreciation of the relevance of aortic involvement in systemic vasculitis and its potential for severe complications. Persistent aortitis observed in some patients by means of imaging or histopathologic examination questions the ability of current therapies to completely suppress the inflammatory process in spite of the clinical remission of the initial symptoms. It remains to be determined whether patients with asymptomatic persistent signs of aortitis would benefit form more intensive therapy since recent data suggest that persistent low-grade subclinical inflammatory activity is not clearly associated with higher frequency of aortic complications. On the other hand, mechanisms involved in aortic dilatation are not completely understood. It is unclear at present whether aortic dilatation results from persistent subclinical activity, abnormal vascular remodelling following the initial injury, hemodynamic influences or a combination of factors. The indication and best method for elective repair of aortic dilatation or stenosis need to be delimitated. Awareness of aortic participation in systemic vasculitis raises a number of important questions and opens an exciting research agenda for coming years that will definitely benefit from multicenter collaboration

6. References

Agard, C., J. H. Barrier, B. Dupas, T. Ponge, A. Mahr, G. Fradet, P. Chevalet et al. 2008. Aortic involvement in recent-onset giant cell (temporal) arteritis: a case-control prospective study using helical aortic computed tomodensitometric scan. *Arthritis Rheum.* 59, no. 5:670-676.

Andrews, J., A. Al-Nahhas, D. J. Pennell, M. S. Hossain, K. A. Davies, D. O. Haskard, and J. C. Mason. 2004. Non-invasive imaging in the diagnosis and management of Takayasu's arteritis. *Ann.Rheum.Dis.* 63, no. 8:995-1000.

Andrews, J. and J. C. Mason. 2007. Takayasu's arteritis--recent advances in imaging offer promise. *Rheumatology.(Oxford).* 46, no. 1:6-15.

Blockmans, D., T. Bley, and W. Schmidt. 2009. Imaging for large-vessel vasculitis. *Curr.Opin.Rheumatol.* 21, no. 1:19-28.

Blockmans, D., W. Coudyzer, S. Vanderschueren, S. Stroobants, D. Loeckx, S. Heye, Ceuninck L. De, G. Marchal, and H. Bobbaers. 2008. Relationship between fluorodeoxyglucose uptake in the large vessels and late aortic diameter in giant cell arteritis. *Rheumatology.(Oxford).* 47, no. 8:1179-1184.

Blockmans, D., Ceuninck L. De, S. Vanderschueren, D. Knockaert, L. Mortelmans, and H. Bobbaers. 2006. Repetitive 18F-fluorodeoxyglucose positron emission tomography in giant cell arteritis: a prospective study of 35 patients. *Arthritis Rheum.* 55, no. 1:131-137.

Bonnin, J.M. and Lander, H. 1956. Giant-cell arteritis; report of a case with autopsy. *J.Pathol.Bacteriol.* 71, no. 2:369-373.

Both, M., K. hmadi-Simab, M. Reuter, O. Dourvos, E. Fritzer, S. Ullrich, W. L. Gross, M. Heller, and M. Bahre. 2008. MRI and FDG-PET in the assessment of inflammatory aortic arch syndrome in complicated courses of giant cell arteritis. *Ann.Rheum.Dis.* 67, no. 7:1030-1033.

Burke, A. P., F. Tavora, N. Narula, J. E. Tomaszewski, and R. Virmani. 2008. Aortitis and ascending aortic aneurysm: description of 52 cases and proposal of a histologic classification. *Hum.Pathol.* 39, no. 4:514-526.

Cardell, B.S. and T. Hanley. 1951. A fatal case of giant-cell or temporal arteritis. *J.Pathol.Bacteriol.* 63, no. 4:587-597.

Chirinos, J. A., L. J. Tamariz, and D. L. Lichtstein. 2004. Large vessel compromise in antineutrophil cytoplasmic antibody-associated systemic vasculitis: comment on the article by Booth et al. *Arthritis Rheum.* 50, no. 10:3398-3399.

Cid, M.C., García-Martínez A, Lozano E, Espígol-frigolé G, Hernández-Rodriguez J. Five clinical conundrums in the management of giant-cell arteritis. 2007. *Rheum. Clin. Dis. North. Am.* ; 33: 819-834.

Cid, M. C., S. Prieto-Gonzalez, P. Arguis, G. Espigol-Frigole, M. Butjosa, J. Hernandez-Rodriguez, M. Segarra, E. Lozano, and A. Garcia-Martinez. 2009. The spectrum of vascular involvement in giant-cell arteritis: clinical consequences of detrimental vascular remodelling at different sites. *APMIS Suppl.*, no. 127:10-20.

Cooke, W.T., Cloake, P.C.P., Govan , A.D.T., Colbeck, J.C. 1946. Temporal arteritis; a generalized vascular disease. *Q.J.Med.* 15:47-75.:47-75.

Domenech, E., E. Garcia-Planella, A. Olazabal, J. Sanchez-Delgado, Y. Zabana, I. Bernal, M. Manosa, A. Olive, and M. A. Gassull. 2005. Abdominal aortitis associated with Crohn's disease. *Dig.Dis.Sci.* 50, no. 6:1122-1123.

Evans, J. M., W. M. O'Fallon, and G. G. Hunder. 1995. Increased incidence of aortic aneurysm and dissection in giant cell (temporal) arteritis. A population-based study. *Ann.Intern.Med.* 122, no. 7:502-507.

Garcia-Martinez, A., J. Hernandez-Rodriguez, P. Arguis, P. Paredes, M. Segarra, E. Lozano, C. Nicolau et al. 2008. Development of aortic aneurysm/dilatation during the followup of patients with giant cell arteritis: a cross-sectional screening of fifty-four prospectively followed patients. *Arthritis Rheum.* 59, no. 3:422-430.

Gelsomino, S., S. Romagnoli, F. Gori, G. Nesi, C. Anichini, C. Sorbara, P. Stefano, and G. F. Gensini. 2005. Annuloaortic ectasia and giant cell arteritis. *Ann.Thorac.Surg.* 80, no. 1:101-105.

Gluth, M. B., K. H. Baratz, E. L. Matteson, and C. L. Driscoll. 2006. Cogan syndrome: a retrospective review of 60 patients throughout a half century. *Mayo Clin.Proc.* 81, no. 4:483-488.

Gonzalez-Gay, M. A., C. Garcia-Porrua, A. Pineiro, R. Pego-Reigosa, J. Llorca, and G. G. Hunder. 2004. Aortic aneurysm and dissection in patients with biopsy-proven giant cell arteritis from northwestern Spain: a population-based study. *Medicine (Baltimore)* 83, no. 6:335-341.

Gornik, H. L. and M. A. Creager. 2008. Aortitis. *Circulation.* 117, no. 23:3039-3051.

Gravanis, M. B. 2000. Giant cell arteritis and Takayasu aortitis: morphologic, pathogenetic and etiologic factors. *Int.J.Cardiol.* 75 Suppl 1:S21-33; discussion S35-6.:S21-S33.

Hall, S., W. Barr, J. T. Lie, A. W. Stanson, F. J. Kazmier, and G. G. Hunder. 1985. Takayasu arteritis. A study of 32 North American patients. *Medicine (Baltimore).* 64, no. 2:89-99.

Hata, A., M. Noda, R. Moriwaki, and F. Numano. 1996. Angiographic findings of Takayasu arteritis: new classification. *Int.J.Cardiol.* 54 Suppl:S155-S163.

Hautzel, H., O. Sander, A. Heinzel, M. Schneider, and H. W. Muller. 2008. Assessment of large-vessel involvement in giant cell arteritis with 18F-FDG PET: introducing an ROC-analysis-based cutoff ratio. *J.Nucl.Med.* 49, no. 7:1107-1113.

Henes, J. C., M. Muller, J. Krieger, B. Balletshofer, A. C. Pfannenberg, L. Kanz, and I. Kotter. 2008. [18F] FDG-PET/CT as a new and sensitive imaging method for the diagnosis of large vessel vasculitis. *Clin.Exp.Rheumatol.* 26, no. 3 Suppl 49:S47-S52.

Heptinstall, R.H., K.A. Porter, and H. Barkley. 1954. Giant-cell (temporal) arteritis. *J.Pathol.Bacteriol.* 67, no. 2:507-519.

Hoffman G.S., Cid M.C., Hellmann D.B., Guillevin L., Stone J.H., Schousboe J. et al. A multicenter, randomized, double-blind, placebo-controlled trial of adjuvant methotrexate treatment for giant cell arteritis. Arthritis.Rheum.2002;46:1309-1318

Hoffman, G.S., Cid, M.C., Rendt-Zagar, K.E., Merkel, P.A., Weyand, C.M., Stone, J.H., et al.2007. Infliximab for maintenance of glucocorticosteroid-induced remission of giant cell arteritis: a randomized trial. *Ann Intern Med*;146:621–30.

Homme, J. L., M. C. Aubry, W. D. Edwards, S. M. Bagniewski, Pankratz Shane, V, C. A. Kral, and H. D. Tazelaar. 2006. Surgical pathology of the ascending aorta: a clinicopathologic study of 513 cases. *Am.J.Surg.Pathol.* 30, no. 9:1159-1168.

Hunder, G. G. 2006. The early history of giant cell arteritis and polymyalgia rheumatica: first descriptions to 1970. *Mayo Clin.Proc.* 81, no. 8:1071-1083.

Kerr, G. S., C. W. Hallahan, J. Giordano, R. Y. Leavitt, A. S. Fauci, M. Rottem, and G. S. Hoffman. 1994. Takayasu arteritis. *Ann.Intern.Med.* 120, no. 11:919-929.

Kerr, L. D., Y. J. Chang, H. Spiera, and J. T. Fallon. 2000. Occult active giant cell aortitis necessitating surgical repair. *J.Thorac.Cardiovasc.Surg.* 120, no. 4:813-815.

Kolvenback , R.R., Karmeli, R., Pinter, L.S., Zhu, Y., Lin, F., Wassiljiew, S., Meyer-Gaessner, M. 2011. Endovascular management of ascending aortic pathology. J Vasc Surg; 53: 1431-7.

Lee, I., S. Park, I. Hwang, M. J. Kim, S. S. Nah, B. Yoo, and J. K. Song. 2008. Cardiac Behçet disease presenting as aortic valvulitis/aortitis or right heart inflammatory mass: a clinicopathologic study of 12 cases. *Am.J.Surg.Pathol.* 32, no. 3:390-398.

Levine, A., S. Kasem, R. Mader, Y. Naparstek, G. Friedman, and A. Ben-Yehuda. Wegener Granulomatosis with back pain, periaortitis, and dural inflammation developing while receiving monthly cyclophosphamide. *J.Clin.Rheumatol.* 12, no. 4:294-297.

Liang, K. P., V. R. Chowdhary, C. J. Michet, D. V. Miller, T. M. Sundt, H. M. Connolly, C. S. Crowson, E. L. Matteson, and K. J. Warrington. 2009. Noninfectious ascending aortitis: a case series of 64 patients. *J.Rheumatol.* 36, no. 10:2290-2297.

Lie, J. T. 1995. Aortic and extracranial large vessel giant cell arteritis: a review of 72 cases with histopathologic documentation. *Semin.Arthritis Rheum.* 24, no. 6:422-431.

Mahr, A.D., Jover, J.A., Spiera, R.F., Hernandez-Garcia, C., Fernandez-Gutierrez, B., Lavalley, M.P., et al. 2007 Adjunctive methotrexate for treatment of giant cell arteritis: an individual patient data meta-analysis. *Arthritis Rheum* 2007;56:2789–97.

Maksimowicz-McKinnon, K., Clark, T.M.,and Hoffman, G.S. 2007. Limitations of therapy and guarded prognosis in an American cohort of Takayasu arteritis patients. *Arthritis Rheum* . 56, 1000-6.

Maksimowicz-McKinnon, K., Clark, T.M., Hoffman, G.S. 2009. Takayasu arteritis and Giant-cell arteritis. A spectrum within the same disease?. Medicine 2009; 88:221-226.

Miller, D. V., P. A. Isotalo, C. M. Weyand, W. D. Edwards, M. C. Aubry, and H. D. Tazelaar. 2006. Surgical pathology of noninfectious ascending aortitis: a study of 45 cases with emphasis on an isolated variant. *Am.J.Surg.Pathol.* 30, no. 9:1150-1158.

Molloy, E.S., Langford, C.A:, Clark, T.M., Gota, C.E., Hoffman, G.S. 2008. Anti-tumour necrosis factor therapy in patients with refractory takayasu arteritis: long-term follow-up. *Ann Rheum Dis* ; 67: 1567-69.

Mukhtyar, C., L. Guillevin, M. C. Cid, B. Dasgupta, Groot K. de, W. Gross, T. Hauser et al. 2009. EULAR recommendations for the management of large vessel vasculitis. *Ann.Rheum.Dis.* 68, no. 3:318-323.

Mwipatayi, B. P., P. C. Jeffery, S. J. Beningfield, P. J. Matley, N. G. Naidoo, A. A. Kalla, and D. Kahn. 2005. Takayasu arteritis: clinical features and management: report of 272 cases. *ANZ.J.Surg.* 75, no. 3:110-117.

Narvaez, J., J. A. Narvaez, J. M. Nolla, E. Sirvent, D. Reina, and J. Valverde. 2005. Giant cell arteritis and polymyalgia rheumatica: usefulness of vascular magnetic resonance imaging studies in the diagnosis of aortitis. *Rheumatology.(Oxford).* 44, no. 4:479-483.

Nesi, G., C. Anichini, S. Tozzini, V. Boddi, G. Calamai, and F. Gori. 2009. Pathology of the thoracic aorta: a morphologic review of 338 surgical specimens over a 7-year period. *Cardiovasc.Pathol.* 18, no. 3:134-139.

Nuenninghoff, D. M., G. G. Hunder, T. J. Christianson, R. L. McClelland, and E. L. Matteson. 2003a. Incidence and predictors of large-artery complication (aortic aneurysm, aortic dissection, and/or large-artery stenosis) in patients with giant cell arteritis: a population-based study over 50 years. *Arthritis Rheum.* 48, no. 12:3522-3531.

Nuenninghoff, D. M., G. G. Hunder, T. J. Christianson, R. L. McClelland, and E. L. Matteson. 2003b. Mortality of large-artery complication (aortic aneurysm, aortic dissection, and/or large-artery stenosis) in patients with giant cell arteritis: a population-based study over 50 years. *Arthritis Rheum.* 48, no. 12:3532-3537.

Nuenninghoff, D. M. and E. L. Matteson. 2003. The role of disease-modifying antirheumatic drugs in the treatment of giant cell arteritis. *Clin.Exp.Rheumatol.* 21, no. 6 Suppl 32:S29-S34.

Ogino, H., H. Matsuda, K. Minatoya, H. Sasaki, H. Tanaka, Y. Matsumura, H. Ishibashi-Ueda et al. 2008. Overview of late outcome of medical and surgical treatment for Takayasu arteritis. *Circulation* 118, no. 25:2738-2747.

Okada, K., K. Eishi, S. Takamoto, M. Ando, Y. Kosakai, K. Nakano, Y. Sasako, and J. Kobayashi. 1997. Surgical management of Behcet's aortitis: a report of eight patients. *Ann.Thorac.Surg.* 64, no. 1:116-119.

Ostberg, G. 1972. Morphological changes in the large arteries in polymyalgia arteritica. *Acta Med.Scand.Suppl.* 533:135-59.:135-159.

Pacini, D., O. Leone, S. Turci, N. Camurri, F. Giunchi, G. N. Martinelli, and Bartolomeo R. Di. 2008. Incidence, etiology, histologic findings, and course of thoracic inflammatory aortopathies. *Ann.Thorac.Surg.* 86, no. 5:1518-1523.

Palazzi, C., C. Salvarani, S. D'Angelo, and I. Olivieri. 2010. Aortitis and periaortitis in ankylosing spondylitis. *Joint Bone Spine.*

Pipitone, N., A. Versari, and C. Salvarani. 2008. Role of imaging studies in the diagnosis and follow-up of large-vessel vasculitis: an update. *Rheumatology.(Oxford).* 47, no. 4:403-408.

Prieto-Gonzalez, S., P. Arguis, A. Garcia-Martinez, G. Espigol-Frigole, M. Butjosa, I. Tavera, J. M. Grau, J. Hernandez-Rodriguez, and M. C. Cid. 2009. Aortic Involvement in Patients with Newly Diagnosed Giant Cell Arteritis (GCA). A Prospective Study Using Computed Tomography (CT) Angiography [abstract]. *Arthritis Rheum.* 60, no. Suppl 10:1971.

Rojo-Leyva, F., N. B. Ratliff, D. M. Cosgrove, III, and G. S. Hoffman. 2000. Study of 52 patients with idiopathic aortitis from a cohort of 1,204 surgical cases. *Arthritis Rheum.* 43, no. 4:901-907.

Salvarani, C., F. Cantini, and G. G. Hunder. 2008. Polymyalgia rheumatica and giant-cell arteritis. *Lancet.* %19;372, no. 9634:234-245.

Sproul, E. E. and J. J. Hawthorne. 1937. Chronic Diffuse Mesaortitis: Report of Two Cases of Unusual Type. *Am.J.Pathol.* 13, no. 2:311-323.

Stone, J. R. 2011. Aortitis, periaortitis, and retroperitoneal fibrosis, as manifestations of IgG4-related systemic disease. *Curr.Opin.Rheumatol.* 23, no. 1:88-94.

Tavora, F. and A. Burke. 2006. Review of isolated ascending aortitis: differential diagnosis, including syphilitic, Takayasu's and giant cell aortitis. *Pathology.* 38, no. 4:302-308.

Tso, E., Flamm, S.D., White, R.D., Schvartzman, P.R., Mascha, E., Hoffman, G.S. 2002. Takayasu arteritis: utility and limitations of magnetic resonance imaging in diagnosis and treatment. *Arthritis Rheum* ;46:1634–42.

Walter, M. A., R. A. Melzer, C. Schindler, J. Muller-Brand, A. Tyndall, and E. U. Nitzsche. 2005. The value of [18F]FDG-PET in the diagnosis of large-vessel vasculitis and the assessment of activity and extent of disease. *Eur.J.Nucl.Med.Mol.Imaging.* 32, no. 6:674-681.

Watts, R. A. and D. G. Scott. 2009. Recent developments in the classification and assessment of vasculitis. *Best.Pract.Res Clin.Rheumatol.* 23, no. 3:429-443.

Webb, M. and A. Al-Nahhas. 2006. Molecular imaging of Takayasu's arteritis and other large-vessel vasculitis with 18F-FDG PET. *Nucl.Med.Commun.* 27, no. 7:547-549.

Weiler, V., S. Redtenbacher, C. Bancher, M. B. Fischer, and J. S. Smolen. 2000. Concurrence of sarcoidosis and aortitis: case report and review of the literature. *Ann.Rheum.Dis.* 59, no. 11:850-853.

Zehr, K. J., A. Mathur, T. A. Orszulak, C. J. Mullany, and H. V. Schaff. 2005. Surgical treatment of ascending aortic aneurysms in patients with giant cell aortitis. *Ann.Thorac.Surg.* 79, no. 5:1512-1517.

Vaglio, A., D. Corradi, L. Manenti, S. Ferreti, G. Garini, and C. Buzio. 2003. Evidende of autoimmunity in chronic periaortitis: a prospective study. *Am.J.Med.* no.114:454-462.

9

Drug-Induced Aortic Aneurysms, Ruptures and Dissections

Olav Spigset
Department of Clinical Pharmacology, St. Olav University Hospital, Trondheim,
Department of Laboratory Medicine, Children's and Women's Disease,
Norwegian University of Science and Technology, Trondheim,
Norway

1. Introduction

Both prescription drugs and illicit substances have been associated with the formation of aortic aneurysms, ruptures of aortic aneurysms, and acute aortic dissections. Most of the clinical information exists as single case reports and case series, but causal relationships have for many drug groups been substantiated on the basis of the known mechanisms of action of the drugs as well as from experimental studies in animals.

For abdominal aneurysms, the most important etiologic factors include systemic hypertension, hyperlipidemia and atherosclerosis. In theory, all drugs having a negative impact of one or more of these factors might increase the risk of aortic aneurysms. On the other hand, drugs positively influencing these factors, such as antihypertensives and cholesterol-lowering drugs, could, at least in theory, have a potentially protective effect on the formation and development of the aneurysms. For aortic dissections, systemic hypertension is a central risk factor, and many drugs known to increase systemic blood pressure abruptly are associated with aortic dissections. In addition, abrupt discontinuation of antihypertensive drugs known to cause rebound hypertension, such as the beta blockers, may precipitate aortic dissections.

The objective of this chapter is to present a comprehensive review of pharmaceutical products and illicit substances associated with the formation and ruptures of aortic aneurysms. Moreover, drugs implicated in acute aortic dissections are also included. Data from case reports and case series are tabulated for completeness. When relevant, these data are also synthesised in order to provide aggregate information, attempting to identify potential drug-specific risk factors. Results from experimental studies are included to provide an understanding of the underlying mechanisms, and treatment options are discussed when they deviate from conventional therapy.

2. Methods

This chapter is a literature review based upon the author's research experience with adverse drug reactions, supplied by a search in the database PubMed, primarily by using the medical subject heading (MeSH) term "aortic aneurysm" with the subheading "chemically induced". Such a search strategy revealed 185 articles, which were scrutinised. The reference lists in the articles were further checked to identify other studies and reports of interest.

3. Drugs associated with aortic aneurysms

3.1 Glucocorticoids

Ruptures of aortic aneurysms are not unknown in autoimmune disorders affecting connective tissue in various organ systems including blood vessels, such as systemic lupus erythematosus (SLE) and rheumatoid arthritis (Smith & Hirst, 1979; Sato et al., 2003; Ohara et al., 2000a, 2000b). In such cases glucocorticoids may have a protective effect by inhibiting the activity of the underlying disorder. However, it has also been suspected that glucocorticoid use could have a precipitating role by increasing blood pressure, blood cholesterol and blood glucose levels, thereby causing atherosclerosis, as well as by increasing the fragility of blood vessels due to its negative effects on collagen formation and connective tissue strength (Smith & Hirst, 1979; Sato et al., 2003; Ohara et al., 2000a, 2000b).

In the literature, a total of 14 cases have been reported after long-term glucocorticoid use in patients with autoimmune disorders affecting connective tissue (Table 1). In these cases, it is by no means obvious whether the rupture is caused by the underlying disease, the treatment with glucocorticoids, or a combination thereof. There are no reports of ruptured aortic aneurysms during long-term treatment with glucocorticoids for disorders and conditions not affecting connective tissue, such as glomerulonephritis, or after organ transplantations. However, there are in addition two cases of ruptures after short-term treatment with glucocorticiods for disorders not causing weakness of connective tissue (Mellingsæter et al., 2009), but on the other hand, these patients also had additional risk factors, such as advanced age (Table 1).

The gender distribution of the 16 cases identified in the literature (Table 1), with 50 % males and 50 % females, seems to reflect the gender distribution of the underlying disorders. As expected, the mean age is also relatively low, 56 years.

Experimental evidence of an association between the use of glucocorticoids and aortic aneurysm rupture is found in an animal study (Reilly et al., 1990). In that study, genetically susceptible mice had a higher risk of developing aortic aneurysms, as well as having a rupture of the aneurysms, when treated with hydrocortisone. When the genetically susceptible mice were given hydrocortisone for 14 days, the mean aortic diameter increased to 1.86 mm, as compared to a stable value of 0.93 mm in a control group of genetically normal mice. In another experiment presented in the same publication (Reilly et al., 1990), nine of the 10 genetically susceptible mice died during the 21-day trial with hydrocortisone (6 with proven aortic rupture, 3 with presumed rupture), and also the 10th mouse in this group had an aneurysm after 21 days. The death risk was dose-dependent, with an average survival of 14 days among mice receiving the two higher hydrocortisone doses, as compared to 18-21 days among mice receiving the two lower doses.

In conclusion, long-term treatment with glucocorticoids has been associated with aortic aneurysm ruptures in numerous case reports, but it is not clear whether the ruptures have been caused by the underlying disease, the drug treatment, or combinations thereof. However, based on the known pharmacological effects of glucocorticoids as well as an experimental study, a causal association is not unlikely, although published evidence implies that this adverse drug reaction is very infrequent.

Reference	Age, gender	Drug, dose, duration of treatment	Location of the aneurysm	Underlying disease/ predisposing factors
Smith et al., 1979	55, male	Prednisolone 10 mg/d for 11 years	Descending thoracal	Rheumatoid arthritis
Smith et al., 1979	68, female	Prednisolone 15 mg/d for "many years"	Descending thoracal	Rheumatoid arthritis
Stehbens et al., 1993	56, male	Glucocorticoids (NS) for 16 years	Infrarenal	SLE
Seyama et al., 1989	54, male	Glucocorticoids (NS) for 1.5 years	Upper abdominal	SLE
Kurata et al., 1985	43, female	Glucocorticoids (NS) for 10 years	Descending thoracal	SLE
Higashina et al., 1990	33, female	Glucocorticoids (NS) for 18 years	Descending thoracal	SLE
Sato et al., 1995[1]	45, female	Glucocorticoids (NS) for 27 years	Infrarenal	Progressive systemic sclerosis
Sato et al., 1995[1,2]	52, female	Glucocorticoids (NS), mean 3.5 mg/d for 16 years	Descending thoracal/ infrarenal	SLE
Sato et al., 1995[1]	73, female	Glucocorticoids (NS) for 15 years	Infrarenal	Rheumatoid arthritis; advanced age
Sato et al., 1995[1,2]	75, female	Glucocorticoids (NS), mean 3.2 mg/d for 32 years	Infrarenal	SLE; advanced age
Sato et al., 1995[1,2]	43, female	Glucocorticoids (NS), mean 2.8 mg/d for 22 years	Infrarenal	SLE
Ohara et al., 2000a[2]	34, male	Glucocorticoids (NS), mean 4.1 mg/d for 21 years	Infrarenal	SLE
Ohara et al., 2000b	73, male	Glucocorticoids (NS), mean 2.5 mg/d for 1 year	Infrarenal	SLE; advanced age
Hussain et al., 1998	40, male	Glucocorticoids (NS) for 15 years	Ascending thoracal	SLE
Melling-sæter et al., 2009	77, male	Prednisolone 40 mg/d for 4 days	Descending thoracal	Pyoderma gangrenosum/ advanced age; previous aorta aneurysm[3]
Melling-sæter et al., 2009	82, male	Prednisolone 60 mg/d for 9 days and 30 mg/d for 5 days	Abdominal	Bullous pemphigoid/ advanced age

Abbreviations: NS = not specified; SLE = systemic lupus erythematosus
[1] The same case is also included in the case series by Ohara et al., 2000a
[2] The same case is also included in the case series by Ohara et al., 2000b
[3] Previously treated with a stent graft in the abdominal part of a thoraco-abdominal aortic aneurysm

Table 1. Published cases of glucocorticoid-associated aortic aneurysm ruptures

3.2 Antihypertensive drugs

Based upon evidence from animal studies, activation of the renin-angoitensin-aldosteron system seems to be a central factor in the development of aortic aneurysms (Daugherty et al., 2006; Lu et al., 2008; Miyake & Morishita, 2009). In a population-based case-control study of more than 15,000 patients with abdominal aortic aneurysms (3,379 with ruptures and 11,974 without ruptures), treatment with angiotensin converting enzyme (ACE) inhibitors before admission was associated with a reduced risk of ruptures (adjusted Odds Ratio [OR] 0.83; 95 % confidence interval [CI] 0.73-0.95). In contrast, protective effects were not found for beta-blockers, calcium antagonists, alpha-blockers or thiazide diuretics. Thus, the beneficial effect of ACE inhibitors on the risk of ruptures seems to be independent of the antihypertensive effect (Hackam et al., 2006). Those who during the last months had discontinued treatment with ACE inhibitors, had on the other hand a marginally higher risk of ruptures (adjusted OR 1.39; 95 % CI 1.09-1.77). In contrast to the above findings, angiotensin receptor blockers (ARBs), which also inhibit the renin-angoitensin-aldosteron system, were not found to have any protective effect (adjusted OR 1.24; 95 % CI 0.71-2.18). However, this apparent discrepancy may be caused by a type II error, as only 132 patients in the entire material used ARBs (Hackam et al., 2006).

Inconsistent with the ACE inhibitor findings cited above, a recent prospective cohort study of 1,701 patients with small abdominal aortic aneurysms found that the growth rate of the aneurysms in fact was higher (3.33 mm/year) in the 169 patients treated with ACE inhibitors than in the remaining patients (2.77 mm/year; p=0.009) (Sweeting et al., 2010). No such associations were found for other groups of antihypertensive drugs.

It should also be noted that in a case-control study, use of calcium antagonists was significantly associated with the occurrence of aortic aneurysms (adjusted OR 2.6; 95 % CI 1.5-4.2), whereas no other antihypertensive drug groups showed an increased risk (Wilmink et al., 2002). In the same study, patients exposed to calcium antagonists also had an increased aortic wall stiffness. Nevertheless, there was no association between calcium antagonists (or with any of the other drug groups) and the growth rate of the aneurysms after they had been detected. The association between calcium antagonist use and the occurrence of aortic aneurysms is consistent with the finding in an animal study in which the calcium antagonist amlodipine accelerated the degradation of elastin (Boyle et al., 1998).

All observational studies, including those cited above, are inevitably subject to bias and confounding. Thus, there is an urgent need for prospective, randomised, controlled trials to elucidate the role of both ACE inhibitors, ARBs, calcium antagonists and other groups of antihypertensives as to whether they have a protective, neutral or provoking effect on the formation and growth of aortic aneurysms and the risk of ruptures.

4. Drugs assosiated with aortic dissections

4.1 Phosphodiesterase-5 inhibitors

The phospodiesterase-5 (PDE-5) inhibitors sildenafil, tadalafil and vardenafil are widely used to cause penile erection in patients with impotence. An association between sildenafil and acute aortic dissection has been suspected in three case reports (Table 2). Hitherto, no cases have been reported for tadalafil and vardenafil.

As all the three patients reported in the literature had predisposing factors for aortic dissection (Table 2), the causal role of sildenafil has been questioned. One patient used isosorbide mononitrate concomitantly. Combinations of PDE-5 inhibitors with nitrates and other nitric oxide donors, including nitroglycerin and isosorbide mono- or dinitrate, are contraindicated due to the risk of excessive increases in systemic blood pressure. Also sexual arousal is associated with increased blood pressure, which could have been a contributing factor. However, at least in one of the patients, the aortic dissection appeared before sexual intercourse took place.

Reference	Age, gender	Drug, dose	Temporal relationship	Predisposing factors	Stanford type [1]
Famularo et al., 2001	42, male	Sildenafil 50 mg	1 hour after intake	Cocaine sniffing 2 hours earlier, heavy smoker	B
Nachtnebel et al., 2006	61, male	Sildenafil 50 mg	30 min after intake	Hypertension, concomitant use of isosorbide mononitrate	A
Tiryakioglu et al., 2009	28, male	Sildenafil 50 mg	2 hours after intake	Bicuspid aortic valve with ascending aortic aneurysm	A

[1] Stanford type A: All dissections involving the ascending aorta, regardless of the site of origin. Stanford type B: All dissections not involving the ascending aorta

Table 2. Published cases of phosphodiesterase-5-associated aortic dissections

In addition to the risk of increasing systemic blood pressure, at least when combined with nitrates and other nitric oxide donors, sildenafil has vasorelaxant and antiproliferative effects on pulmonary vascular smooth muscle cells. Due to these effects it is also used in patients with pulmonary hypertension. Although not substantiated experimentally, it has been speculated that a similar antiproliferative effect in the aorta as in the pulmonary artery might cause a thinner media due to smooth muscle cell loss, rendering the aortic wall more vulnerable to dissections (Nactnebel et al., 2006).

In conclusion, sildenafil and possibly also other PDE-5 inhibitors have the potential to increase systemic blood pressure in certain situations, thus being able to provoke aortic dissections in vulnerable individuals.

4.2 Vascular endothelial growth factor inhibitors

Vascular endothelial growth factor (VEGF) inhibitors are a drug group inhibiting vascular proliferation and promoting apoptosis of cells participating in the formation of new blood vessels. As VEGF expression is increased in a variety of tumors, VEGF inhibitors are primarily used in the treatment of malignant diseases. An association between acute aortic dissection and treatment with the VEGF inhibitors sorafenib, sunitinib and bevacizumab has been suspected on the basis of three case reports, summarised in Table 3.

Hypertension is one of the major adverse drug reactions of VEGF inhibitors. For sorafenib and sunitinib, overall incidences of 23.4 and 22.5 % have been reported in meta-analyses (Wu et al., 2008). For bevacizumab, the incidence of hypertension in studies included in a meta-analysis ranged from 2.7 % to 32 % during low-dose treatment and between 17.6 % and 36 % during high-dose treatment (Zhu et al., 2007). In most cases, the increased blood pressure can be treated with antihypertensive drugs, but a minority of patients will not respond to antihypertensive therapy and the VEGF inhibitor has to be discontinued.

Reference	Age, gender	Drug	Temporal relationship	Predisposing factors	Stanford type[1]
Aragon-Ching et al., 2008	70, male	Bevaci-zumab	After 28 cycles of be-vacizumab for 21 days	Hypertension for 25 years, increased considerably after 10 months of bevacizumab treatment	B
Edeline et al., 2010	58, male	Sunitinib	After 4 cycles of sunitinib for 28 days	None; no increase in systemic blood pressure observed during sunitinib treatment	B
Serrano et al., 2010	77, female	Sorafenib	After 3 cycles of sorafenib for 21 days	Advanced age	B

[1] Stanford type A: All dissections involving the ascending aorta, regardless of the site of origin. Stanford type B: All dissections not involving the ascending aorta

Table 3. Published cases of vascular endothelial growth factor inhibitor-associated aortic dissections

The pathogenetic mechanism behind VEGF inhibitor-induced hypertension remains uncertain. It has been suggested that as VEGF inhibitors also block the effects of other growth factors including platelet-derived growth factor (PDGF), and as PDGF plays a role in blood vessel tonus regulation and microvascularisation, this could be a possible mechanism (Edeline et al., 2010). However, closely related protein kinase inhibitors such as imatinib, dasatinib and nilotinib, which inhibits PDGF without inhibiting VEGF, are not particularly linked to hypertension. On this basis, a direct effect via VEGF inhibition seems more likely. The involvement of VEGF in the formation of normal blood vessels during embryonic development and in the carcinogenesis is well studied, but its possible function in normal blood vessels in adults is unclear. Suggested mechanisms include impaired angiogenesis at the microcirculation level, endothelial dysfunction associated with decreased levels of the vasodilator nitric oxide which is normally stimulated by VEGF, and alterations in the renin-angiotensin-aldosteron system (Sica, 2006).

Based upon the high incidence of hypertension during treatment with VEGF inhibitors, patients treated with these drugs should be closely followed with blood pressure measurements. If hypertension develops, it should be treated adequately. Obviously, as hypertension is a well-known risk factor for aortic dissection, also VEGF inhibitor-induced hypertension will increase the risk of aortic dissection.

4.3 Antihypertensive drugs

Antihypertensive drugs are known to protect a vulnerable aorta from dissections, and discontinuation of such drugs could therefore be expected to increase the risk of acute dissections. In particular antihypertensive drugs for which rebound hypertension occur after abrupt discontinuation, such as beta-blockers and clonidine, would be expected to increase the risk of aortic dissections.

One single case of acute aortic dissection has been reported within a short time interval after abrupt discontinuation of antihypertensive drug treatment (Eber et al., 1993). A 60-year-old man treated with beta-blockers for hypertension for 20 years developed a Stanford type A dissection two days after stopping metoprolol. It is not explicitly stated in the report whether the drug was tapered down before discontinuation or stopped abruptly, but is seems likely that treatment ceased directly from a dose of 50-100 mg/day. In such cases rebound effects including increased blood pressure, tachycardia and cardiac arrhythmias, and in some cases even cardiac infarction and sudden cardiac death, may occur (Houston & Hodge, 1988; Psaty et al., 1990). Therefore, current recommendations state that beta-blockers (and clonidine) should be tapered over at least 1-2 weeks before discontinuation.

4.4 Other drugs

Anticoagulants and fibrinolytic drugs have in two case reports been associated with aortic dissections and ruptures of thoracic aortic aneurysms. The first case was an 80-year-old woman who developed a Stanford type B aortic dissection during treatment with warfarin (Blunt & Impallomeni, 2004). Notably, her International Normalised Ratio (INR) was 4.8, indicating a considerably increased bleeding risk. The authors speculate that the underlying mechanism was a bleeding into an atheromatous plaque in the thoracic aorta. The second case was a 67-year-old man who was treated with the tissue plasminogen activator (t-PA) nateplase due to an acute ischemic stroke and who developed a rupture of a thoracic aortic aneurysm (Hayashi et al., 2004). The authors suggest that the t-PA infusion caused the rupture, based upon some evidence that plasminogen activators are able to degrade abdominal aortic aneurysms (Reilly, 1996).

A single case report of aortic dissection exists in a patient receiving chemotherapy for cancer (Golden et al., 1997). The patient was a 42-year-old man treated with cyclophosphamide, vincristine, procarbazine, prednisolone, bleomycin and vinblastine for Hodgkin's disease. As many of these agents are known to cause endothelial cell damage, the authors postulate that a toxic effect to endothelial cells in the aortic wall was the underlying mechanism. However, the patient also had other risk factors, including hypercholesterolemia and tobacco smoking. Thus, a causal relationship between the cytotoxic drugs and the aortic dissection remains obscure, and, if the suggested underlying mechanism is correct, it is remarkable that no more reports are found in the literature.

Numerous other drugs than those presented earlier in this review have the ability of causing hypertension. Consequently, these drugs might, at least in theory, increase the risk of aortic dissections. Common for these drugs is that there are no published case reports of aortic dissections related to their use. Whether the reason for the lack of such reports is that the relationship has not been recognised, or it is that the excess risk is so low that it can be considered negligible, is unknown. Drugs known to increase systemic blood pressure include sympathomimetic substances like adrenaline, noradrenaline, dopamine, metaraminol and phenylephrine, which might cause excessive elevations in blood pressure when the dose or, when given as an infusion, the rate of infusion, is not carefully controlled. Other drugs known to cause hypertension as an adverse drug reaction include non-steroidal antiinflammatory drugs (NSAIDs), ciclosporin and venlafaxine, just to mention a few. Moreover, monoamine oxidase inhibitors induce excessive hypertension when indirectly acting sympathomimetic drugs or tyramine-rich food or beverages are ingested concomitantly (Davies & Davies, 1998).

4.5 Illicit drugs

4.5.1 Cocaine

The association between cocaine abuse and aortic dissection is well documented. In some case series of patients with aortic dissection the proportion caused by cocaine abuse is relatively high. For example, in a material from a US urban hospital, 14 of the 38 cases of aortic dissection registered between 1981 and 2000 (37 %) were related to cocaine use (Hsue et al., 2002). In another US study, (Singh et al., 2007), 13 of 46 cases (28 %) diagnosed between 1996 and 2005 were associated with cocaine. Finally, in a chart review for the period 1990-2006, 16 of 163 patients (9.8 %) had used cocaine the last 24 hours before symptom onset (Daniel et al., 2007). In contrast, only 0.5 % of the cases in the International Registry for Aortic Dissection were found to be related to cocaine (Eagle et al., 2002). The proportion found to be caused by cocaine abuse will clearly depend on the frequency of cocaine use in the population from which the subjects originate. Moreover, cases associated with cocaine use will not be revealed if the patients are not explicitly asked about cocaine use or preferably tested for the presence of the cocaine metabolite benzoylecgonine in urine.

In addition to these four more systematic studies (Hsue et al., 2002; Eagle et al., 2002; Daniel et al., 2007; Singh et al., 2007), numerous single cases, summarised in Table 4, are reported in the literature.

Based on the 16 cases detailed by Daniel et al. (2007) and the 19 cases presented in Table 4, subjects with cocaine-related aortic dissections seem to be younger than average. All were younger than 60 years of age, three of four were younger than 50, and the mean age was 44 years. In total, 77 % were males. Almost all were long-term users, many had a history of uncontrolled hypertension, and the dissections occurred shortly after intake of cocaine. In some cases, symptoms appeared during or within the first few minutes after ingestion, but there could also be a lag-time of up to 24 hours – with one possible exception; an apparent lag-time of 3 days is reported in one case (Divakaran et al., 2007). In both the studies by Hsue et al. (2002) and by Daniel et al. (2007), the mean lag-time was 12 hours. However, based upon the 19 single cases (Table 4), the median lag-time could be estimated to about 1.5-2 hours, only.

It has been suggested that Stanford type B dissections are more common among cocaine users than in the average population (Singh 2007). However, according to Daniel et al. (2007), it was not apparent that type B dissections were more common. Of the 16 cases presented by Daniel et al. (2007) plus the 19 case reports (Table 4), 54 % were of type A whereas 46 % were of type B. As a comparison, 62 % were of type A and 38 % of type B in a general material consisting of 464 patients with acute aortic dissection (Ince et al., 2007).

It has been claimed that both the recurrence risk and the mortality of aortic dissections could be higher among cocaine users than among subjects with dissections unrelated to cocaine use (Hsue et al., 2002). The most likely reason for a possibly increased recurrence risk is continued cocaine use after discharge; there is no data available indicating that the recurrence risk would be increased in patients able to seize cocaine abuse after the first episode of dissection.

The effects of cocaine on the cardiovascular system are caused by its sympathomimetic properties. Cocaine predominantly exerts its pharmacological effects by blocking the reuptake of noradrenaline and dopamine from the synaptic cleft into presynaptic neurons. Increased levels of noradrenaline in the synaptic cleft activate postsynaptic alpha-adrenergic and beta-adrenergic receptors. An enhanced release of noradrenaline into the synaptic cleft by cocaine may also take place, causing further receptor activation. Activation of alpha-1 receptors in blood vessels causes elevation of the systemic blood pressure through vasoconstriction. Activation of beta-1 receptors in the heart promotes ventricular contractility and increases heart rate, thereby contributing to the effects on blood pressure.

Reference	Age, gender	Route of administration	Interval between intake and symptom onset	Predisposing factors	Stanford type[1]
Barth et al., 1986	45, male	Inhalation	Hours	Hypertension	A
Edwards & Rubin, 1987	41, male	Insufflation	30 min	Hypertension	B
Grannis et al., 1988	46, male	Insufflation	1.5 hours	Hypertension	B
Gadaleta et al., 1989	45, male	Insufflation	Unknown	Hypertension	A
Fischer & Holroyd, 1992	58, male	Subcutaneously	5 min	Hypertension	B
Om et al., 1992	47, male	Intravenously	Unknown; died before surgery	Hypertension	A
Cohle & Lie, 1992	35, male	Inhalation	Unknown; found dead	NR	A
Simons et al., 1992	26, female	Insufflation	Unknown	NR	A
Adkins et al., 1993	43, male	Inhalation	During smoking	NR	A
McDermott et al., 1993	37, male	Inhalation	12-18 hours	Hypertension	B
Sherzoy et al., 1994	50, female	Inhalation	2 hours	Hypertension	B
Rashid et al., 1996	42, male	Inhalation	40 min	Hypertension	A
Perron & Gibbs, 1997	33, male	Inhalation	Unclear	None	A
Hohm, 1995	28, male	NR	Unclear	None	A
Baumgartner & Omari, 1997	40, female	NR	NR	NR	A
Madu et al., 1999	34, female	Inhalation	2 hours	Hypertension	B
Divakaran et al., 2007	45, male	NR	3 days?	NR	A
Johnson et al., 2008	48, male	Inhalation	"Short"	Hypertension	A
Szeberin et al., 2009	35, male	NR	NR	NR	B

Abbreviations: NR = not reported
[1] Stanford type A: All dissections involving the ascending aorta, regardless of the site of origin. Stanford type B: All dissections not involving the ascending aorta

Table 4. Published cases of cocaine-associated aortic dissections

The sudden and considerable increase in blood pressure shortly after intake of cocaine obviously will increase shear stress in the aorta, sometimes causing a disruption of the intima and a dissection. More infrequently, the stress may produce an intramural hematoma that subsequently may rupture into the lumen (Scherzoy et al., 1994; Singh et al., 2010). In addition, long-term cocaine use may impair the elastic properties of the aorta, thereby reducing the ability of the aortic wall to withstand fluctuations in blood pressure and shear stress (Bigi et al., 2008).

As for aortic dissection of other causes, the immediate treatment of cocaine-induced dissections is to lower the blood pressure. In general, beta-blockers are most often used for this purpose. However, for cocaine-related dissections, beta-blockers should be avoided because they do not antagonise the alpha-adrenergic effects and may thus exacerbate, or at least not counteract, cocaine-related vasoconstriction of the coronary and visceral arteries (Lange et al., 1990; Hollander, 2008; Singh et al., 2010). The combined alpha- and beta-blocker labetalol would therefore, at least in theory, be a better choice. However, labetalol does not reverse the vasoconstriction of the coronary arteries fully, most likely because its alpha-antagonistic properties are too weak (Boehrer et al., 1993; Hollander, 2008). Nevertheless, some authors still recommend the use of labetalol. Alternative treatments include nitroglycerin, which reverse the cocaine-induced vasoconstriction of the coronary arteries to a sufficiently high degree, and verapamil (Lange & Hills, 2001). Also nitroprusside and hydralazine have been suggested, although these drugs, which do not exert beta-blocking properties, in fact may increase the shear stress of the aorta further due to reflex tachycardia with a subsequent increase in cardiac output (Hollander, 2008; Singh et al., 2010).

4.5.2 Methamphetamine, amphetamine and 3,4-methylenedioxymethamphetamine (MDMA; ecstasy)

There are numerous case reports of acute aortic dissection related to methamphetamine, and a few case reports exist for the closely related agents amphetamine and 3,4-methylenedioxymethamphetamine (MDMA; ecstasy) (Table 5). For simplicity, these three substances are described as "amphetamines" in this chapter. Among the 13 cases published in detail in the literature (Table 5), all were males. Their mean age was 38 years, and none were older than 52, thus resembling the situation for cocaine users and reflecting the characteristics of the population using these illicit drugs. In nine of the 11 cases where the type of dissection was reported (81 %), the dissections were Stanford type A.

In a systematic review of 35 deceased patients with aortic dissection screened for drug use in California during the years 1987-1996, seven (20 %) tested positive for methamphetamine (Swalwell & Davis, 1999). Whereas the mean age in the total group was 52 years, the mean age among those who tested positive for methamphetamine was 41 years. In six of the seven cases (86 %), the dissection was of type A. Thus, the characteristics of this group are similar to those of the 13 cases published in detail (Table 5).

In a population-based study of 3,116 aortic dissections in subjects aged 18 to 49 years (Westover & Nakonezny, 2010), abuse and dependence of amphetamines were significantly associated with aortic dissections (OR 3.33, 95 % CI 2.37-4.69). Interestingly, the OR for abuse and dependence of amphetamines was lower than for Marfan syndrome (OR = 374), cardiovascular syphilis (OR = 106), bicuspid aorta valve (OR = 45), Takayashu disease (OR = 31), Turner syndrome (OR = 22), Ehlers-Danlos syndrome (OR = 13), giant cell arthritis (OR = 6.5), hypertension (OR = 7.7), coarctation of the aorta (OR = 4.6) and motor vehicle accidents (OR = 3.6), but higher than for cocaine abuse/dependence (OR = 1.6), tobacco use (OR = 1.4), and age (OR = 1.1). The higher risk for the amphetamines than for cocaine is somewhat surprising on the basis of the number of published cases in the literature. One possible explanation for the increased risk might be that the amphetamines most likely have a prolonged effect on the blood pressure increments as compared to cocaine, due to a slower elimination from the body.

Reference	Age, gender	Drug	Temporal relationship	Predisposing factors	Stanford type[1]
Davis & Swalwell, 1994	52, male	Methamphetamine	Not known[2]	Hypertension, also positive for cocaine	A
Davis & Swalwell, 1994	42, male	Methamphetamine	Not known[2]	Hypertension	NR
Davis & Swalwell, 1994	28, male	Methamphetamine	Not known[2]	None	NR
Kim et al., 1999	37, male	Methamphetamine	Not known	None	A
Wako et al., 2007	39, male	Methamphetamine	Not known[3]	None	A
Wako et al., 2007	37, male	Methamphetamine	Not known[3]	Hypertension	B
Wako et al., 2007	38, male	Methamphetamine	Not known[3]	Hypertension	B
Wako et al., 2007	35, male	Methamphetamine	Not known[3]	None	A
Wako et al., 2007	44, male	Methamphetamine	Not known[3]	Hypertension	A
Wako et al., 2007	44, male	Methamphetamine	Not known[3]	Hypertension	A
Obioha, 2009	42, male	Methamphetamine	2 days	None	A
Dihmis et al., 1997	27, male	Amphetamine	Not known[2]	NR	A
Duflou & Mark, 2000	29, male	MDMA (ecstasy)	Possibly 12 hours[2]	None	A

Abbreviations: MDMA = 3,4-methylenedioxymethamphetamine; NR = not reported

[1] Stanford type A: All dissections involving the ascending aorta, regardless of the site of origin. Stanford type B: All dissections not involving the ascending aorta

[2] Patient deceased, intake detected by post-mortem toxicological screening

[3] Intake identified by drugs-of-abuse screening in urine

Table 5. Published cases of aortic dissections associated with methamphetamine, amphetamine and 3,4-methylenedioxymethamphetamine (ecstasy)

Like cocaine, the amphetamines exert their stimulating effects by increasing available noradrenaline and dopamine in the brain synapses. However, in contrast to cocaine, the effect is predominantly mediated by enhancing the release of neurotransmitters from presynaptic neurons rather than by inhibiting the reuptake. Nevertheless, the final common pathway for cocaine and the amphetamines is activation of adrenergic alpha and beta receptors, thereby causing elevation of systemic blood pressure through vasoconstriction and increased ventricular contractility and heart rate, respectively (see also section 4.5.1).

It has not been stated in the literature whether specific antihypertensive drugs should be preferred for dissections caused by amphetamines. However, based on the mechanism of action, it seems reasonable to consider the same treatments for amphetamine- as for cocaine-related dissections. Thus, beta-blockers should be avoided because they would be expected to exacerbate, or at least not counteract, the tendency to cause vasoconstriction of the coronary and visceral arteries (see also section 4.5.1). The beta-blocker esmolol has nevertheless been suggested as the drug of choice in a recent case report (Obioha et al., 2009), but the authors of this report have, somewhat surprisingly, not discussed the potential risks with beta-blocker treatment in these patients.

5. Conclusions

The only drug group for which relatively clear-cut evidence of involvement in the formation and rupture of aortic aneurysms exists, is the glucocorticoids. In addition, there is inconsistent evidence from epidemiological studies regarding whether the various antihypertensive drug classes protect against or in fact may precipitate growth and ruptures of aortic aneurysms. Prospective controlled clinical trials in this area are urgently needed to elucidate this issue.

Drug groups implicated in aortic dissection include those known to increase systemic blood pressure, such as phosphodiesterase-5 inhibitors like sildenafil, and vascular endothelial growth factor inhibitors like sorafenib, sunitinib and bevacizumab. Moreover, abrupt discontinuation of antihypertensive drugs known to cause rebound hypertension after cessation of therapy, such as beta-blockers, may also cause aortic dissection. In addition, single case reports exist for a few other drugs. Finally, illicit drugs such as cocaine, amphetamine, methamphetamine and ecstasy are associated with acute aortic dissections, with relative risk increases in the order of magnitude of about 2-3. Thus, the increased risk of aortic dissection for these substances is presumably considerably higher than for legal medicines.

6. References

Adkins, M.; Gaines, W.; Anderson, W.; Laub, G.; Fernandez, J. & McGrath L. (1993). Chronic type A aortic dissection: an usual complication of cocaine inhalation. *Ann Thorac Surg*, Vol. 56, pp. 977-979

Aragon-Ching, J.B.; Ning, Y.-M. & Dahut WL. (2008). Acute aortic dissection in a hypertensive patient with prostate cancer undergoing chemotherapy containing bevacizumab. *Acta Oncol*, Vol. 47, pp. 1600-1601

Barth, C.W.; Bray, M. & Roberts, W. (1986). Rupture of the ascending aorta during cocaine intoxication. *Am J Cardiol*, Vol. 57, p. 496

Baumgartner, F.J. & Omari, B.O. (1997). Method of repair of cocaine-induced chronic type A aortic dissection. *Ann Thorac Surg*, Vol. 64, pp. 1518-1519

Bigi, M.A.; Aslani, A. & Mehrpour M. (2008). Effect of chronic cocaine abuse on the elastic properties of the aorta. *Echocardiography*, Vol. 25, pp. 308-311

Blunt, D.M. & Impallomeni, M.G. (2004). Warfarin-associated thoracic aortic dissection in an elderly woman. *Age Ageing*, Vol. 33, pp. 199-201

Boehrer, J.D.; Moliterno, D.J.; Willard, J.E.; Hills, L.S. & Lange, R.A. (1993). Influence of labetalol on cocaine-induced coronary vasoconstriction in humans. *Am J Med*, Vol. 94, pp. 608-610

Boyle, J.; Loftus, I. & Goodall, S. (1998). Amlodipine potentiates metalloproteinase activity and accelerates elastin degradation on a model of aneurysmal disease. *Eur J Vasc Endovasc Surg*, Vol. 16, pp. 408-414

Cohle, S.D. & Lie, T.J. (1992). Dissection of the aorta and coronary arteries associated with acute cocaine intoxication. *Arch Pathol Lab Med*, Vol. 10, pp. 723-727

Daniel, J.C.; Huynh, T.T.; Zhou, W.; Kougias, P.; El Sayed, H.F.; Huh, J.; Coselli, J.S. & Lin H. (2007). Acute aortic dissection associated with the use of cocaine. *J Vasc Surg*, Vol. 46, pp. 427-433

Daugherty, A.; Rateri, D.L. & Cassis, L.A. (2006). Role of the renin-angiotensin-aldosteron system in the development of abdominal aortic aneurysms in animals and humans. *Ann N Y Acad Sci*, Vol. 1085, pp. 82-91

Davies, C.J. & Davies, D.M. (1998). Disorders of the peripheral vascular system. In: *Davies's textbook of adverse drug reactions*, Davies, D.M.; Ferner, R.E. & de Glanville, H. (Eds.), pp. 169-189, Chapman & Hall Medical, London

Davis, G.G. & Swalwell, C.I. (1994). Acute aortic dissections and ruptured berry aneurysms associated with methamphetamine abuse. *J Forensic Sci*, Vol. 39, pp. 1481-1485

Dihmis, W.C.; Ridley, P.; Dhasmana, J.P. & Wisheart, J.D. (1997). Acute dissection of the arota with amphetamine misue. *BMJ*, Vol. 314, p. 1665

Divakaran, V.; Mungee, S.; Salciccioli, L. & Clark, L.T. (2007). Bedside ultrasound diagnosis of aortic dissection in a cocaine abuser. *Eur J Intern Med*, Vol. 18, pp. 595-596

Duflou, J. & Mark, A. (2000). Aortic dissection after ingestion of "ecstacy" (MDMA). *Am J Forensic Med Pathol*, Vol.21, pp. 261-263

Eagle, K.A.; Isselbacher, E.M. & DeSanctis, R.W. (2002). Cocaine-induced aortic dissection in perspective. *Ciculation*, Vol. 105, pp. 1529-1530

Eber, B.; Tscheliessnigg, K.-H.; Anelli-Monti, M.; Kaumann, P.; Lueger, A., Delgado, P.; Kullnig, P. (1993). Aortic dissection due to discontinuation of beta-blocker therapy. *Cardiology*, Vol. 83, pp. 128-131

Edeline, J.; Laguerre, B.; Rolland, Y.; Patard, J.-J. (2010). Aortic dissection in a patient treated by sunitinib for metastatic renal carcinoma. *Ann Oncol*, Vol. 21, pp. 186-187

Edwards, J. & Rubin, R.N. (1987). Aortic dissection and cocaine abuse. *Ann Intern Med*, Vol. 107, pp. 779-780

Famularo, G.; Polchi, S.; Di Bona, G.; Manzara, C. (2001). Acute aortic dissection after cocaine and sildenafil abuse. *J Emerg Med*, Vol. 21, pp. 78-79

Fischer, A. & Holroyd, P.R. (1992). Cocaine-associated dissection of the thoracic aorta. *J Emerg Med*, Vol. 10, pp. 723-727

Gadaleta, D.; Hall, M.H. & Nelson, R.L. (1989). Cocaine-induced aortic dissection. *Chest*, Vol. 96, pp. 1203-1206

Golden, M.A.; Vaughn, D.J.; Crooka, G.W.; Holland, A. & Bavaria, J.E. (1997). Aortic dissection in a patient receiving chemotherapy for Hodgkin's disease. *Angiology*, Vol. 48, pp. 1063-1065

Grannis, F.W. Jr.; Bryant, C.; Caffaratti, J.D. & Turner, A.F. (1988). Acute aortic dissection associated with cocaine abuse. *Clin Cardiol*, Vol. 11, pp. 572-574

Hackam, D.G.; Thiruchelvam, D. & Redelmeier, D.A. (2006). Angiotensin converting enzyme inhibitors and aortic rupture: a population-based case-control study. *Lancet*, Vol. 368, pp. 659-665

Hayashi, H.; Kawamata, H.; Ichikawa, K.; Tajima, H. & Kumazaki, T. (2004). Rupture of a thoracic aneurysm: a rare adverse reaction following systemic tissue plasminogen activator infusion. *Heart Vessels*, Vol. 19, pp. 208-211

Higashina, M.; Watanabe, H. & Hashimoto, H. (1990). A successfully treated case of thoracic aneurysm during the course of SLE. *Systemic vascular research committee of Japan, Annual report 1990*, pp. 87-90

Hohm, S.P. (1995). A 28-year-old man with an aortic dissection and history of cocaine abuse. *J Emerg Nurs*, Vol. 21, pp. 199-201

Hollander, J.E. (2008). Cocaine intoxication and hypertension. *Ann Emerg Med*, Vol. 51 (suppl.), pp. S18-S20

Houston, M.C. & Hodge, R. (1988). Beta-adrenergic blocker withdrawal syndromes in hypertension and other cardiovasular diseases. *Am Heart J*, Vol. 116, pp. 515-523

Hsue, P.Y.; Salinas, C.L.; Bolger, A.F.; Benowitz, N.L. & Waters, DD. (2002). Acute aortic dissection related to crack cocaine. *Circulation*, Vol. 105, pp. 1592-1595

Hussain, K.M.A.; Chandna, H.; Santhanam, V.; Sehgal, S.; Jain, A. & Denes, P. (1998). Aortic dissection in a young corticosteroid-treated patient with systemic lupus erythematosus. *Angiology*, Vol. 49, pp. 649-652

Ince, H. & Nienaber, C.A. (2007). Diagnosis and management of patients with aortic dissections. *Heart*, Vol. 93, pp. 266-270

Johnson, J.A.; Callison, C. & Miller, A.N. (2008). A 48-year-old man with paralysis and hypotension. *Chest*, Vol. 134, pp. 862-865

Kim, M.J.; Kim, M.S.; Han, S.W. & Han, S.B. (1999). A case of acute dissection of the aorta associated with methamphetamine abuse [in Korean]. *Journal of the Korean Society of Echocariography*, Vol. 7, pp. 75-79

Kurata, N.; Tanai, K.; Kinashi, S. & Irino, S. (1985). An autopsy case of systemic lupus erythematosus complicated by thoracic aortic aneurysm. *Systemic vascular research committee of Japan, Annual report 1985*, pp. 313-316

Lange, R.A.; Cigarroa, R.G.; Flores, E.D.; McBride, W.; Kim, A.S.; Wells, P.J.; Bedotto, J.B.; Danziger, R.S. & Hills, L.D. (1990). Potentiation of cocaine-induced coronary vasoconstriction by beta-adrenergic blockade. *Ann Intern Med*, Vol. 112, pp. 897-903

Lange, R.A. & Hills, D. (2001). Cardiovascular complications of cocaine use. *N Engl J Med*, Vol. 345, pp. 351-358

Lu, H.; Rateri, D.L.; Cassis, L.A. & Daughtery, A. (2008). The role of the renin-angiotensin system in aortic aneurysmal diseases. *Curr Hypertens Rep*, Vol. 10, pp. 99-106

Madu, E.C.; Shala, B. & Baugh, D. (1999). Crack-cocaine-associated aortic dissection in early pregnancy – a case report. *Angiology*, Vol. 50, pp. 163-168

McDermott, J.; Schuster, M.; Crummy, A. & Archer, C. (1993). Crack and aortic dissection. *Wis Med J*, Vol. 92, pp. 453-455

Mellingsæter, T.C.; Rørdam, O.M. & Spigset, O. (2009). Association between aortic aneurysm rupture and short-term prednisolone use in two patients with dermatological disorders. *J Europ Acad Dermatol Venerol*, Vol. 23, pp. 585-586

Miyake, T. & Morishita, R. (2009). Pharmacological treatment of abdominal aortic aneurysm. *Cardiovas Res*, Vol. 83, pp. 436-443

Nactnebel, A.; Stöllberger, C.; Ehrlich, M. & Finsterer, J. (2006). Aortic dissection after sildenafil-induced erection. *South Med J*, Vol. 99, pp. 1151-1152

Obioha, C.C.; Engel, R.A. & Ingall T. (2009). 42-year-old male methamphetamine user with dysarthria and facial drop. *Mayo Clin Proc*, Vol. 84, pp. 912-915

Ohara, N.; Miyata, T.; Sato, O.; Osihiro, H. & Shigematsu, H. (2000a). Aortic aneurysm in patients with autoimmune diseases treated with corticosteroids. *Int Angiol*, Vol. 19, pp. 270-275

Ohara, N.; Miyata, T.; Kurata, A.; Oshiro, H.; Sato, O. & Shigematsu, H. (2000b). Ten years' experience of aortic aneurysm associated with systemic lupus erythematosus. *Eur J Vasc Endovasc Surg*, Vol. 19, pp. 288-293

Om, A.; Porter, T. & Mohanty, P.K. (1992). Transesophagal echocardiograpic diagnosis of acute aortic dissection complicating cocaine abuse. *Am Heart J*, Vol. 123, pp. 532-534

Perron, A.D. & Gibbs, M. (1997). Thoracic aortic dissection secondary to crack cocaine ingestion. *Am J Emerg Med*, Vol. 15, pp. 507-509

Psaty, B.M.; Koepsell, T.D.; Wagner, E.H.; LoGerfor, J.P. & Inui, T.S. (1990). The relative risk of incident coronary heart disease associated with recently stopping the use of beta-blockers. *JAMA*, Vol. 263, pp. 1653-1657

Rashid, J.; Eisenberg, M.J. & Topol, E. (1996). Cocaine-induced aortic dissection. *Am Heart J*, Vol. 132, pp. 1301-1304

Reilly, J.M.; Savage, E.B.; Brophy, C.M. & Tilson, M,D. (1990). Hydrocortisone rapidly induces aortic rupture in a genetically susceptible mouse. *Arch Surg*, Vol. 125, pp. 707-709

Reilly, J.M. (1996). Plasminogen activators in abdominal aortic aneurismal disease. *Ann N Y Acad Sci*, Vol. 800, pp. 151-156

Sato, O.; Takagi, A.; Miyata, T. & Takayama, Y. (1995). Aortic aneurysm in patients with autoimmune disorders treated with corticosteroids. *Eur J Vasc Endovasc Surg*, Vol. 10, pp. 366-369

Serrano, C.; Suárez, C.; Andreu, J. & Carles, J. (2010). Acute aortic dissection during sorafenib-containing therapy. *Ann Oncol*, Vol. 21, pp. 181-182

Seyama, K.; Muto, J. & Furua, H. (1989) A case of upper abdominal aortic aneurysm associated with systemic lupus erythematosus. *Jin To Touseki*, Vol. 27, pp. 1139-1141

Sherzoy, A.; Sadler, D. & Brown, J. (1994). Cocaine-related aortic dissection diagnosed by transesophagal echocardiography. *Am Heart J*, Vol. 128, pp. 641-643

Sica, D.A. (2006). Angiogenesis inhibitors and hypertension: an emerging issue. *J Clin Oncol*, Vol. 24, pp. 1329-1331

Simons, A.J.; Arazoza, E.; Hare, C.L.; Smulyan, H.; Lighty, G.W. Jr. & Parker. F.B. Jr. (1992). Circumferential aortic dissection in a young woman. *Am Heart J*, Vol. 123, pp. 1077-1079

Singh, S.; Trivedi, A.; Adhikari, T.; Molnar, J.; Arora, R. & Khosla, S. (2007). Cocaine-related acute aortic dissection: patient demographics and clinical outcomes. *Can J Cardiol*, Vol. 23, pp. 1131-1134

Singh, A.; Khaja, A. & Alpert, M.A. (2010). Cocaine and aortic dissection. *Vasc Med*, Vol. 15, pp. 127-133

Smith, D.C. & Hirst, A.E. (1979). Spontaneous aortic rupture associated with chronic steroid therapy for rheumatoid arthritis in two cases. *AJR Am J Roentgenol*, Vol.132, pp. 271-273

Sthebens, W.E.; Delahunt, B.; Shirer, W.C. & Naik, D.K. (1991) Aortic aneurysm in systemic lupus erythematosus. *Histopathology*, Vol. 22, pp. 275-277

Swalwell, C.I. & Davis, G.G. (1999). Methamphetatmine as a risk factor for acute aortic dissection. *J Forensic Sci*, Vol. 44, pp. 23-26

Sweeting, M.J.; Thompson, S.G.; Brown, L.C.; Greenhalgh, R.M. & Powell, J.T. (2010). Use of angiotensin converting enzyme inhibitors is associated with increased growth rate of abdominal aortic aneurysms. *J Vasc Surg*, Vol. 52, pp. 1-4

Szeberin, Z.; Firneisz, G.; Biro, G.; Szabo, G.V.; Sotonyi, P.; Windisch, M.; Krepuska, M.; Sipos, F.; Mihaly, E. & Ascady, G. (2009). Surgical treatment of acute type B aortic dissection associated with use of cocaine [in Hungarian]. *Orv Hetil*, Vol. 150, pp. 129-131

Tiryakioglu, S.K.; Tiryakioglu, O.; Turan, T. & Kumbay, E. (2009). Aortic dissection due to sildenafil abuse. *Interactive Cariovasc Thorac Surg*, Vol. 9, pp. 141-143

Veronese, M.L.; Mosenkis, A.; Flaherty, K.T.; Gallagher, M.; Stevenson, J.P.; Townsend, R.R. & O'Dwyer, P.J. (2006). Mechanisms of hypertension associated with BAY- 43-9006 treatment. *J Clin Oncol*, Vol. 14, pp. 1363-1369

Wako, E.; LeDoux, D.; Mitsumori, L.; Aldea, G.S. (2007) The emerging epidemic of methamphetamine-induced aortic dissection. *J Cardiac Surg*, Vol. 22, pp. 390-393

Westover, A.N. & Nakonezny, P.A. (2010). Aortic dissection in young adults who abuse amphetamines. *Am Heart J*, Vol. 160, pp. 315-321

Wilmink, A.B.M.; Vardulaki, K.A.; Hubbard, C.S.; Day, N.E.; Ashton, H.A.; Scott, A.P. & Quick, C.R.G. (2002). Are all antihypertensive drugs associated with abdominal aortic aneurysms? *J Vasc Surg*, Vol. 36, pp. 751-757

Wu, S.; Chen, J.J.; Kudeka, A.; Lu, J. & Zhu, X. (2008). Incidence and risk of hypertension with sorafenib in patients with cancer: a systematic review and meta-analysis. *Lancet Oncol*, Vol. 9, pp. 117-123

Zhu, X.; Wu, S.; Dahut, W.L. & Parikh, C.R. (2007). Risks of proteinuria and hypertension with bevacizumab, an antibody against vascular endothelial growth factor: systematic review and meta-analysis. *Am J Kidney Dis*, Vol. 49, pp. 186-193

10

Pathophysiology of Abdominal Aortic Aneurysm Rupture and Expansion: New Insight on an Old Problem

Efstratios Georgakarakos[1] and Christos V. Ioannou[2]
[1]*"Democritus" University of Thrace Medical School, Alexandroupolis,*
[2]*University of Crete Medical School, Iraklion,*
Greece

1. Introduction

The infrarenal aorta is a region of variable hemodynamics, with low mean and oscillating shear stress, variable secondary flow patterns with vortex formations and consequent high particle residence time (Tang et al, 2006, Dua & Dalman, 2010). Among the biomechanical parameters, wall stress holds a fundamental role, since its distribution and maximum values have been associated with the risk of Abdominal Aortic Aneurysms (AAA) rupture (Fillinger et al, 2003 and Venkatasubramaniam et al, 2004). Rupture can occur where the mechanical forces per unit area of the aortic wall (stress) exceed the local strength, so that reliable rupture risk estimation should take into account both the local distribution of stress and wall strength. Furthermore, high values of wall stress in transition areas of AAAs, ie inflection site between the neck and the AAA sac have been recently reported to differentiate those small AAAs with rapid expansion rate, possibly rendering them amenable to early intervention (Li et al, 2010a).

Computer-enhanced geometric modeling and Finite Element Analysis (FEA) have been used to study the biomechanical behavior of the aorta and the aortic aneurysms (Steinman et al, 2003), contributing in the development of measures to assess AAA rupture risk (Malkawi et al, 2010) and expansion (Li et al, 2010b). This chapter reviews from the clinical point of view the role of wall stress in AAA rupture risk models.

2. Reconstructing the AAA models

Many research groups have evaluated AAA rupture risk with estimation of PWS using the FEA technique, which utilizes small subsections (elements) of a 3-dimentional AAA model, created by segmentation (**Figure 1**) and meshing (**Figure 2**). The stress computations rely on the principles of conservation of mass and momentum for all finite elements of the model. Most researchers acquire information on the 3D AAA realistic geometric configuration using contrast-enhanced high-resolution spiral CT angiography. The acquisition of the two-dimensional CT images for each case is followed in principle by the creation of outlines of the outer and the inner surface of the AAA. Consequently, a stack of contours is reconstructed including the common iliac arteries and the neck of the AAA as fixation points are required in essential boundary conditions. The latter are needed for the solution the conservation laws. The result is a detailed map of the wall stress values throughout the aneurysm (**Figure 3**).

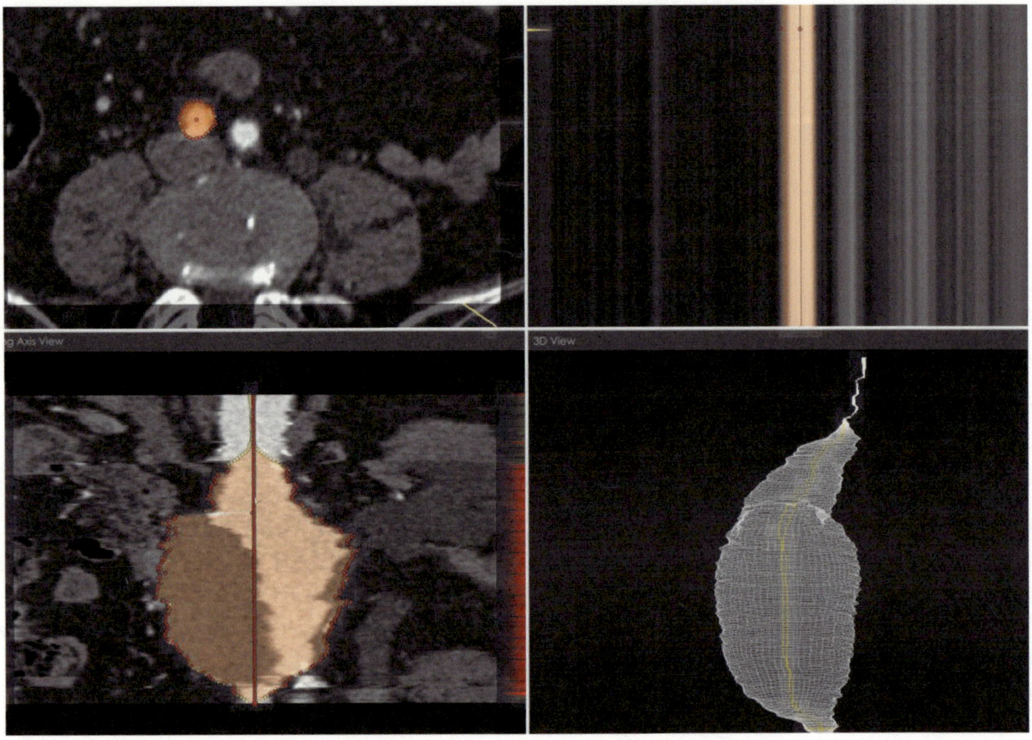

Fig. 1. Reconstructed images of the aneurysm are created from contrast enhanced CT images using purpose-developed software.

3. Role of wall stress in AAA rupture and expansion

Rupture remains the most threatening outcome of an AAA and is related to maximum diameter (Brewster et al, 2003) (**Table 1**).

Max. Diameter (cm)	Annual rupture risk (%)
<4	0
4-5	0.5-5
5-6	3-15
6-7	10-20
7-8	20-40
>8	30-50

Table 1. Annual rupture risk according to diameter (Brewster et al, 2003)

In current clinical practice, aneurysm diameter is one of the primary criteria used to decide when to treat a patient with an abdominal aortic aneurysm (AAA). The current threshold for treatment is 5.5 cm; however, many surgeons have come across gigantic AAAs (e.g., 11 or 12 cm) that have not yet ruptured, as well as small aneurysms <5.5 cm that have. There is evidence that the simple association of aneurysm diameter with the probability of rupture is not sufficient, and presumably other parameters play a role in causing an aneurysm to rupture or protecting it from rupture. This problem has spawned a need for new methods to reliably predict the actual risk of AAA rupture in the clinical setting.

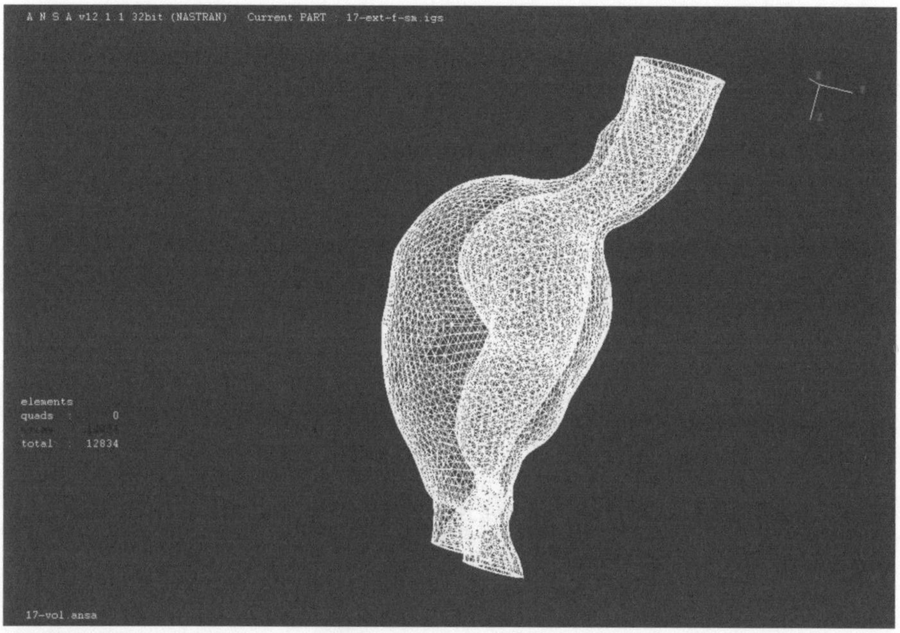

Fig. 2. Creation of the mesh

According to the biomechanical approach, rupture occurs when the stress on the aneurysm wall exceeds its failure strength. Laplace's law can estimate the stress values in ideally thin-walled shapes of simple geometry. However, these assumptions are rarely met in daily routine, since the patent-specific AAA models present variable asymmetry. Therefore, patient-specific knowledge of the magnitude and distribution of AAA wall stress and failure strength are useful measures in assessing the susceptibility to rupture. Stress is a measure of the internal forces induced on a material due to blood pressure and flow (Raghavan et al, 2005). Peak wall stress reflects the mechanical load sustained by the AAA wall during maximal systolic pressurization and depends on the mechanical properties and the geometric configuration of the wall (Raghavan et al, 2005). Arterial wall stress distributions for uniform wall loading, as well as flow-induced non-uniform pressure wall loading, are presented using the von Mises stress, a scalar measure of the stress tensor, proportional to the strain energy density at each point. Von Mises stress is expressed as σ_{VM}:

$$\sigma_{VM} = \sqrt{\frac{1}{2}\left[(\sigma_1 - \sigma_2)^2 + (\sigma_1 - \sigma_3)^2 + (\sigma_2 - \sigma_3)^2\right]}$$

where σ_1, σ_2, σ_3 are the principal stresses (Papaharilaou et al, 2007). PWS refers to the mechanical load sustained by the AAA wall during maximal systolic pressurization. Its value depends on arterial systolic pressure and the mechanical properties and geometric configuration of the material under study. Scotti et al (Scotti et al, 2005) studied virtual aneurysm models of variable asymmetry and wall thickness distribution. They showed that the variability in wall thickness can increase the PWS by 4 times compared with AAA models of uniform thickness. Moreover, they showed that variable thickness and asymmetry affect not only the magnitude but also the distribution of the stress values. Therefore, it is important for modern patient-specific rupture risk assessment to reproduce the specific AAA geometry and wall thickness. Decreasing of wall thickness by 25% causes a 20% increase in PWS and vice versa (Venkatasubramaniam et al, 2004). Therefore, the abovementioned observations depict the limitations of Laplace's law in accurate stress estimation.

Stress analysis has three main components, the study of the geometry under evaluation, the material model that characterizes the mechanical behavior of the aneurysmal tissue and the study of the boundary conditions under observation, eg blood pressure. Peak Wall Stress (PWS) estimation with the Finite element analysis (FEA) technique has been extensively used through the last decade, utilizing a well known mathematical model that describes the biomechanical properties of the AAA wall (Raghavan & Vorp, 2000).

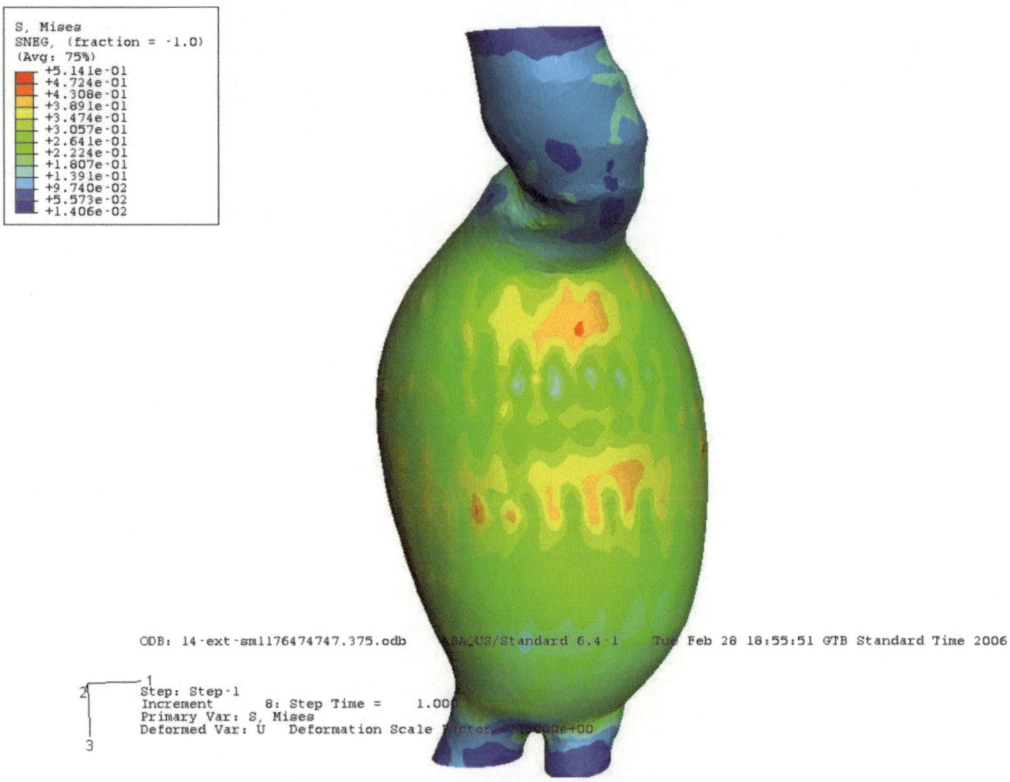

Fig. 3. The detailed map of the wall stress values throughout the aneurysm wall, after Finite Element Analysis. Wall stress values representation is based on a color-scaled climax. The red color depicts the Peak Wall Stress location, whereas blue color represents the sites of lowest wall stress.

The possible relation of PWS to the risk and the site of rupture in AAAs have been delineated in many studies. PWS has been estimated in ruptured and nonruptured, diameter-matched AAAs and was found to be significantly higher in the rupture group near the time of rupture (Fillinger et al, 2002, 2003, Heng et al, 2008; Venkatasubramaniam et al, 2004; Truijers et al, 2007; Vande Geest et al, 2008, Raghavan et al, 2005a). Moreover, a large prospective study by Fillinger et al (Fillinger et al, 2003) showed that PWS could differentiate AAAs that required urgent repair better than the maximum diameter criterion. In this study, Low-stress aneurysms presented a lower rupture rate whether they were small or large, with high stress aneurysms having a higher rupture rate regardless of size. The PWS values could differentiate more sufficiently than maximum diameter those AAAs prone to rupture over time. The conclusion was that the ruptured AAAs had higher values than the non-ruptured ones and that the elevated values were not simply an acute or incidental event near the time of rupture, but rather a characteristic that could be early recognized, thus gaining a predictive value with respect to the risk of rupture. Though the computational evaluation of PWS with FEA can be a strenuous and time-consuming effort (Leung et al, 2006), the intra- and interobserver variation for PWS is acceptable (Heng et al, 2008), making reliable in studies the utilization of PWS for rupture risk evaluation.

The expansion of the small AAAs is a multifactorial process, where biomechanical and biological factors interact (Dua & Dalman, 2010). It is well documented that cells along the aortic wall can respond biochemically to mechanical stress (Nakahashi et al, 2002). In early stages of AAA enlargement the elastin degradation induced by the wall shear stress (ie. the tangential force exerted by the movement of blood along the axis of flow) elevates the wall stress but accelerates sac enlargement, despite the stress-mediated collagen turnover (Sheidaei et al, 2011).

Slow growth rate in smaller AAAs has been proven to be associated with low stress values, whereas a rapid growth rate in this category seems to depend on the amount of intaluminal thrombus (ILT) rather than on the level of wall stress, which is decreased (Speelman et al, 2010). The presence of ILT promotes elastolytic activity with consequent structural degradation of the adjacent AAA wall (Kazi at al, 2003 and Wiernicki et al, 2010). These findings have been also confirmed recently by Parr et al (Parr et al, 2011), who reported a strong correlation of AAA rapid growth rate with the initial AAA diameter ($r = 0.44$, $P = .006$) and thrombus volume ($r = 0.50$, $P = 0.001$).

4. Evaluating the AAA geometry

PWS has been clearly associated with the risk of rupture. Wall stress has been found to be 12% more specific and 13% more sensitive in rupture prediction than maximum diameter alone and may differentiate ruptured and symptomatic small AAAs from the asymptomatic ones (Truijers et al, 2007; Vande Geest et al, 2008; Fillinger et al, 2003). Its values depend on the mechanical properties and the geometric configuration of the aneurysm wall (Raghavan et al, 2005). PWS estimation requires highly experienced personnel in a process that can require considerable power to run (Leung et al, 2006). Therefore, a useful adjunct tightly related to PWS assessment could provide great help regarding the rupture risk or growth rate estimation. The association of certain geometric parameters with high values of PWS has been demonstrated in many studies. This paragraph summarizes the most important of these studies, underscoring the importance of geometric parameters as potential adjunctive parameters along with maximum diameter and elevated PWS in rupture risk assessment.

Nathan et al (Nathan et al, 2010) studied the differences between saccular and fusiform descending thoracic aortic aneurysms. Although the saccular aneurysms in his study were of smaller diameter than the fusiform ones, the mean PWS was equivalent between the two groups. Since the elevated rupture risk of saccular aneurysms has been well defined in the literature, the abovementioned findings could imply that factors such as aneurysm shape influence the PWS values more effectively than maximum diameter, thus predisposing smaller AAAs having a rupture risk comparable to that of larger AAAs. Complex geometry contributes to equivalently complex stress distribution, with regions of high curvature being associated with high stress values (Sacks et al, 1999). The actual, individualized AAA geometry is the main reason for the non-uniform distribution of stress in the wall. Local anatomy can influence the AAA growth rate 1.5-fold greater than the traditional risk factors (e.g. gender, age, hypertension, heart disease, hypercholesterolemia, renal failure, chronic obstructive pulmonary disease (COPD), smoking, diabetes mellitus and peripheral disease) (Helderman et al, 2010). Furthermore, Pappu et al suggested that an increase in mean tortuosity of the centerline correlated better with rupture of small AAA than an increase in mean transverse diameter (Pappu et al, 2008).

Advanced patient-specific computational models can be used to assess the correlation between PWS and 3D geometric features. Giannoglou et al (Giannoglou et al, 2006) reported a strong relationship between PWS values and the centerline curvature in AAA models, whereas Doyle et al (Doyle et al, 2010) advocated a correlation between PWS and centerline asymmetry. Both studies were based on computational models without taking into account the presence of thrombus. Others have reported a correlation between PWS and centerline tortuosity in AAA models with ILT (Georgakarakos et al, 2010). While the major difference in the abovementioned studies is whether or not ILT was integrated into the model, they all agree that geometric features will play a significant role in prospective studies estimating the risk of AAA expansion or rupture. While the correlation of these 3D geometric features with maximum diameter (making them dependent variables) reduces the impact of these findings, they may be used as adjuncts to diameter.

Geometric parameters can affect the hemodynamic behavior of AAAs, which in turn could have an important implication regarding the prognosis of rupture or the estimation of the aneurysm distension rate. Li and Kleinstreuer showed that an AAA neck angle substantially impacts flow fields, causing strong irregular vortices in the AAA sac, remarkably influencing wall stress distribution (Li & Kleinstreuer, 2006). Furthermore, Xenos et al (Xenos et al, 2010a) showed that the peak value of von Mises stress increases as the iliac angle increases. Specifically, the increase in the iliac bifurcation angle is associated with constantly high stress values of Von Mises stress values in this area; yet, when these blood stagnation points were exluded, an overall decrease of the mean stress values in the rest of the AAA wall (ie. sac wall) was revealed.

As small AAAs enlarge, a variety of geometrical changes can take place, including the length and angulation of AAA neck, the asymmetry of the centerline, the tortuosity of iliac arteries and the angulation of the iliac bifurcation (Georgakarakos et al, 2011b). Certain geometric changes, especially in the iliac bifurcation, have been postulated to mirror an adaptation response during the aneurysmal progression disease, in an attempt to alter the wall stress distribution patterns and decline the stress values, in favor of rupture risk attenuation and AAA growth deceleration. The increase in iliac angulation seems to lower the stress values in the AAA wall with instantaneous increase in iliac bifurcation stress values (blood stagnation site), trying to re-distribute the mechanical load at sites less prone to rupture (**Figure 4**), being the iliac site (Xenos et al, 2010).

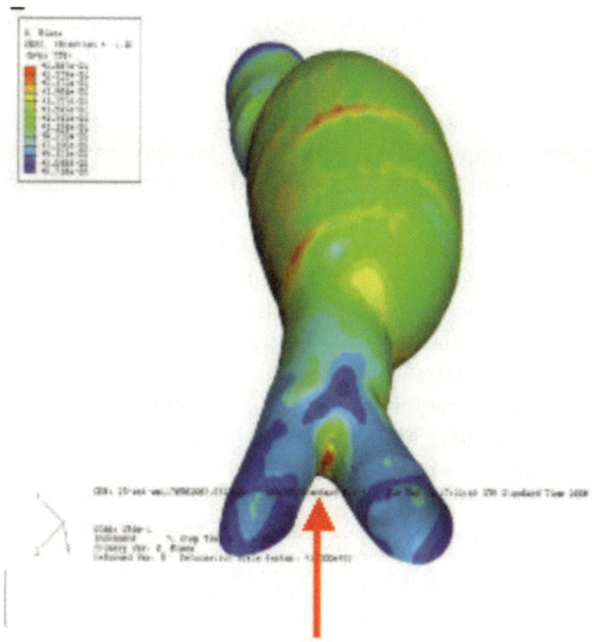

Fig. 4. The iliac bifurcation is generally assumed to be a site less susceptible to rupture. In the early stages of AAA enlargement, accumulation of high stress values in this area by certain geometrical adaptations can be considered as an adaptation response, in order to reduce stress in other wall areas.

5. Association of mechanical stress and biomarkers

Mechanical and biological factors have been implicated in the growth rate of the small AAAs, apart from the aforementioned clinical factors. Increased levels of Metalloproteinase-2 (MMP-2) have been implicated in the degradation of elastine in the small AAAs wall, leading to their generation and expansion, whereas the increased expression of MMP-9 leads to accelerated expansion of the larger AAAs and rupture (Choke et al, 2005).
AAA wall degeneration or alteration of integral properties induced by biochemical factors such as metalloproteinases (MMPs) and mechanical loading constitute a field to focus on, since there has been growing evidence of pathogenic correlation between these factors. The mechanical loading of the AAA wall, as expressed by PWS, has been implicated in the expansion of small AAAs, since a relative low wall stress was associated with a lower aneurysm rate, as reported by Speelman et al (Speelman et al, 2010a). The ratio of wall stress to the maximum diameter of the AAA has been postulated to be a valuable index for predicting AAA growth. Interestingly, the latter study reconfirmed also the positive relation of MMP-9 to increased growth rate, despite the fact that no correlation between MMP-9 and wall stress was found, implying that AAAs in patients with high wall stress/max Diameter values may undergo more rapid growth and wall damage than those with low wall stress/max Diameter values. AAA growth is most likely a multifactorial phenomenon, possibly combining biological and mechanical effects, as well as dynamic flow effects through the AAA (Khanafer et al, 2007).

Rahman et al studied the levels of MMPs in areas of low and high wall stress values in the AAA wall (Rahman et al, 2011). Finite Element Analysis was used to estimate the values and distribution areas of low and peak wall stress (PWS) on the wall of AAAs before surgery. These areas were accordingly mapped out and excised intraoperatively, providing tissue samples for MMPs analysis. Elevated levels of MMP levels were detected at areas of PWS compared to areas of low stress, despite that fact that no statistical significance was reached (possibly attributed to type 2 statistical error). Moreover, small AAAs with rapid growth rate can be differentiated from small ones of slower growth rate by the high values of wall stress at the area of inflection between the neck and the AAA sac (Li, 2010a and Li et al, 2010b). Localized geometric abnormalities correlate with high PWS values (Sacks et al, 1999) which can induce an increased inflammatory reaction (Xu et al, 2010) and overexpression of MMPs, thus attenuating the structural integrity of the sac wall. The abovementioned findings underscore the importance of interconnection between biomechanical factors and bioengineering tools for the study, identification and prediction of small AAAs prone to rapid growth and/or rupture.

6. Mechanical properties of the wall

The computational estimation of PWS with Finite Element Analysis models relies strongly on the material properties data input into these models. In most studies the AAA wall has been assumed to be hyperelastic, incompressible and isotropic material (Georgakarakos et al, 2011a). The values of these parameters represent mean data derived from large-scale population tissue mechanical studies. However, there is increasing evidence of the anisotropic properties of the AAA wall, ie the preferential stiffness of the wall in one plane compared to the other, as a result of heterogeneous mechanical behavior of the structural substrate, depended on the orientation of the collagen fibers (Rissland et al, 2009 and Rodríguez et al, 2008, 2009). Whether the adaptation of the anisotropic wall properties in the computational models yields statistically significant difference in the evaluation of the PWS values and distribution, thus affecting the rupture risk computation, remains to be delineated in large-scale studies.

Moreover, rupture risk estimates or expansion-rate predictions should be obtained in a patient-specific basis, since mechanical parameters in AAAs such as segmental dilation and compliance, stiffness and pressure strain elastic modulus vary among AAAs from different patients and variable maximum diameters (Long et al, 2004, 2005; Wilson et al, 2003). AAA rupture is associated with aortic wall weakening as a result of discordant repair / remodeling mechanisms, mirrored by an increase in thickness and a decrease in stiffness, correlated with decreased strength (Di Martino et al, 2006). Since different AAA of the same maximum diameter can have different strength levels, it seems that noninvasive techniques to estimate mechanical properties of the AAA wall would be a helpful adjunct for prediction of AAA rupture risk.

Strength is calculated from a mathematical type which takes into account the square root of the ILT thickness, the presence of positive family history, the gender, smoking status and age of the patient and the normalized diameter (Vande Geest et al, 2006a), strength = $71.9 - 37.9\ (ILT^{1/2} - 0.81) - 15.6\ (NORD - 2.46) - 21.3\ HIST + 19.3\ SEX$, where ILT is the local attached ILT thickness in cm; NORD is the local diameter normalized to the diameter of the non-aneurysmal aorta (infrarenal) estimated form the patient's age and sex (Raghavan et al, 2000); HIST is the family history (1/2 with history, -1/2 without history); and SEX is patient's gender (1/2 male, -1/2 female).

Since the wall strength presents a spatial distribution along the AAA wall, an accurate method to estimate rupture-risk on a patient-specific model should take into account not only PWS, but also the local wall strength variation (Vorp et al, 2005). The Rupture Potential Index (RPI) estimates the ratio of local PWS to local wall strength, RPI = Local wall stress (N/cm^2) / Local wall strength (N/cm^2). The importance of simultaneous incorporation of the wall strength in the rupture risk prediction is underscored in a recent retrospective study, where the rupture risk indices between 15 men and 15 women were compared. Taken into account the reported higher rupture risk for women, it was interesting to note that though PWS values did not differ between the 2 groups, the difference in peak wall rupture risk between the groups almost approached statistical significance ($P = .06$), suggesting also that differences in biomechanical properties could contribute to the higher rupture risk reported for women.

Small patient series have provided promising results regarding the utility of RPI in the prediction of rupture as well as the detection of the rupture site (Xenos et al, 2010b). Larger-scale prospective clinical trials are needed for validation of RPI as a predictive tool for rupture, before this tool can be sufficiently incorporated into routine clinical practice.

7. The intraluminal thrombus

ILT is generated by activated platelets that aggregate toward the AAA wall. For the generation of ILT the following seem to be essential a) a proximal recirculating zone, with b) high values of wall shear stress (WSS), so that the platelets can sustain the WSS long enough, to get activated and aggregate (Biasetti et al, 2010). The aggregation sites are preferably located in areas of low WSS. The frequently observed asymmetric ILT distribution (**Figure 5A**) can be attributed to the asymmetry and complexity of the flow in asymmetric AAAs (**Figure 5B**), (Ekaterinaris et al, 2006 and Bluestein et al, 2009).

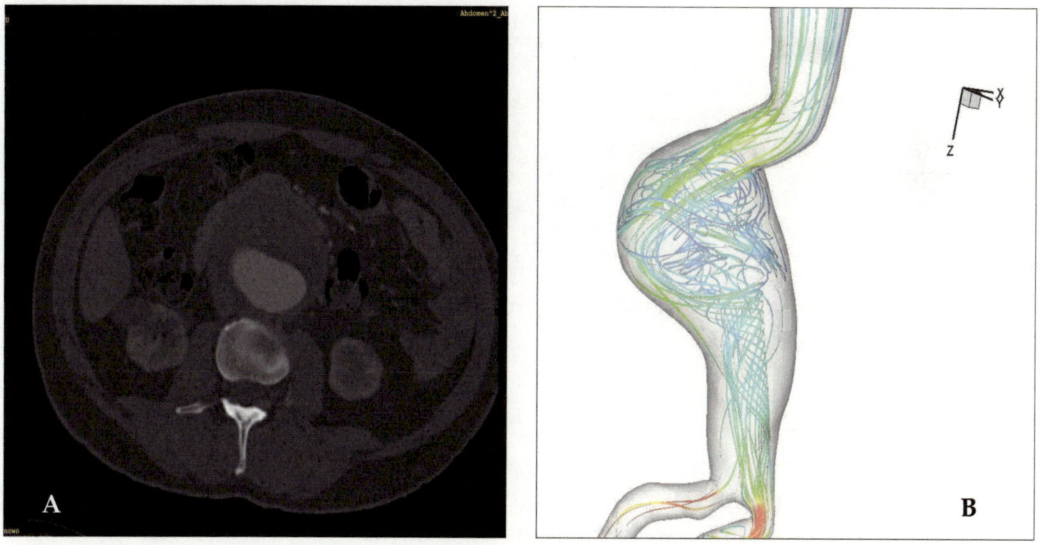

Fig. 5. A) Aneurysm sac with asymmetric distribution of intraluminal thrombus (eccentric, anterior). B) Complex flow ribbons in the AAA lumen. The inferiorly-anteriorly located thrombus causes narrowing of the lower sac, which in turn, induces the complex flow pattern above.

The integration of intraluminal thrombus (ILT) on the FEA models plays a crucial role in the estimation of wall stress values and stress distribution (Georgakarakos et al, 2009 and Wang et al, 2002). ILT consists of 3 layers (abluminal, medial and luminal) with marked differences in mechanical properties and structure (**Figure 6A**). The luminal layer (**Figure 6B**) consists of a network of fibrin fibers, with Young's modulus values 54 and 57 N/cm^2 in the longitudinal and circumferential directions, respectively (van 't Veer et al, 2008). The medial layer shows some degree of degeneration of the fibrin fibers and presents a 33 and 27 N/cm^2 in the longitudinal and circumferential directions, respectively (Wang et al, 2001). Finally, the abluminal layers appear too degenerated (**Figure 6C**) to be tested on vitro for determination of the mechanical properties. Vande Geest et al performed planar biaxial testing on the luminal layer of ILT and estimated the maximum tangential modulus to be 23.1 and 20.1 N/cm^2 in the longitudinal and circumferential directions, respectively (Vande Geest et al, 2006b). Di Marino et al (Di Marino et al, 1998) estimated the range of ILT Young's modulus to be 5-20 N/cm^2, whereas Hinnen et al (Hinnen et al, 2007) 1.3-5.9 N/cm^2.

It is clear that there is a wide variation in the mechanical properties of ILT. The mechanical properties of the thrombus vary not only within the ILT volume of a given AAA but also between different ILTs (Ashton et al, 2009; van Dam et al, 2008). Consequently, the hemodynamic load on the AAA wall can be modified by the variations in local thickness, shear modulus and volume of ILT (Speelman et al, 2010b). Moreover, the varying mechanical properties of the thrombus account for the large variability in its compressibility (Truijers et al, 2009), which could influence its protective role against AAA rupture or sac enlargement. Furthermore, fissures in ILT can breach the ILT "cushion" effect, resulting in increase in wall stress in the underlying AAA wall (Polzer et al, In Press).

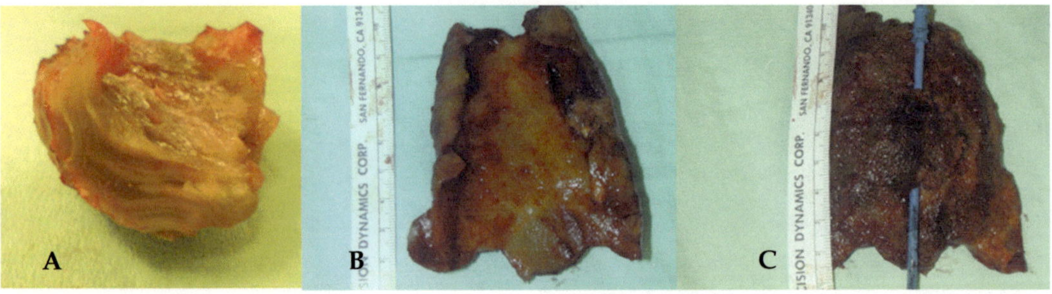

Fig. 6. A) The different layers of intraluminal thrombus (ILT), B) The luminal surface of ILT, C) The abluminal surface of ILT.

8. Conclusion

AAA rupture is a matter of deficient wall strength and increased hemodynamic loading. Therefore, reliable rupture risk estimation should take into account both the local distribution of wall stress and wall strength. Refinements in computational methods of these parameters could lead to identification of high-risk aneurysms, patient-specific risk assessment, detailed geometric characterization of AAAs and precise follow-up of aneurysm growth. The development of hybrid models that would take into account the geometric, biomechanical and biologic factors in a patient-specific basis is awaited with great interest. Furthermore, advances in ultrasound and dynamic MRI imaging are expected to provide us with important information regarding the material properties of ILT over the cardiac cycle, the spatial variance of compliance, stiffness and distensibility of the AAA wall and, finally a detailed mapping of the AAA wall thickness. The aforementioned elements are necessary for improvement of accurate, reliable patient-specific prediction models of rupture risk.

9. References

Ashton JH, VandeGeest JP, Simon BR & Haskett DG. (2009). Compressive mechanical properties of the intraluminal thrombus in abdominal aortic aneurysms and fibrin-based thrombus mimics. *J Biomech.*;42:197-201.

Biasetti J, Gasser TC, Auer M, Hedin U & Labruto F. (2010). Hemodynamics of the normal aorta compared to fusiform and saccular abdominal aortic aneurysms with emphasis on a potential thrombus formation mechanism. *Ann Biomed Eng.*; 38:380-90.

Bluestein D, Dumont K, De Beule M, Ricotta J, Impellizzeri P, Verhegghe B & Verdonck P. (2009). Intraluminal thrombus and risk of rupture in patient specific abdominal aortic aneurysm - FSI modelling. *Comput Methods Biomech Biomed Engin.*; 12:73-81.

Brewster DC, Cronenwett JL, Hallett JW, Johnston KW, Krupski WC, & Matsumura JS. (2003). Guidelines for the treatment of abdominal aortic aneurysms. Report of a subcommittee of the Joint Council of the American Association for Vascular Surgery and Society for Vascular Surgery. *J Vasc Surg*; 37:1106-17.

Di Martino E, Bohra A, Vande Geest JP, Gupta N, Makaroun MS & Vorp DA. (2006). Biomechanical properties of ruptured versus electively repaired abdominal aortic aneurysm wall tissue. *J Vasc Surg.*; 43:570-576.

Choke E, Cockerill G, Wilson WRW, Sayed S, Dawson J, Loftus I & Thompson MM. (2005). A review of biological factors implicated in abdominal aortic aneurysm rupture. *Eur J Vasc Endovasc Surg*; 30:227-244.

Di Martino E, Mantero S, Inzoli F, Melissano G, Astore D, Chiesa R & Fumero R. (1998). Biomechanics of abdominal aortic aneurysm in the presence of endoluminal thrombus: experimental characterisation and structural static computational analysis. *Eur J Vasc Endovasc Surg.*; 15:290-9.

Doyle BJ, Callanan A, Burke PE, Grace PA, Walsh MT, Vorp DA & McGloughlin TM. (2009). Vessel asymmetry as an additional diagnostic tool in the assessment of abdominal aortic aneurysms. *J Vasc Surg.*; 49:443-454.

Dua MM & Dalman RL. (2010). Hemodynamic influences on abdominal aortic aneurysm disease: Application of biomechanics to aneurysm pathophysiology. *Vascul Pharmacol.*; 53:11-21.

Ekaterinaris JA, Ioannou CV & Katsamouris AN. (2006). Flow dynamics in expansions characterizing abdominal aorta aneurysms. *Ann Vasc Surg.*; 20:351-9.

Fillinger MF, Raghavan ML, Marra SP, Cronenwett JL & Kennedy FE. (2002). In vivo analysis of mechanical wall stress and abdominal aortic aneurysm rupture risk. *J Vasc Surg.*; 36:589-597.

Fillinger MF, Marra SP, Raghavan ML & Kennedy FE. (2003). Prediction of rupture risk in abdominal aortic aneurysm during observation: wall stress versus diameter. *J Vasc Surg.*; 37:724-732.

Georgakarakos E, Ioannou CV, Volanis, Y Papaharilaou, J Ekaterinaris & Katsamouris AN. (2009). The Influence of Intraluminal Thrombus on Abdominal Aortic Aneurysm Wall Stress. *Int Angio*l; 28:325-333.

Georgakarakos E, Ioannou CV, Kamarianakis Y, Papaharilaou Y, Kostas T, Manousaki E & Katsamouris AN. (2010). The Role of Geometric Parameters in the Prediction of Abdominal Aortic Aneurysm Wall Stress. *Eur J Vasc Endovasc Surg*; 39: 42-48.

Georgakarakos E, Ioannou CV, Papaharilaou Y, Kostas T & Katsamouris AN. (*2011a*). Computational evaluation of airtic aneurysm rupture risk: what have we learned so far? *J Endovasc Ther.; 18:* 214-25.

Georgakarakos E, Ioannou CV, Georgiadis GS, Kapoulas K, Schoretsanitis N & Lazarides M. (*2011b*). Expanding Current EVAR Indications to Include Small Abdominal Aortic Aneurysms: A Glimpse of the Future. *Angiology;* In Press, doi: 10.1177/0003319711398651.

Giannoglou G, Giannakoulas G, Soulis J, Chatzizisis Y, Perdikides T, Melas N, Parcharidis G & Louridas G. (2006). Predicting the risk of rupture of abdominal aortic aneurysms by utilizing various geometrical parameters: revisiting the diameter criterion. *Angiology.*; 57:487-494.

Larsson E, Labruto F, Gasser TC, Swedenborg J & Hultgren R. (In Press) Analysis of aortic wall stress and rupture risk in patients with abdominal aortic aneurysm with a gender perspective. *J Vasc Surg*; doi:10.1016/j.jvs.2010.12.053.

Helderman F, Manoch IJ, Breeuwer M, Kose U, Boersma H, van Sambeek MR, Pattynama PM & Schouten O. (2010). Predicting patient-specific expansion of abdominal aortic aneurysms. *Eur J Vasc Endovasc Surg.*; 40:47-53.

Heng MS, Fagan MJ, Collier JW, Desai G, McCollum PT & Chetter IC. (2008). Peak wall stress measurement in elective and acute abdominal aortic aneurysms. *J Vasc Surg.*; 47:17-22.

Hinnen JW, Rixen DJ, Koning OH, van Bockel JH & Hamming JF. (2007). Development of fibrinous thrombus analogue for in-vitro abdominal aortic aneurysm studies. *J Biomech.*; 40:289-95.

Kazi M, Thyberg J, Religa P, Roy J, Eriksson P, Hedin U & Swedenborg J. (2003). Influence of intraluminal thrombus on structural and cellular composition of abdominal aortic aneurysm wall. *J Vasc Surg.*; 38:1283-92.

Khanafer KM, Bull JL, Upchurch GR Jr & Berguer R. (2007). Turbulence significantly increases pressure and fluid shear stress in an aortic aneurysm model under resting and exercise flow conditions. *Ann Vasc Surg*; 21:67-74.

Leung JH, Wright AR, Cheshire N, Crane J, Thom SA, Hughes AD & Xu Y. (2006). Fluid structure interaction of patient specific abdominal aortic aneurysms: a comparison with solid stress models. *Biomed Eng Online.*; 5:33.

Li Z & Kleinstreuer C. (2006). Effects of blood flow and vessel geometry on wall stress and rupture risk of abdominal aortic aneurysms. *J Med Eng Technol.*; 30:283-297.

Li ZY, Sadat U, U-King-Im J, Tang TY, Bowden DJ, Hayes PD & Gillard JH. (2010a). Association between aneurysm shoulder stress and abdominal aortic aneurysm expansion: a longitudinal follow-up study. *Circulation*; 122:1815-22.

Li ZY. (2010). Computed wall stress may predict the growth of abdominal aortic aneurysm. Conf *Proc IEEE Eng Med Biol Soc.* 2010b;: 2626-9.

Long A, Rouet L, Bissery A, Goeau-Brissonniere O & Sapoval M. (2004). Aortic compliance in healthy subjects: evaluation of tissue Doppler imaging. *Ultrasound Med Biol.*; 30:753-9.

Long A, Rouet L, Bissery A, Rossignol P, Mouradian D & Sapoval M. (2004). Compliance of abdominal aortic aneurysms: evaluation of tissue Doppler imaging. *Ultrasound Med Biol.*; 30:1099-108.

Long A, Rouet L, Bissery A, Rossignol P, Mouradian D & Sapoval M. (2005). Compliance of abdominal aortic aneurysms evaluated by tissue Doppler imaging: correlation with aneurysm size. *J Vasc Surg.*; 42:18-26.

Malkawi AH, Hinchliffe RJ, Xu Y, Holt PJ, Loftus IM & Thompson MM. (2010). Patient-specific biomechanical profiling in abdominal aortic aneurysm development and rupture. *J Vasc Surg.*; 52:480-8.

Nakahashi TK, Hoshina K, Tsao PS, Sho E, Sho M, Karwowski JK, Yeh C, Yang RB, Topper JN & Dalman RL. (2002). Flow loading induces macrophage antioxidative gene expression in experimental aneurysms. Arterioscler Thromb Vasc Biol.; 22:2017-22.

Nathan D, Xu C, Brinster C, Gorman R, Gorman III J, Desjardins B, Wang G, Woo E, Fairman R & Jackson B. (2010). Rupture risk of saccular descending thoracic aortic aneurysms by stress modeling. J Am Coll Surg.; 211; Suppl 1, S143-S144.

Papaharilaou Y, Ekaterinaris J, Manousaki E & Katsamouris AN. (2007). A decoupled fluid structure approach of estimating wall stress in abdominal aortic aneurysms. *J Biomech.*; 40:367–377.

Pappu S, Dardik A, Tagare H & Gusberg RJ. (*2008*). Beyond fusiform and saccular: a novel quantitative tortuosity index may help classify aneurysm shape and predict aneurysm rupture potential. *Ann Vasc Surg.*; 22:88-97.

Parr A, McCann M, Bradshaw B, Shahzad A, Buttner P & Golledge J. (2011). Thrombus volume is associated with cardiovascular events and aneurysm growth in patients who have abdominal aortic aneurysms. *J Vasc Surg.*; 53:28-35.

Polzer S, Gasser TC, Swedenborg J & Bursa J. (In Press). The Impact of Intraluminal Thrombus Failure on the Mechanical Stress in the Wall of Abdominal Aortic Aneurysms. Eur J Vasc Endovasc Surg., doi:10.1016/j.ejvs.2010.12.010.

Raghavan ML, Fillinger MF, Marra SP, Naegelein BP & Kennedy FE. (*2005a*). Automated methodology for determination of stress distribution in human abdominal aortic aneurysm. *J Biomech Eng.*; 127:868-71.

Raghavan ML, Kratzberg JA & Golzarian J. (2005b). Introduction to biomechanics related to endovascular repair of abdominal aortic aneurysm. *Tech Vasc Interv Radiol.*; 8:50-5.

Raghavan ML & Vorp DA. (2000). Toward a biomechanical tool to evaluate rupture potential of abdominal aortic aneurysm: identification of a finite strain constitutive model and evaluation of its applicability, *J Biomech*; 33:475-482.

Rahman MN, Khan JA, Mazari FA, Mockford K, McCollum PT & Chetter IC. (2011). A randomized placebo controlled trial of the effect of preoperative statin use on matrix metalloproteinases and tissue inhibitors of matrix metalloproteinases in areas of low and peak wall stress in patients undergoing elective open repair of abdominal aortic aneurysm. Ann Vasc Surg.; 25:32-8.

Rissland P, Alemu Y, Einav S, Ricotta J & Bluestein D. (2009). Abdominal aortic aneurysm risk of rupture: patient-specific FSI simulations using anisotropic model. *J Biomech Eng.*; 131:031001.

Rodríguez JF, Ruiz C, Doblaré M & Holzapfel GA. (2008). Mechanical stresses in abdominal aortic aneurysms: influence of diameter, asymmetry, and material anisotropy. *J Biomech Eng.*; 130:021023.

Rodríguez JF, Martufi G, Doblaré M & Finol EA. (2009). The effect of material model formulation in the stress analysis of abdominal aortic aneurysms. *Ann Biomed Eng.*; 37:2218-21.

Sacks MS, Vorp DA, Raghavan ML, Federle MP & Webster MW. (*1999).* In vivo three-dimensional surface geometry of abdominal aortic aneurysms. *Ann Biomed Eng.*; 27:469-79.

Scotti CM, Shkolnik AD, Muluk SC & Finol EA. (2005). Fluid-structure interaction in abdominal aortic aneurysms: effects of asymmetry and wall thickness. *Biomed Eng Online.*; 4:64.

Sheidaei A, Hunley SC, Zeinali-Davarani S, Raguin LG & Baek S. (2011). Simulation of abdominal aortic aneurysm growth with updating hemodynamic loads using a realistic geometry. *Med Eng Phys.*; 33(1):80-8.

Speelman L, Hellenthal FA, Pulinx B, Bosboom EM, Breeuwer M, van Sambeek MR, van de Vosse FN, Jacobs MJ, Wodzig WK & Schurink GW. (2010a). The influence of wall stress on AAA growth and biomarkers. Eur J Vasc Endovasc Surg.; 39: 410-6.

Speelman L, Schurink GW, Bosboom EM, Buth J, Breeuwer M, van de Vosse FN & Jacobs MH. (2010b). The mechanical role of thrombus on the growth rate of an abdominal aortic aneurysm. J Vasc Surg.; 51:19-26.

Steinman DA, Vorp DA & Ethier CR. (2003). Computational modeling of arterial biomechanics: insights into pathogenesis and treatment of vascular disease. J Vasc Surg.; 37:1118-28.

Tang BT, Cheng CP, Draney MT, Wilson NM, Tsao PS, Herfkens RJ & Taylor CA. (2006). Abdominal aortic hemodynamics in young healthy adults at rest and during lower limb exercise: quantification using image-based computer modeling. *Am J Physiol Heart Circ Physiol.*; 291:668-76.

Truijers M, Fillinger MF, Renema KW, Marra SP, Oostveen LJ, Kurvers HA, Schultzekool LJ & Blankensteijn JD. (2009). In-vivo imaging of changes in abdominal aortic aneurysm thrombus volume during the cardiac cycle. J Endovasc Ther.; 16:314-319.

Truijers M, Pol JA, Schultzekool LJ, van Sterkenburg SM, Fillinger MF & Blankensteijn JD. (2007). Wall stress analysis in small asymptomatic, symptomatic and ruptured abdominal aortic aneurysms. *Eur J Vasc Endovasc Surg.*; 33:401-407.

van Dam EA, Dams SD, Peters GW, Rutten MC, Schurink GW, Buth J & van de Vosse FN. (2008). Non-linear viscoelastic behavior of abdominal aortic aneurysm thrombus. *Biomech Model Mechanobiol.*; 7:127-37.

Vande Geest JP, Di Martino ES, Bohra A, Makaroun MS & Vorp DA. (2006a). A biomechanics-based rupture potential index for abdominal aortic aneurysm risk assessment: demonstrative application. *Ann N Y Acad Sci.*; 1085:11-21.

Vande Geest JP, Sacks MS & Vorp DA. (2006b). A planar biaxial constitutive relation for the luminal layer of intra-luminal thrombus in abdominal aortic aneurysms. *J Biomech.*; 39:2347-54.

Vande Geest JP, Schmidt DE, Sacks MS & Vorp DA. (2008). The effects of anisotropy on the stress analyses of patient-specific abdominal aortic aneurysms. *Ann Biomed Eng.*; 36:921-932.

van 't Veer M, Buth J, Merkx M, Tonino P, van den Bosch H, Pijls N & van de Vosse F. (2008). Biomechanical properties of abdominal aortic aneurysms assessed by simultaneously measured pressure and volume changes in humans. *J Vasc Surg.*; 48:1401-7.

Venkatasubramaniam AK, Fagan MJ, Mehta T, al KJ, Ray B, Kuhan G, Chetter IC &, McCollum PT. (2004). A comparative study of aortic wall stress using finite element analysis for ruptured and non-ruptured abdominal aortic aneurysms. *Eur J Vasc Endovasc Surg.*; 28:168-176.

Vorp DA & Vande Geest JP. (2005). Biomechanical determinants of abdominal aortic aneurysm rupture. *Arterioscler Thromb Vasc Biol.*; 25:1558-66.

Wang DH, Makaroun M, Webster MW & Vorp DA. (2001). Mechanical properties and microstructure of intraluminal thrombus from abdominal aortic aneurysm. *J Biomech Eng.*; 123:536-9.

Wang DH, Makaroun MS, Webster MW & Vorp DA. (2002). Effect of intraluminal thrombus on wall stress in patient-specific models of abdominal aortic aneurysm. *J Vasc Surg.*; 36:598-604.

Wiernicki I, Stachowska E, Safranow K, Cnotliwy M, Rybicka M, Kaczmarczyk M & Gutowski P. (2010). Enhanced matrix-degrading proteolytic activity within the thin thrombus-covered wall of human abdominal aortic aneurysms. *Atherosclerosis.*; 212:161-5.

Wilson KA, Lee AJ, Lee AJ, Hoskins PR, Fowkes FG & Ruckley CV, Bradbury AW. (2003). The relationship between aortic wall distensibility and rupture of infrarenal abdominal aortic aneurysm. *J Vasc Surg.*; 37:112-7.

Xenos M, Alemu Y, Zamfir D, Einav S, Ricotta JJ, Labropoulos N, Tassiopoulos A & Bluestein D. (2010a). The effect of angulation in abdominal aortic aneurysms: fluid-structure interaction simulations of idealized geometries. *Med Biol Eng Comput.*; 48:1175-90.

Xenos M, Rambhia SH, Alemu Y, Einav S, Labropoulos N, Tassiopoulos A, Ricotta JJ & Bluestein D. (2010b). Patient-based abdominal aortic aneurysm rupture risk prediction with fluid structure interaction modeling. *Ann Biomed Eng.*, 38:3323-37.

Xu XY, Borghi A, Nchimi A, Leung J, Gomez P, Cheng Z, Defraigne JO & Sakalihasan N. (2010). High levels of 18F-FDG uptake in aortic aneurysm wall are associated with high wall stress. *Eur J Vasc Endovasc Surg.*; 39:295-301.

11

An Analysis of Blood Flow Dynamics in AAA

Bernad I. Sandor[1], Bernad S. Elena[2],
Barbat Tiberiu[1], Brisan Cosmin[2] and Albulescu Vlad[2]
[1]*Romanian Academy – Timisoara Branch,*
[2]*University of Medicine and Pharmacy "Victor Babes" Timisoara,*
Romania

1. Introduction

The current standard for determination of AAA disease progression is external aneurysm diameter measurement (Vainas et al., 2003), where the diameter enlargement is an indirect cumulative indicator of disease progression.
Generally, the maximum diameter and expansion rate of the AAAs, obtained from ultrasound or CT scans is used to assess the risk of rupture. Surgical treatment is recommended when the maximum diameter of AAA measures 55 mm or above (Katz & Cronenwett, 1994; Lederle et al., 2002).
The untreated AAAs, tend to grow and may rupture or dissect upon reaching a diameter of 6–7 cm (Katz & Cronenwett, 1994). At this stage, it is likely that the arterial wall will no longer withstand the blood pressure, and surgical intervention is usually recommended for aneurysms 0.5 cm below than the critical diameter (Lederle et al., 2002).
Various past numerical and experimental studies were conducted to investigate blood flow patterns in the AAAs. Disturbance in blood flow influence physiological parameters and processes, pressure, wall shear stress (WSS), wall remodelling and inflammation (Fillinger et al., 2003).
In this work we describe the complexity of the blood flow using a time dependent analisys, to determine the effects of aneurysm asymmetry, wall shear stress distribution and vortex dynamics inside the aneurysm.

2. Patient and methods

The study subject was male (62 year old), and the AAA maximum transverse diameter was 6.4 cm. The total length of the AAA was 11.6 cm. Patient-specific computed tomography (CT) scans were obtained, in order to investigate the AAAs' wall shear stress.

2.1 Anatomical model reconstruction

To produce a realistic three-dimensional model of a patient anatomy, spiral CT (Somatom Sensation 64 Scanner - Siemens Medical Systems, Erlangen, Germany) data was then used to reconstruct the infrarenal section of the aorta. The selected patient had an anterior-posterior asymmetric aneurysm in the infrarenal aorta with a maximum diameter of approximately 6.4 cm (Figure 1). Digital files in Digital Imaging and Communications in Medicine

(DICOM) file format, containing cross-sectional information were then imported to CFD software package for reconstruction.

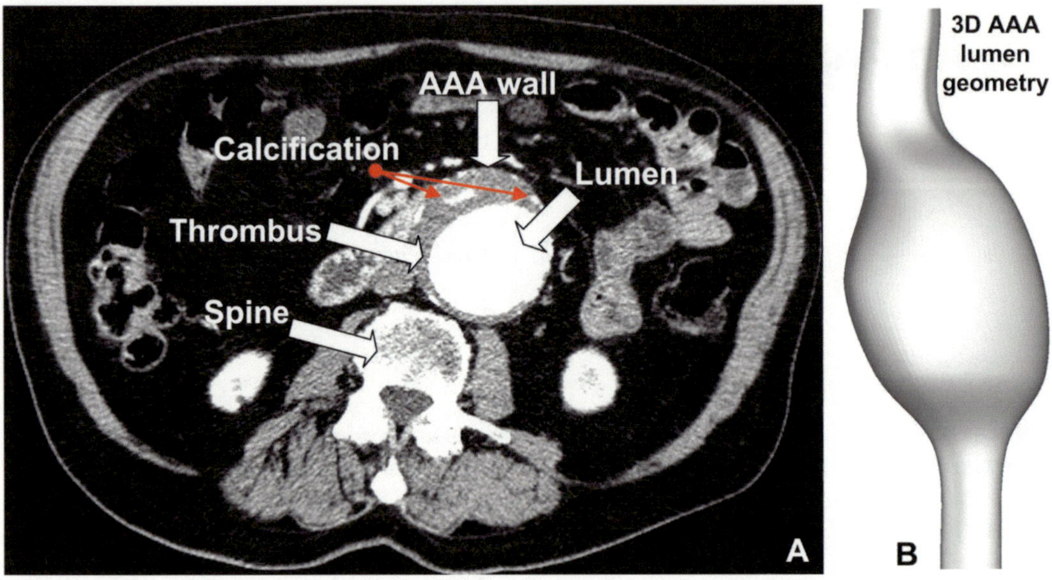

Fig. 1. CT scan and 3D reconstruction of the investigated section of the abdominal aorta. Axial cross-section CT slices are used for the three-dimensional reconstructions (A). 3D reconstruction of examined AAA (B). Anterior-posterior asymmetric AAA model result from the CT-scan.

The reconstructed aneurysm model is shown in Figure 2. The asymmetry parameter β (Figure 3) is defined as the ratio of the maximum posterior and anterior wall dimensions (Kleinstreuer & Vorp, 2006). Asymmetry parameter for the investigated patient are β =0.37.

The corresponding finite-element computational domain is composed of 574,280 hexahedral linear elements, for a total of 596,181 nodes. The software Gambit v2.4 (Ansys Fluent, Ansys Inc., 2006) was used for the mesh generation (Figure 4).

A fine resolution near the wall, with the height of the wall boundary cells (y+ < 2) and a minimum of at least 7 grid nodes inside the boundary layer was ensured for the geometry owing to the requirements of the numerical model.

Mesh independence study we performed in order to determine the optimum number of mesh elements. The optimum mesh size was determined once the peak wall shear stress does not increase by more than 2%.

2.2 Boundary conditions

At the inlet, a spatial velocity profile was imposed (Figure 5). These waveforms are triphasic pulses appropriate for normal hemodynamics conditions in the infrarenal segment of the human abdominal aorta first reported by Mills (Mills et al., 1970). The use of an input transient velocity based on normal physiology is justified by the fact that the inlet boundary condition is applied in the section of undilated segment of the abdominal aorta anterior the proximal neck of the aneurysm (Finol et al., 2003).

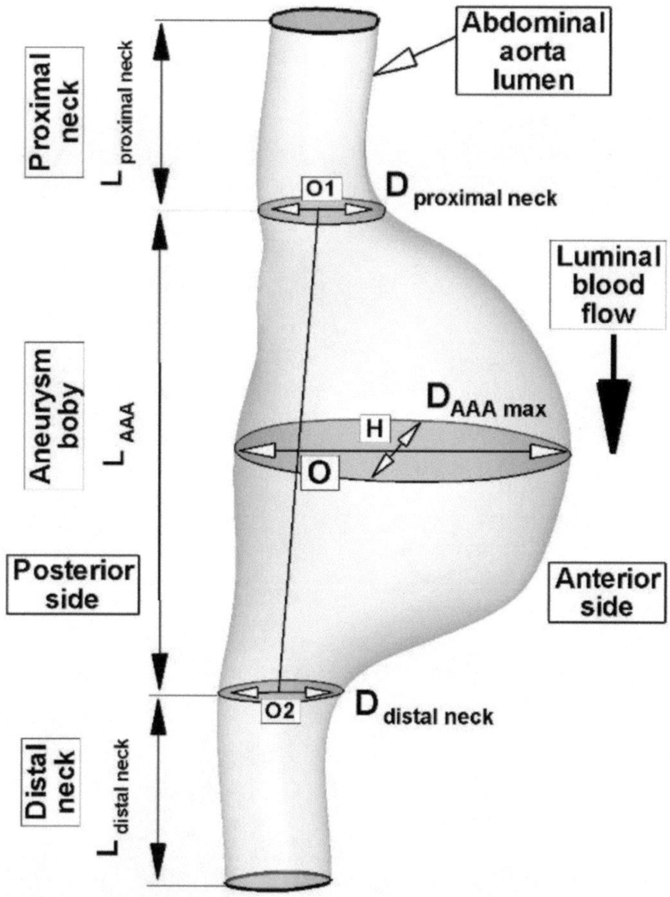

Fig. 2. Computational domain for asymmetry parameter β =0.37. Geometrical parameters used for AAA rupture risk evaluation.

In order to prevent overestimating the wall shear stress, a zero pressure state AAA has been used in present numerical simulations (Marra et al., 2005). No slip condition was applied at the fluid-wall interface. The cardiac cycle period was 1 s, with peak systolic flow occurring at 0.302s, and peak diastolic flow at 0.7s (Figure 5b). The length of the systolic and diastolic periods were 0.32s and 0.68s respectively. Blood was treated as a incompressible Newtonian fluid, an acceptable assumption for large arteries (Perktold et al., 1991).

Hemodynamic parameters are considered to be responsible for aneurysm initiation and growth. In majority of the computational studies, non Newtonian viscosity of blood, wall elasticity, blood particle composition and temperature effects are neglected, due to their secondary importance. The hemodynamic factors play a vital role in regulating the structure and functions of the endothelial layer.

We considered the dynamic viscosity of 0.004 Pas and density of 1050 kg/m3 for the blood (Table 1). The shear stress induced by blood flow was neglected in this study (Raghavan et al., 2000; Raghavan & Vorp, 2000; Thubricar et al., 2001), although the effects of blood flow have been shown to reduce wall stress by 10% in uniformly thick walled ideal models and by up to 30% in variable wall thickness models (Scotti et al., 2005).

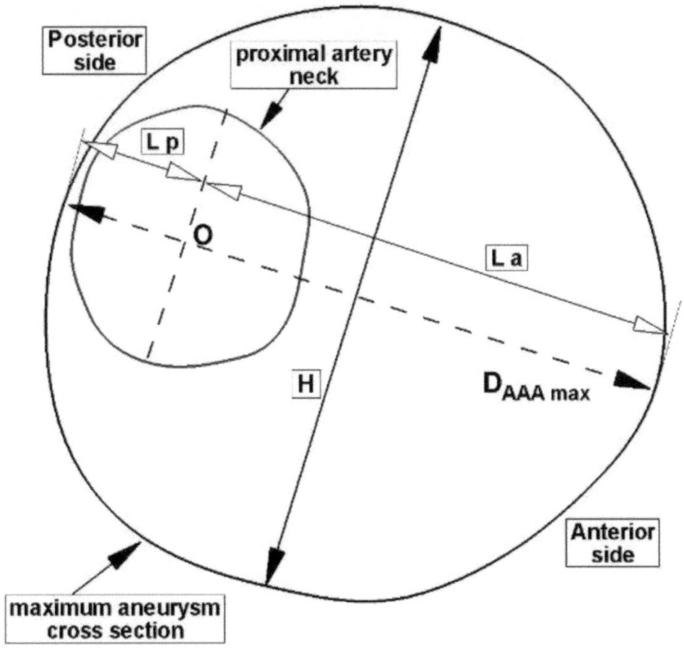

Fig. 3. Artery neck projected onto the plane of maximum aneurysm cross section.

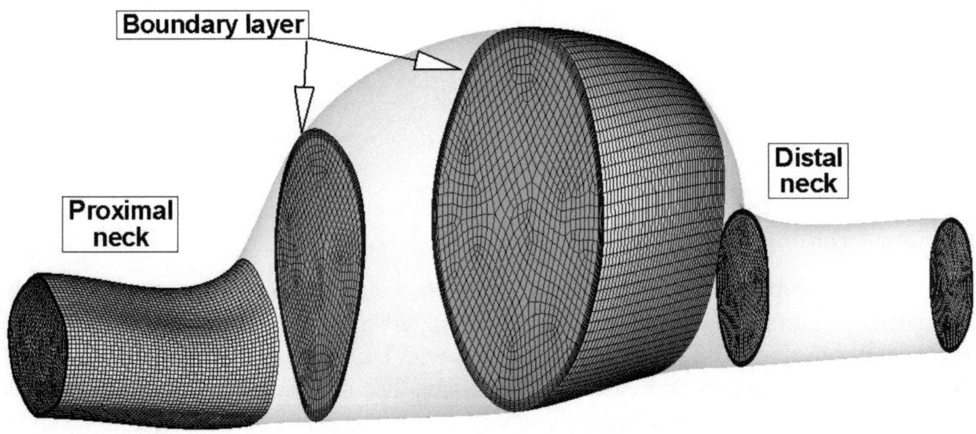

Fig. 4. Computational model for the patient specific reconstructed AAA. Intraluminal fluid mesh. Boundary layer contained 7 grid modes.

Incompressible, Newtonian flow is simulated for average resting conditions at a heart rate of 65 bpm. The governing equations are solved with the software Ansys FLUENT v6.3 (Ansys Inc.), which uses the finite volume method (FVM) for the spatial discretization. The workstations used to perform the simulations in this work is TYANPSC 600 (Tyan Computer Corporation) personal supercomputer with Intel® Xeon™ 5100 Dual Core, 40.0 GB RAM memory, and running on Windows® Compute Cluster Server 2003 operating system. The run time for a single simulation (on 8 processors) based on 3 consecutive pulsatile flow cycles was approximately 5 days real time.

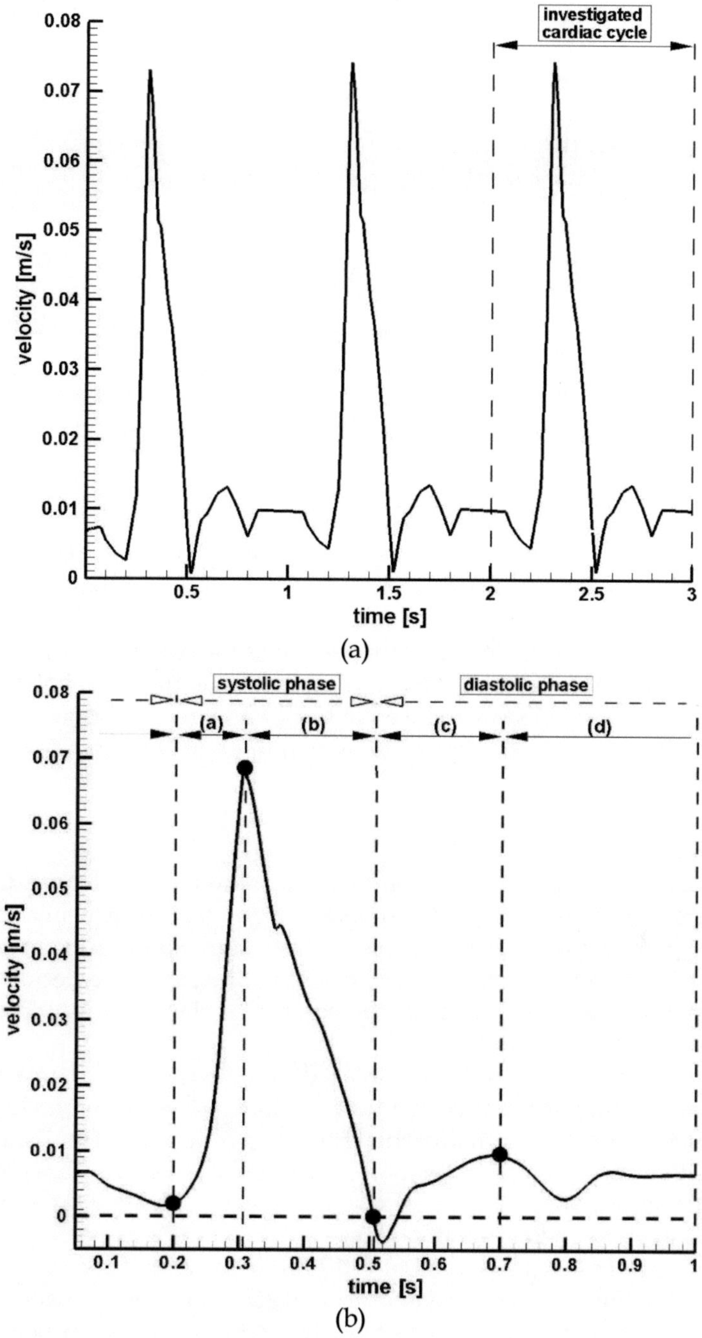

Fig. 5. Pulsatile velocity waveform reproduced from Scotti (Scotti et al., 2005). Enlarged view of the first three cardiac cycle (a). Peak systolic flow occurs at t=0.302 s and diastolic phase begins at t=0.52 s (b). In figure (b), we have: a - systolic acceleration, b - systolic deceleration, c - early diastole, d - late diastole.

Parameters	Normal artery[a]	Aneurysm[b]	Current simulation
Wall thickness	1.5 mm	0.5-2.0 mm	1.5 mm
Inner diameter	20 mm	40-80 mm	30-64 mm
Length	Inlet: 200 mm Outlet: 60 mm	80 mm	116 mm
Density	1120 kg/m^3	1120 kg/m^3	1050 kg/m^3
Others		Asymmetry: $0.45 \leq \beta \equiv L_p / L_a \leq 1$	Asymmetry: $\beta \equiv L_p / L_a \equiv 0.37$ (See Figure 4)

[a]Reference (Raghavan & Vorp, 2000),
[b]Reference (Di Martino et al., 2001).

Table 1. Parameters used in the numerical simulation

3. Results

Based on the AAA pulsatile flow (Figure 5b), the following four flow phases summarize the aneurysm's size and the asymmetry parameter both dependent of the flow dynamics (Finol et al., 2003):

1. *Systolic acceleration* involves downstream ejection of the residual vortices.
2. *Systolic deceleration* is characterized by flow separation in the proximal neck.
3. *Early diastole* is characterized by reduced in size of flow recirculation.
4. *Late diastole* is characterized by recirculation regions present downstream of the aneurysm midsection.

3.1 Velocity profiles

Aneurysm sac diameter, aspect ratio, aneurysm shape and parent artery diameter are the parametric factors known to influence the nature of blood flow within an aneurysm. In CFD as well as in experimental studies, the researchers studied intra aneurismal flow as a function of these geometric parameters. For example, the neck size decide the amount of flow entering in the aneurysm sac and the volume of the aneurysm deciding on how sluggish the flow in the aneurysm sac.

The investigated AAAs demonstrates complex flow patterns over the cardiac cycle. The effect of aneurysm asymmetry in pulsatile flow dynamics is depicted in Figures 6, 7 and 8. At peak flow t=0.3s (Figure 6a), a characteristic attached flow pattern is obtained throughout the aneurysm with nearly stagnant flow, present along the anterior wall where the diameter is the greatest (cross-section B-B). During systolic deceleration, flow separation occurs and the vortex begins to travel in the aneurysm sac.

The complex flow pattern was observed at t=0.7s near the exit of the proximal neck of the aneurysm, where the flow is intensified and recirculation zones are present (Figure 7b). This stage is depicted with significant and asymmetric flow recirculation near the aneurysm proximal neck (Figure 7b, cross-section A-A).

In Figure 7, we see an internal jet of fluid surrounded by a recirculating vortex. At the end of the systolic deceleration phase, a small recirculating vortex develops at the end of the proximal neck. During systolic deceleration and early diastole a large recirculating flow region fills the aneurysm sac.

Figures 6 and 7 illustrates secondary velocity vectors in the cross section of the aneurysm. At the time t=0.3s near the proximal neck of the aneurysm exhibits no significant secondary flow, but one large secondary vortice is obtained along the proximal neck of the aneurysm at the time t=0.7 s (Figure 7b).

We can see in Figures 6, 7 and 8 the flow in investigated AAA presents two regimes. The first regime with no vortex formation is presented in Figures 6 and 8a, and the second regime is with vortical structures (Figures 7 and 8b). These flow regimes, depend on the different phases of the cardiac cycle and on the aspect ratio of the aneurysm.

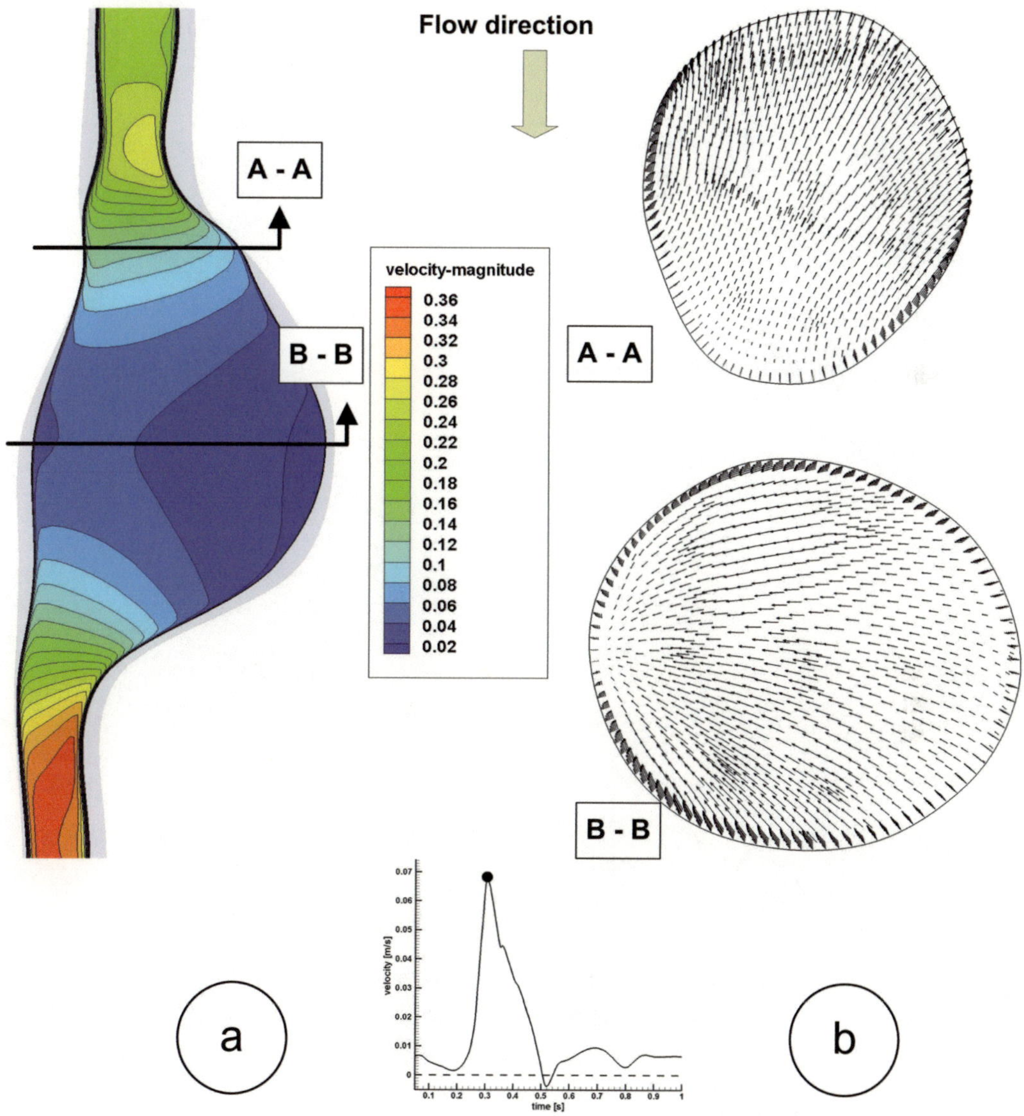

Fig. 6. Velocity field at the time t=0.3s, peak systole in the AAA. a) longitudinal section, velocity magnitude contour plot; b) velocity vector plot in cross-section; A-A in proximal neck and B-B in the maximum diameter region

The flow in the aneurysm decelerates and becomes unstable. This leads to flow separation, recirculation and possible transition to turbulence (Khanafer et al., 2007). Turbulence is induced by sudden expansion of the flow in the proximal neck (Figure 8b). This flow expansion generates recirculation region which produce additional wall shear stresses, increasing the rate of wall dilation (Khanafer et al., 2007).

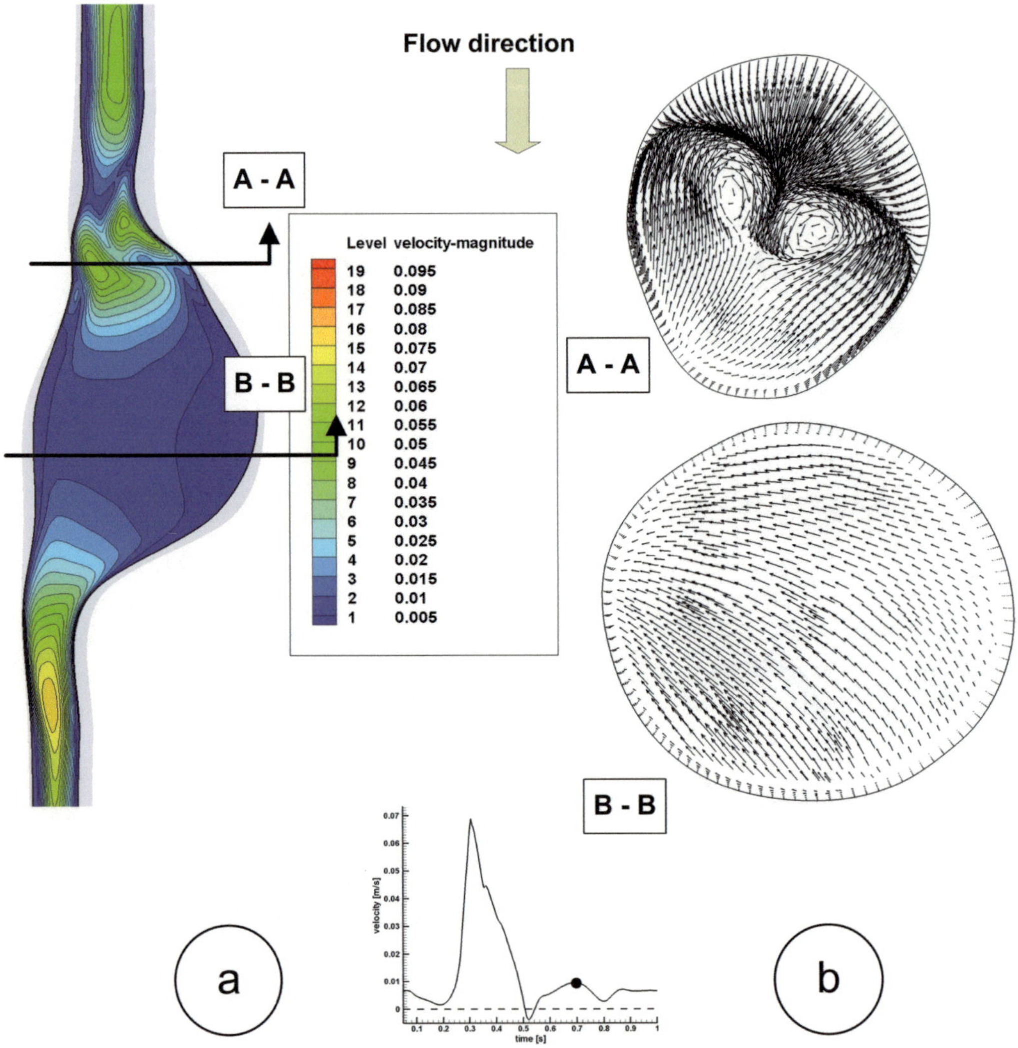

Fig. 7. Velocity magnitude b) Cross-section velocity vectors in proximal neck and maximum diameter region at the time t=0.7 s of the cardiac cycle. Vortical flow through the proximal neck.

3.2 Wall shear stress analysis

Throughout the cardiac cycle the wall shear stress distribution corresponds to the velocity gradients. Fluid shear stress is defined as a measure of the tangential forces per unit area generated by the flow stream on the walls of the AAA.

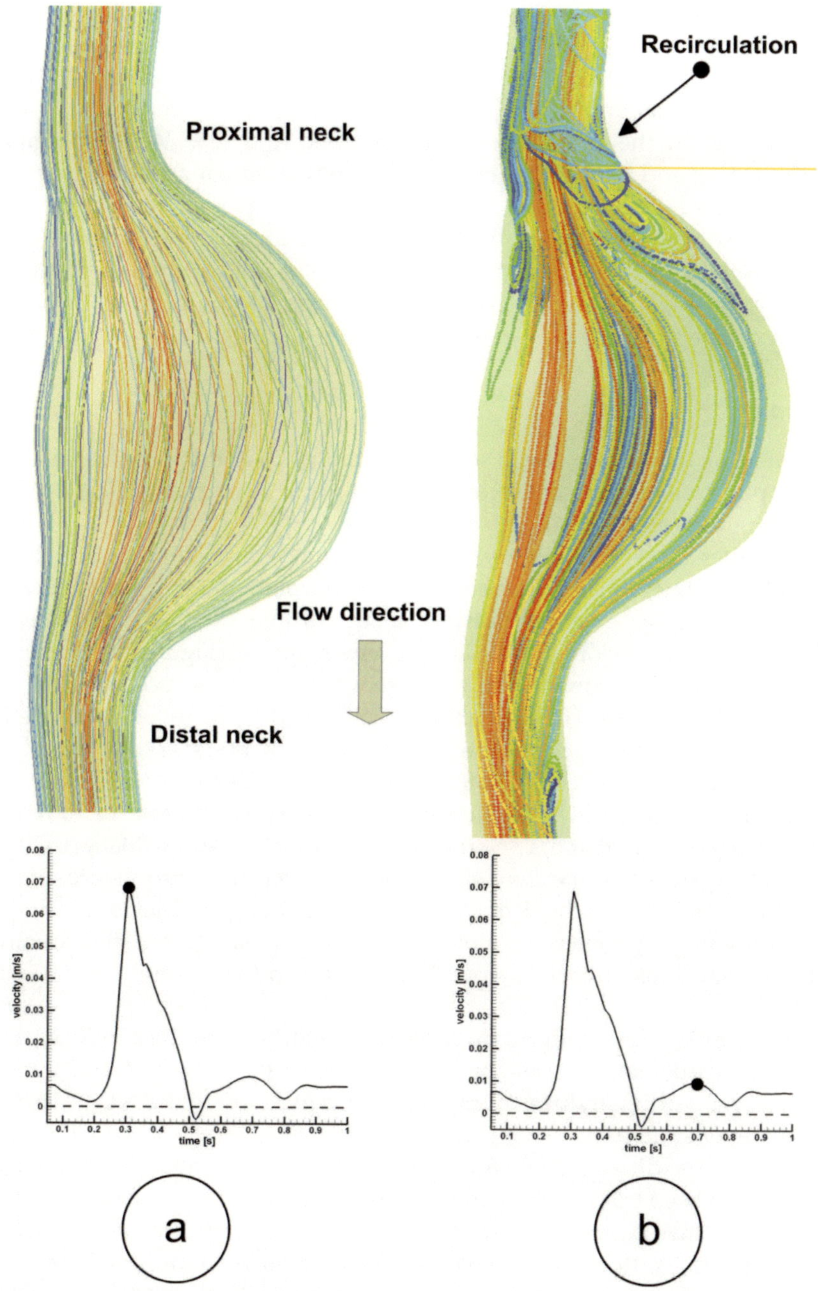

Fig. 8. a) 3D flow patern in the investigated AAA. b) Strong recirculation is present in the proximal neck and in the end of the distal neck. Helical flow is show inside to the aneurysm sac.

Along the maximum transversal diameter of the aneurysm, a slow recirculating flow exists, where the WSS is low. This flow pattern increase the residence time of blood along the aneurysm sac resulting in enhanced mass transfer.

Low wall shear stress in the range of ± 0.4 Pa plays a vital role in degenerating the endothelial layer, and resulting in an inflammatory cell response by initiating vascular wall remodeling (Malek 1999). We can see in Figure 9, that the WSS less than 0.4 Pa covered a wide area of the aneurysm body.

High WSS occurres in the proximal aneurysm neck, and low WSS in regions of flow separation (Figures 9 and 7). Sudden changes in cross-sectional area or in curvature cause local increment and adverse pressure gradient which creates low WSS in the aneurysm body (Figure 9). Regions of high WSS are likely to lead to matrix degradation by expression of plasmin, matrix-metalloproteinases and smooth muscle cells apoptosis (Ekaterinas et al., 2006). This may cause degenerative lesions of aneurysmal wall, altering the wall thickness and eventually causing rupture (Tan et al., 2008).

4. Discussion

Previous numerical studies in the literature, pointed that the flow in an aneurysm is complex with presence of vortices, secondary flows and strong amplification of instability (Venkatasubramaniam et al., 2004).

The velocity profiles showed highly disturbed flow and recirculation within the aneurysm sac. At the end of systole, the flow is a combination of rotational and recirculated secondary flows (Figures 7 and 8). Cross-sectional velocity profiles showed disturbed flow and recirculation in proximal neck region and in the aneurysm sac (Figure 7b).

During diastole the flow became instable and recirculation occurred almost everywhere in the aneurysm sac (Figure 8b). The flow patterns observed here, are characterized by helical flow and large recirculation zone. Same results found in literature for the blood flow in presence of the aneurysm (Tan et al., 2008; Boutsianis et al., 2009).

Disturbed flow induced by sudden expansion of the flow stream, results in additional stresses acting on the aneurysm wall that may be responsible for further aortic dilation. Dilation results in further radial expansion of the flow stream and in intensified turbulence. The latter then becomes a self-perpetuating mechanism for aneurysm dilation (Doyle et al., 2007).

Recirculation presented by the vector plot in aneurysm sac, suggested that certain disturbed flow conditions may cause injury to endothelium and induce stimuli for inflammation or degradation.

Consequently, complex flow pattern, by increasing wall tension may induce dilation of an aneurysm. Cyclic turbulent stresses are known to alter the structure and integrity of the arterial wall. Large eddies induce vibrations at frequencies which cause the dilation of arteries (Khanafer et al., 2007).

Due to the highly three-dimensional nature of blood flow in the abdominal aneurysm, it can be a difficult task to keep track of the paths of fluid particles within the flow field.

An effective way to investigate these fluid motions is to numerically inject a passive or non-interactive tracer into the flow, and we have carried out such an investigation in the present work. We have introduced a tracer, which serves as a visualization tool to analyze the flow characteristics. Figure 10 presents the tracer distribution inside to the aneurysm's body.

Further, in a large recirculating flow region the particles residence time is large and could be a contributing factor for thrombosis in the aneurysm.

The obtained results for WSS are in agreement with published data from the investigations considering the physiological aorta (Doyle et al., 2007) as well as with data from patient-specific fluid-solid interaction simulations (Leung et al., 2006).

Pressure contours at the peak systole (time t=0.3s) and peak diastole (t=0.7s) are presented in Figure 9. Pressure gradient generally decreases in the flow direction. Highest pressure of about 15.4 kPa (115.5 mmHg) at the time t=0.3s is found in the exit region of the AAA.

Therefore the highest pressure difference between inlet and outlet is about 1.3kPa (9.75 mmHg) at the time t=0.3s and about 0.6 kPa (4.5 mmHg) at the time t=0.7s . In diastolic flow, the inlet velocity begins to decelerate, reducing the overall pressure gradient.

As the cardiac cycle continues, pressure drop is expected to decrease and recirculation regions dominate of the aneurysm sac (Cheng et al., 2010).

4.1 Wall shear stress analysis

The blood flow dynamics in aneurysm models is governed by the compliance of the vessel. The velocity vectors illustrate a streamlined profile absent of vortices, a flow path customarily associated with a condition of systolic acceleration (Figure 8a).

The vortices are developed in the proximal neck and are dissipated in the aneurysm (Figure 8b). Vortex growth inside the AAA sac creates favorable conditions for increased platelet deposition rates and an increased risk of rupture (Thubrikar et al., 2003).

Geometry has been well established as a contributing factor to aneurysm expansion and rupture potential, independently of the heterogenity of the wall (Di Martino et al., 2001).

Significant gradients occur at the inflection points of the aneurysm curvature. For the investigated aneurysm, the changes in curvature lead to higher displacements and increased wall shear stress, suggestive for the effect of flow through the gradual expansions and contractions of the geometry (Figures 7 and 8).

Figures 7 and 9 present the area prone to vascular remodeling increases with decrease the blood velocity. In this case the flow along the aneurysm body is sluggish and the WSS along the maximum transversal diameter of the aneurysm drops, increasing the risk of leukocyte adhesion.

4.2 Study limitation

The study presented here is not without limitations. Firstly, it is known that calcifications occur in almost all AAAs. Intraluminal trombus - ILT and calcification were not included in the present study.

Another important limitation of the present study is the assumed uniform wall thickness. It has been shown that ILT can reduce the strain and the rate of dilation by up to 15% (Thubrikar et al., 2003).

The major assumptions used in the present study include the rigid wall approximation. These assumptions represent a reasonable first approximation for the blood flow in the abdominal aorta.

5. Conclusion

Based on a recent article describing how the aneurysm can induce a considerable increase in wall shear stress during flow systole in the region of aneurysm sac, we have used the CFD technique to investigate the relation between the blood hemodynamics and WSS during the cardiac cycle.

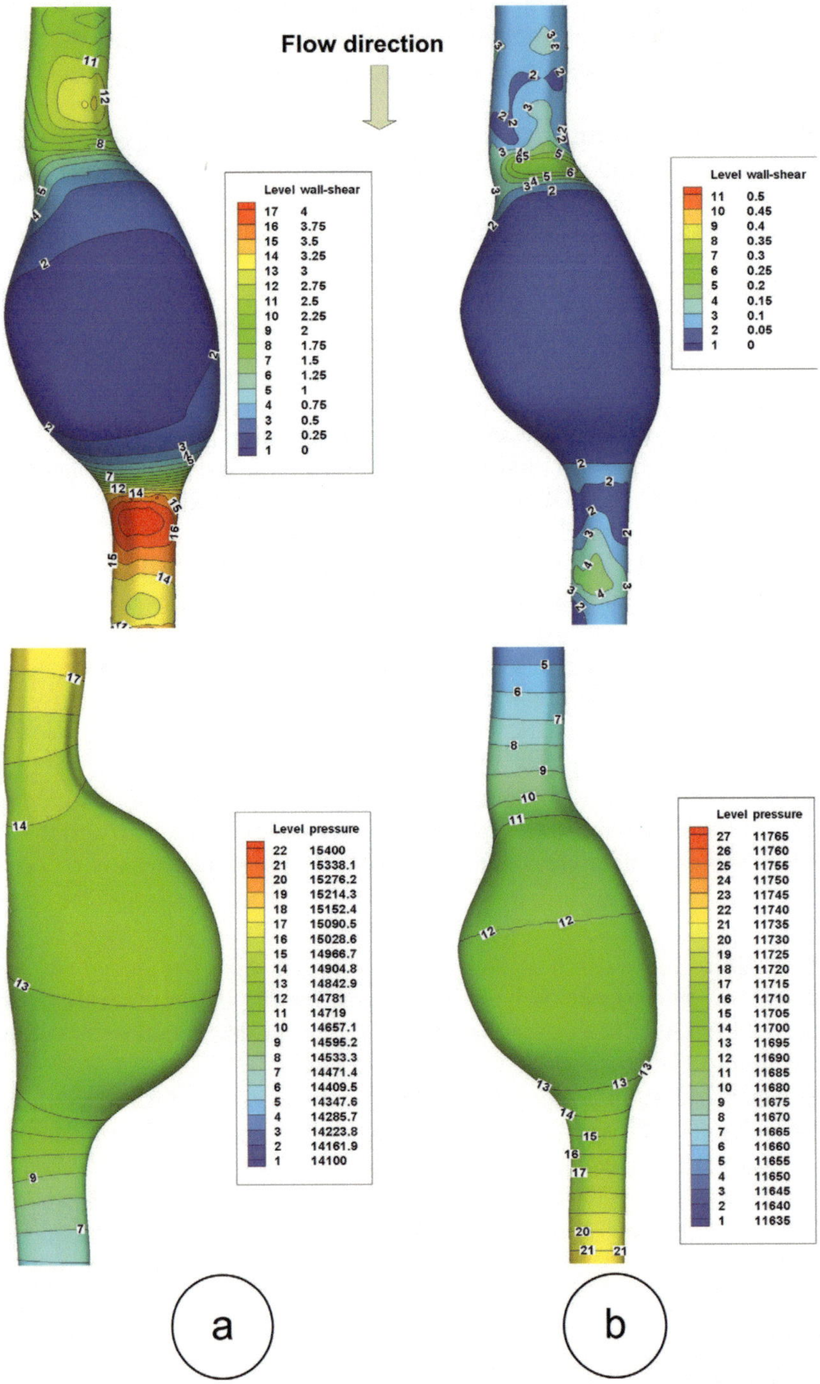

Fig. 9. Pressure and wall shear stress magnitude distributions on the anterior side of the aortic wall for different stages of the cardiac cycle: a) peak systole t=0.3 s and b) peak diastole t=0.7 s.

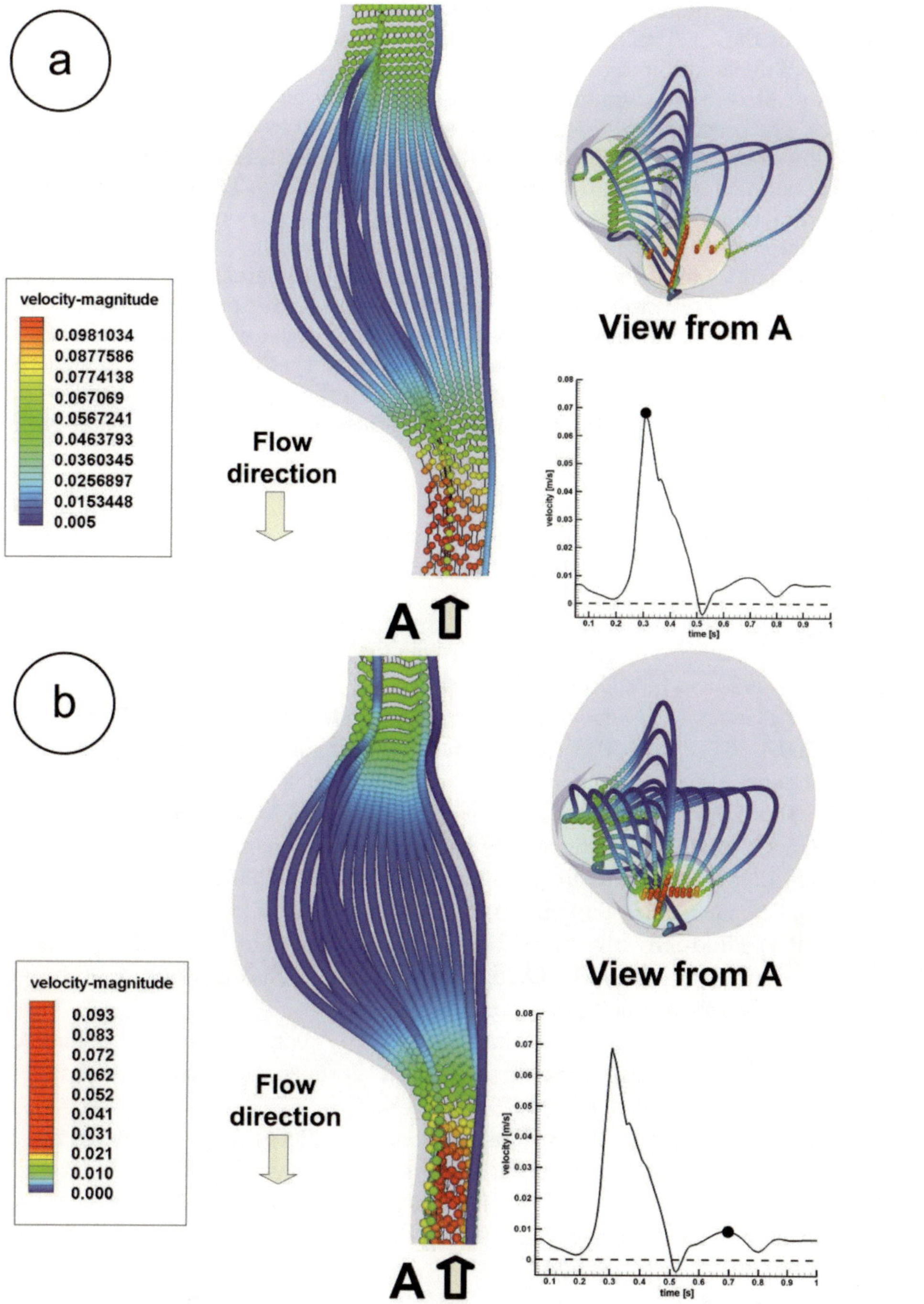

Fig. 10. Particles' motion inside the aneurysm colored by velocity magnitude at the different moment of the cardiac cycle: a) t=0.3 s and b) t=0.7 s. In order to compare the blood velocity in the different moment of the cardiac cycle, both velocity fields are represented for the same velocity range.

The virtual AAA models presented in this work provide a fundamental baseline for application of the CFD methodology as a non-invasive tool for rupture risk prediction in individual patients, outlining the importance of aneurysm asymmetry. This approach takes into account blood flow dynamics, which is inherently transient, and its effect on the wall mechanics. The present study demonstrates the relationship between the fluid velocity field and the flow-induced wall stresses. During the cardiac cycle, the instantaneous fluid forces acting on the inner wall will deform and expand the artery. From this study result that a complete understanding of the variation of intra aneurysmal hemodynamics with variations in the cardiac cycle is a critical tool for physician.
The fluid dynamics in a asymmetric aneurysm model is characterized by the development of vortices during the systolic deceleration phases. The distortion energy stored in the vessel as it expands during the cardiac cycle contributes to the early formation of recirculation regions in the aneurysm. This yields high velocity gradients at the distal end of the aneurysm. These flow patterns, in combination with the geometrical features of the model, determine the distribution of flow-induced wall stresses.

6. Acknowledgment

The present research has been supported by the Romanian National Authority for Scientific Research through the CNCSIS 798/2008 project, contract no: 590/2009.

7. References

Ansys FLUENT, Ansys Inc., User guide, 2006.

Boutsianis, E.; Guala, M.; Olgac, U.; Wildermuth, S.; Hoyer, K.; Venticos, Y. & Poulikakos, D. (2009). CFD and PTV steady flow investigation in an anatomically accurate abdominal aortic aneurysm. *Journal of Biomechanical Engineering*, Vol.131, p. 011008-15.

Cheng, Z.; Tan, F.P.P.; Riga, C.V.; Bicknell, C.D.; Hamady, M.S.; Gibbs, R.G.J.; Wood, N.B. & Xu, X.Y. (2010). Analysis of flow patterns in a patient-specific aortic dissection model. *Journal of Biomechanical Engineering*, Vol.132, No.5, 051007.

Di Martino, E.S.; Guadagni, G.; Fumero, A.; Ballerini, G.; Spirito, R.; Biglioli, P. & Redaelli, A. (2001). Fluid-Structure Interaction Within Realistic Three-Dimensional Models of the Aneurysmatic Aorta as a Guidance to Assess the Risk of Rupture of the Aneurysm. *Med. Eng. Phys.*, Vol.23, p. 647–655.

Doyle, B.J.; Callanan, A. & McGloughlin, T.M. (2007). A comparison of modelling techniques for computing wall stress in abdominal aortic aneurysms. *BioMedical Engineering OnLine*, Vol.6, doi:10.1186/1475-925X-6-38.

Ekaterinaris, J.A.; Ioannou, C.V. & Katsamouris, A.N. (2006). Flow dynamics in expansions characterizing abdominal aorta aneurysms. *Ann Vasc Surg*, Vol.20, No.3, pp.351–359.

Fillinger, M.F.; Marra, S.P.; Raghavan, M.L. & Kennedy, F.E. (2003). Prediction of rupture risk in abdominal aortic aneurysm during observation: wall stress versus diameter. *J Vasc Surg*, Vol.37, No.4, pp. 724–732.

Finol, E.A.; Keyhani, K. & Amon, C.H. (2003). The effect of asymmetry in abdominal aortic aneurysms under physiologically realistic pulsatile flow conditions. *Journal of Biomechanical Engineering*, Vol.125, pp. 207-217 .

Lederle, A.; Wilson, S.E.; Johnson, G.R.; Reinke, D.B.; Littooy, F.N.; Acher, C.W.; Ballard, D.J.; Messina, L.M.; Gordon, I.L.; Chute, E.P.; Krupski, W.C.; Busuttil, S.J.; Barone, G.W.; Sparks, S.; Graham, L.M.; Rapp, J.H.; Makaroun, M.S.; Moneta, G.L.; Cambria, R.A.; Makhoul, R.G.; Eton, D.; Ansel, H.J.; Freischlag, J.A. & Bandyk, D. (2002). Immediate repair compared with surveillance of small abdominal aortic aneurysms. *N Engl J Med*, Vol.346, No.19, pp. 1437-1444.

Leung, J.H.; Wright, A.R.; Cheshire. N.; Crane, J.; Thom, S.A.; Hughes, A.G. & Xu, Y. (2006). Fluid structure interaction of patient specific abdominal aortic aneurysms: a comparison with solid stress models, *BioMedical Engineering OnLine*, Vol.5. p. 33.

Katz, D.A. & Cronenwett, J.L. (1994). The cost-effectiveness of early surgery versus watchful waiting in the management of small abdominal aortic aneurysms. *Journal of Vascular Surgery*, Vol.19, pp. 980-990.

Kleinstreuer C. & Zhonghua L. (2006). Analysis and computer program for rupture-risk prediction of abdominal aortic aneurysms, *BioMedical Engineering OnLine*, Vol.5, p:19.

Khanafer, K.M.; Bull, J.L.; Upchurch, G.R. Jr.; Berguer, R. & Arbor, A. (2007). Turbulence Significantly Increases Pressure and Fluid Shear Stress in an Aortic Aneurysm Model under Resting and Exercise Flow Conditions. *Ann Vasc Surg.*, Vol.21, p. 67-74.

Malek, A.M.; Alper, S.L. & Izumo, S. (1999). Hemodynamic shear stress and its role in atherosclerosis. *Journal of the American Medical Association*, Vol.282, No.21, pp. 2035.

Marra, S.P.; Raghavan, M.L.; Whittaker, D.R.; Fillinger, M.F.; Chen, D.T.; Dwyer, J.M.; Tsapakos, M.J. & Kennedy, F.E. (2005). Estimation Of The Zero-Pressure Geometry Of Abdominal Aortic Aneurysms From Dynamic Magnetic Resonance Imaging. *Proceedings of the ASME 2005 Summer Bioengineering Conference*, Vail, Colorado, USA, June 22 - 26, 2005.

Mills, C.; Gabe, I.; Gault, J.; Mason, D. & Ross, JJr.; Braunwald, E. & Shillingford, J. (1970). Pressure-flow relationships and vascular impedance in man. *Cardiovascular Research*, Vol.4, pp. 405-417.

Perktold, K.; Resch, M. & Florian, H. (1991). Pulsatile non-Newtonian flow characteristics in a three-dimensional human carotid bifurcation model. *J Biomech Eng*, Vol.113, No.4, pp. 464-475.

Raghavan, M.L.; Vorp, D.A.; Federle, M.P.; Makaroun, M.S. & Webster, M.W. (2000). Wall stress distribution on three-dimensionally reconstructed models of human abdominal aortic aneurysm. *J Vasc Surg*, Vol.31, pp. 760-769.

Raghavan, M.L. & Vorp, D.A. (2000). Toward a Biomechanical Tool to Evaluate Rupture Potential of Abdominal Aortic Aneurysm: Identification of a Finite Strain Constitutive Model and Evaluation of its Applicability. *J. Biomech.*, Vol.33, p. 475–482.

Scotti, C.M.; Shkolnik, A.D.; Muluk, S.C. & Finol, E. (2005). Fluid-structure interaction in abdominal aortic aneurysms: effect of asymmetry and wall thickness. *Biomed Eng Online*, Vol.4, p: 64.

Tan, F.P.P.; Borghi, A.; Mohiaddin, R.H.; Wood, N.B.; Thom, S. & Xu, X.Y. (2008). Analysis of flow patterns in a patient-specific thoracic aortic aneurysm model. *Comput Struct*, doi:10.1016/j.compstruc.2008.09.007.

Thubrikar, M.J.; Robicsek, F.; Labrosse, M.; Chervenkoff, V. & Fowler, B.L. (2003). Effect of thrombus on abdominal aortic aneurysm wall dilation and stress. *J Cardiovasc Surg*, Vol.44, No.1, p. 67-77.

Thubrikar, M.J.; Al-Soudi, J. & Robicsek, F. (2001). Wall stress studies of abdominal aortic aneurysm in a clinical model. *Ann Vasc Surg*, Vol.15, pp. 355-366.

Vainas, T.; Lubbers, Y.; Stassen, F.R.M., *et al.* (2003). Serum C-reactive protein level is associated with abdominal aortic aneurysm size and may be produced by aneurysmal tissue. *Circulation*, Vol.107, pp. 1103–1105.

Venkatasubramaniam, A.K.; Fagan, M.J.; Mehta, T.; Mylankal, K.J.; Ray, B.; Kuhan, G.;, et al. (2004). Comparative study of aortic wall stress using finite element analysis for ruptured and non-ruptured abdominal aortic aneurysms. *Eur J Vasc Endovasc Surg*, Vol.28, No.2, pp. 168–176.

12

Numerical Simulation in Aortic Arch Aneurysm

Feng Gao[1], Aike Qiao[2] and Teruo Matsuzawa[3]
[1]*Tokyo University of Science,*
[2]*Beijing University of Technology,*
[3]*Japan Advanced Institute of Science and Technology,*
[1,3]*Japan*
[2]*China*

1. Introduction

The aorta, acting as the main conduit through which cardiac output is delivered to the systemic arterial bed, is continuously exposed to high pulsatile pressure and shear stress, making it prone to mechanical injury. It is also more prone to rupture than other vessels, particularly with the development of aneurysmal dilation. Fifty percent of patients who experience a rupture of a aortic aneurysm die before reaching the hospital (Bengtsson & Bergqvist, 1993). The incidence increases with age and has been reported as 6 per 100,000 person-years (Knowles & Kneeshaw, 2004). Aneurysmal degeneration that occurs in the aortic arch is termed a aortic arch aneurysm. Patients who have aortic arch aneurysm have multiple aortic lesions or aneurysmal disease which involves segment of aorta (Crawford et al., 1984). Aortic arch aneurysms represent only 10% of aneurysms of the thoracic aorta and it has higher risk of rupture than other aneurysm (Knowles & Kneeshaw, 2004).
Blood flow through the aorta is one of the most complex flow situations found in the cardiovascular system. Blood flow is pulsatile and pressure inside aortic aneurysm is non-uniform. The dynamics interaction between blood flow and wall may influence the wall stress. Computer modeling has made impressive progress in scientific, engineering, biological and medical applications in recent years and it offers the prospect of providing both a better insight into a range of biomechanical problems and improved tools for the design of medical devices and the diagnosis of pathologies. Computational methods such as mathematical modeling methods (Rideout, 1991; Rupnic & Runvovc, 2002; Abdolrazaghi et al., 2008), computational fluid dynamics methods, (Botnar et al., 2000; Shahcheraghi et al., 2002; Morris et al., 2005; Tokuda et al. 2008) loosely coupled methods (Di Mrrtino et al., 2001; Gao et al., 2006abc) have been used to simulate the biomechanical problems in arotic arch and aortic arch aneurysm. The aim of this chapter is to describe the numerical simulation and computer modeling work in aortic arch aneurysm.

2. Aorta, aortic arch and structure of aortic wall

Arteries are vessels that carry blood away from the heart. The aorta is the largest artery in the body (Fig. 1). It arises from the left ventricle of the heart, forms an arch, and then extends down to the abdomen where it branches off into two smaller arteries. It consists of the ascending aorta, the aortic arch, and the descending aorta. Ascending aorta extends upward from the aortic root to the point where the innominate artery branches off the aorta, and the aorta begins to form an arch. Aortic arch represents the curved portion at the top of the aorta. Descending aorta begins just beyond the arch as the aorta bends down into the body. It carries and distributes oxygen rich blood to all arteries.

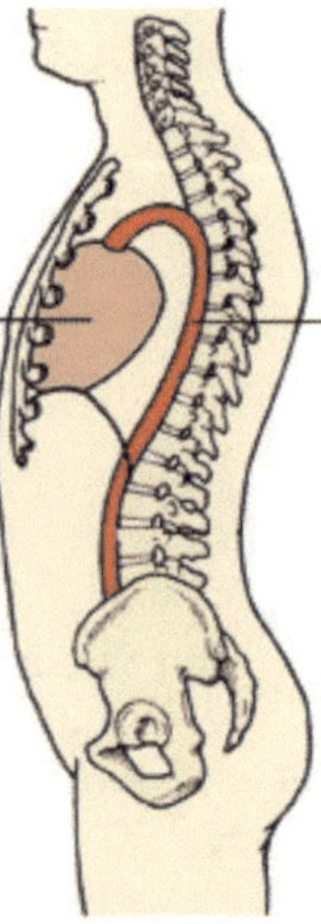

Fig. 1. Aorta in the human body. It arises from the left ventricle of the heart, forms an arch, and then extends down to the abdomen.

The aorta is distinguished by their great elasticity. This helps them smooth out the large fluctuations in blood pressure created by the heartbeat. In order to understand the properties of aorta, the three types of arteries should first be mentioned. These are elastic arteries, medium muscular arteries, small arteries and arterioles. For aorta, large arteries and small arteries, the typical radius, typical length, and typical numbers are shown in Table 1.

Vessel	Typical radius (mm)	Typical length (mm)	Typical number
Aorta	12	500	1
Large arteries	3	250	50
Small arteries	1	50	$2x10^3$

Table 1. The typical radius, length, and numbers for aorta, large arteries and small arteries.

Elastic arteries experience the greatest pressures and are closest to the heart. The aorta is the largest elastic artery that delivers blood from the left ventricle of the heart to the rest of the body. Aorta is described as arteries that contain more elastin than smooth muscle content in the media. The elastin is necessary to allow the vessel to expand and recoil during pulsatile flow (Benjamin Cummings, 1996). The current investigation will work with the elastic artery, such as the aorta (throracic and abdominal) and carotid arteries (Yamada, 1970). The innermost layer is the tunica intima. The middle layer is the tunica media and the outermost layer is the tunica adventitia.

In general, the overall mechanical properties of the arterial wall are determined by how different compositions of collagen, elastin and protein are linked. The general rule is that when the elastin ratio is higher than the collagen ratio, the elastic modulus decreases and distensibility increases and vice versa (Doublin & Rovick, 1969). The Young's modulus of three layers of the aorta wall is different. Xie et al. (1995) did the bending experiments of blood vessel wall and found that the Young's modulus of the inner layer (intima and media) was three to four times larger than that of the outer layer (adventitia). The elastic modulus of arterial wall became a little higher after de-endothelization in Fischer's experiments (Fischer et al., 2002) and this means the elasticity of intima is lower than the mean elasticity of vessel wall since the intima layer mainly consists of endothelial cells.

3. Computational geometric reconstruction of aortic arch aneurysm

The geometric modeling is the fundamental part of the aorta modeling analysis. Owing to the complex geometry of the aorta, three-dimensional models of aorta and aortic aneurysm are considerably important. Advances in imaging are being introduced initially as research tools and subsequently as clinical diagnostic tests. The reconstruction of aorta structures involves the use of sets of clinical data (MRI or CT) that are processed to extract the vessel morphology.

3.1 STL format of aortic arch aneurysm model

Stereo lithography (STL) describes a raw unstructured triangulated surface by unit normal and vertices (ordered by the right-hand rule) of the triangles using a threedimensional Cartesian coordinate system. The surface is logically tessellated or broken down into a series of small triangles (facets). Each facet is described by a perpendicular direction and three points representing the vertices (corners) of the triangle. Point cloud and connectivity matrix data written in this format can be imported into a variety of CAD or grid generation software. A patient-specific aortic arch aneurysm model in STL format was reconstructed from CT medical images (Fig. 3). This model is a surface model in geometry, which cannot be used for numerical simulation directly (Fu et al., 2008). Reverse engineering software Geomagic and Pro/E were used to process the surface model of STL format to rebuild a patient-specific model of aortic arch aneurysm that can be used in numerical simulation.

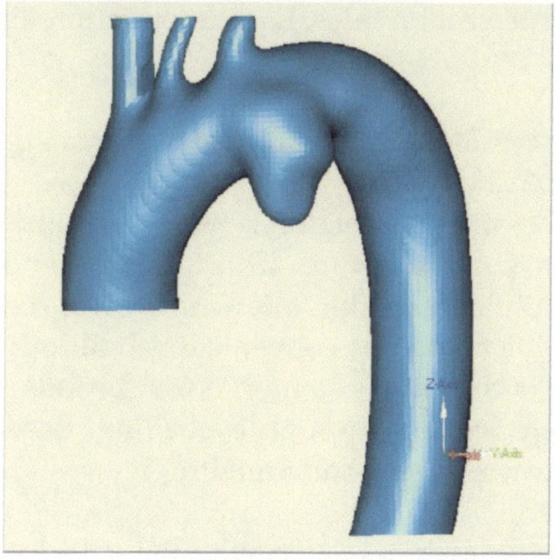

Fig. 3. A patient-specific aortic arch aneurysm model of STL format

3.2 Method of aortic arch aneurysm model reconstruction

3.2.1 Processing STL surface model

Because the boundaries of the three branches will impact the integration of patch arrangement and lead to the failure of creating NURBS (Non-Uniform Rational B-Splines) surface, the main purpose of this study is also to find a way to construct the aneurysm model, it is necessary to simplify the three branches.

1. Simplifying surface

Opening the STL formatted surface model of the aortic arch aneurysm in Geomagic. First, cut the three branches using the "section by plane" mode. Then erase red boundaries (the boundary line after intersecting) of the incisions using the "sandpaper" and "relax" function, thus the simplified surface model is composed of closed areas with only two closed boundaries at the ends.

2. Dividing areas

To regularly arrange patches, the method of "section by plane" was applied to divide the model into several orbicular areas. There are some rules to obey when locating the cutting plane: to preserve the changing information of geometry as much as possible; to divide more annulus at the place where shapes change sharply; approximately keeping the normal vector of the cutting plane and the trend of vessel's growth in the same direction.

3. Rectifying arrangement of the patches

Create triangle patches under the curvature level 0.3 by using "detect curvature" in "detect curvature" mode. Delete extra orange boundaries (panel-demarcation line) and rectify arrangement of the patches manually to make sure each red boundary with only four keypoints. The arrangement of each opposite keypoints must vary with the changed area to avoid torsion around the direction of the bloodstream.

4. Checking and output

After checking and repairing the arrangement of quadrilateral patches with "repair patches" function, NURBS surface fitted with 48 pieces of quadrilateral patches was finally created. Then export this NURBS surface model in IGES format.

3.2.2 Reconstructing solid model

1. Preprocessing areas

Open the NURBS surface model in Pro/E. Create planes that are parallel to the former red closed boundaries and get intersection lines. Each intersection line is composed of four lines connected end to end.

2. Creating solid part

Based on the former intersection lines, a solid model was created by blended drawing.

3. Reconstructing three branches

Because the shape near the three branches is very complicated and irregular, precise measurement is difficult in CAD software. Considering some small differences are not important and have little influence on the following works, therefore, it is viable to make some hypotheses and simplifications for convenient rebuilding of branches. Branches and aortic arch were connected with round chamfer; cross sections were simplified as circle or ellipse; and the centers were located through eyeballing. Based on these simplifications, three branches were reconstructed using software Pro/E.

4. Creating boundary layer

The thickness of the boundary layer is related with the velocity, factor of friction, location, shape, etc. Even at the same place, the thickness of the boundary layer may be different at different times. To gradually obtain finer grids in the boundary layer in the following meshing procedure, a solid shell was primarily constructed to approximately imitate the boundary layer. Because the thickness of the boundary layer is extremely thin and uncertain, an assumed layer thickness not less than 10% of the maximal diameter is sufficient for the boundary layer and easy to construct. Create circle and ellipse lines in the former planes that are parallel to the former red closed boundaries. Place centers near the centroid. Choose inner diameter not more than 80% of the maximal distance of the section. To avoid the situation where stents cross the boundary layer, properly move some centers away from the aneurysm and reduce the inner diameter to about 20%-60% of the maximal distance of the section. A shell remained after cutting a hollow by blended drawing (Fig. 4).

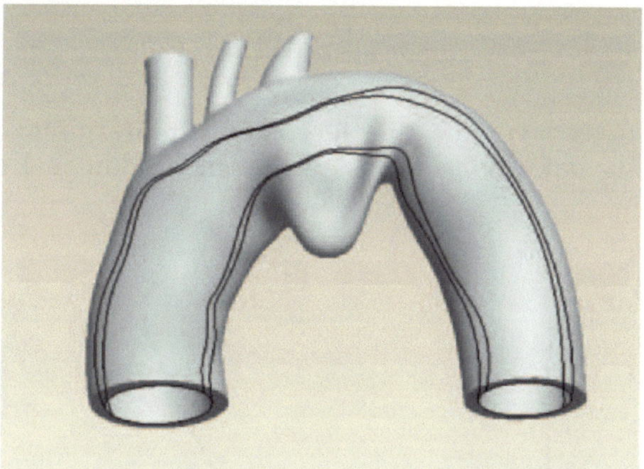

Fig. 4. Reconstructed solid model of aortic arch aneurysm for numerical simulation

4. Simulation in aortic arch and aortic arch aneurysm

4.1 Mathematical modeling on aortic aneurysm

It was Stephen Hales in his Statistical Essays who considered arterial elasticity and postulated its buffering effect on the pulsatile nature of blood flow (Hales, 1733). He likened the depulsing effect to the fire engines of his day, in which a chamber with an air-filled dome acted to cushion the bolus from the inlet water pump so that "a more nearly equal spout" flowed out the nozzle. This analogy became the basis of the first modern cardiovascular models. In the translation from English to German, Hales' s inverted globe became a windkessel (air kettle); his idea later became known as the Windkessel theory when it was more formally developed and propounded by the German physiologist Otto Frank near the beginning of our century (Noordergraaf, 1978).

A short segment of aorta can be modeled by an elastic, isobaric chamber attached to a rigid inlet and outlet tube. The ability of the chamber to store fluid depends on its compliance, C, which is defined as

$$C = \frac{dV_c}{dP_c} \tag{1}$$

where *Vc* is total segment (chamber) volume and *Pc* is chamber pressure. Many modelers prefer to use the reciprocal of compliance (termed stiffness, *S*, or elastance, *E*). Here, viscoelastic (stress relaxation) effects are assumed negligible, so that compliance is not an explicit function of time. Thus, compliance becomes an instantaneous variable which can be obtained from the experimentally determined, steadystate pressure-volume (*P-V*) relationship of the segment. Furthermore, model order can be reduced, as pressure can be mathematically represented as an empirical function of volume, either by a piecewise linear approximation, a polynomial quotient, or some other function fit to the *P-V* relationship. A typical *P-V* curve is illustrated in Fig. 5, along with its piecewise liner approximation. In arteries, pressure is usually positive with small oscillations about a nominal operating point (point a in Fig. 5). Hence the piecewise linear approximation can be reduced to a single line with constant slope $1/C$:

$$P_c = \frac{\left(V_c - V_{c_0}\right)}{c} \tag{2}$$

where V_{c0} is the unstressed volume (the idealized zero-pressure volume intercept). Of course, if pressure fluctuates outside this region, then additional straight-line sections should be included.

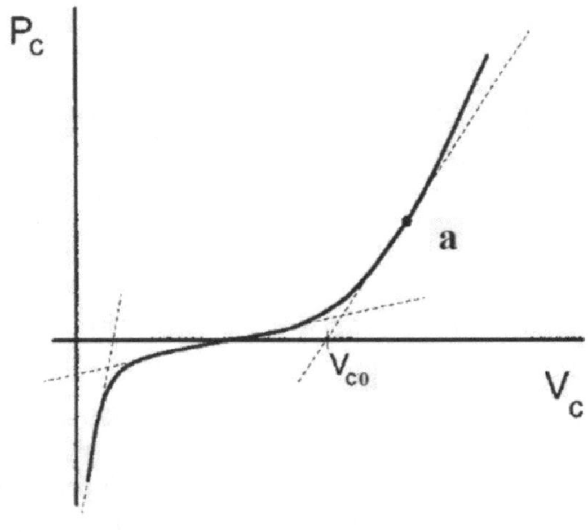

Fig. 5. Pressure-volume relationship of aorta

Assuming that blood is incompressible and newtonian, that the flow profile is parabolic and unchanging with axial distance along a straight rigid tube, then flow (poisenillean) is linearly proportional to the pressure gradient across the ends of the tube. Hence, flow into and out of the chamber may be calculated given P_{in} and P_{out} (the inlet and outlet pressures); P_c; L_{in} and L_{out} (the inertances due to fluid mass); and R_{in} and R_{out} (the resistances due to viscous drag)

$$L_{in}\frac{df_{in}}{dt} + R_{in}f_{in} = P_{in} - P_c \tag{3}$$

$$L_{out}\frac{df_{out}}{dt} + R_{out}f_{out} = P_c - P_{out} \tag{4}$$

where f_{in} and f_{out} are the flows into and out of the segment. Volume can now be calculated from the difference between the inlet and outlet flows: P_c, V_c, f_{in}, and f_{out} can now be uniquely determined at any time given P_{in}, P_{out}, and the initial conditions of the segment. Determination of the parameters L and R are more problematic. They can be derived analytically, although probably because the modeling assumptions are not completely correct, an empirical fit generally produces better segmental properties.

$$\frac{dV_c}{dt} = f_{in} - f_{out} \tag{5}$$

The mathematical modeling method has been applied to the cardiovascular system for the study of system pathologies (Rideout, 1991; Rupnic & Runvovc, 2002). The aortic aneurysm has primarily been probed and the compliance of aortic aneurysms was investigated and the effects of the pathology were observed (Long et al., 2004; Morris-Stiff et al., 2005). The cardiac pressure-volume loops for aortic aneurysms has been presented by utilizing electronic cardiovascular modeling (Abdolrazaghi et al., 2008). The electronic parameters are correlated to their mechanical parameters as follows: voltage is analogous to pressure, capacitance to compliance, and inductance to inertance. The aortic aneurysm with different diameters were applied and left ventricle pressure-volume with aortic aneurysm increased. There is significant increase in pressure both in thoracic and abdominal aortic aneurismal condition, therefore it can be understood that the hypertension could be principal symptom of these disease (Abdolrazaghi et al., 2008).

4.2 Hemodynamics simulation in aortic arch and aortic aneurysm

Blood flow through the aorta is one of the most complex flow situations found in the cardiovascular system. This is mainly due to the strong curvature effects, irregular geometry, tapering and branching. The human aortic arch has a characteristic configuration. One of its characteristics is that the centerline of the arch does not lie in a plane. Another is that there are major branches at the top of the arch. Kilner et al. (1993) observed a characteristic helical blood flow pattern in the human aortic arch using magnetic resonance measurements, and showed the qualitative flow structure in the arch. However, it is difficult to obtain distribution and transient change in the wall shear stress from measuring clinical images. Instead of experimental methods, the detailed flow in human arteries can be studied by using computational fluid dynamics methods (Botnar et al., 2000). The highly disturbed flow patterns that have been reported in regions of arterial branching and curvature are attributable to a large degree to the combined effects of complex arterial geometry and flow pulsatility. One vascular site within which the fluid mechanical environment is especially complex is the region of the aortic arch and its major branches. The arch is characterized by extensive curvature, which would be expected to lead to velocity profile skewness as well as to complex secondary flow motion. Furthermore, the three aortic arch branches which emerge in different planes are likely to have a large impact on the flow field.

A few computational studies have been made of steady and unsteady blood flow in the human aortic arch (Shahcheraghi et al., 2002; Morris et al., 2005; Tokuda et al., 2008). The simulation results demonstrate that the primary flow velocity is skewed towards the inner aortic wall in the ascending aorta, but this skewness shifts to the outer wall in the descending thoracic aorta. Within the arch branches, the flow velocities were skewed to the distal walls with flow reversal along the proximal walls. Extensive secondary flow motion was observed in the aorta, and the structure of these secondary flows was influenced considerably by the presence of the branches. Within the aorta, wall shear stresses were highly dynamic, but were generally high along the outer wall in the vicinity of the branches and low along the inner wall, particularly in the descending thoracic aorta. Within the branches, the shear stresses were considerably higher along the distal walls than along the proximal walls. Wall pressure was low along the inner aortic wall and high around the branches and along the outer wall in the ascending thoracic aorta.

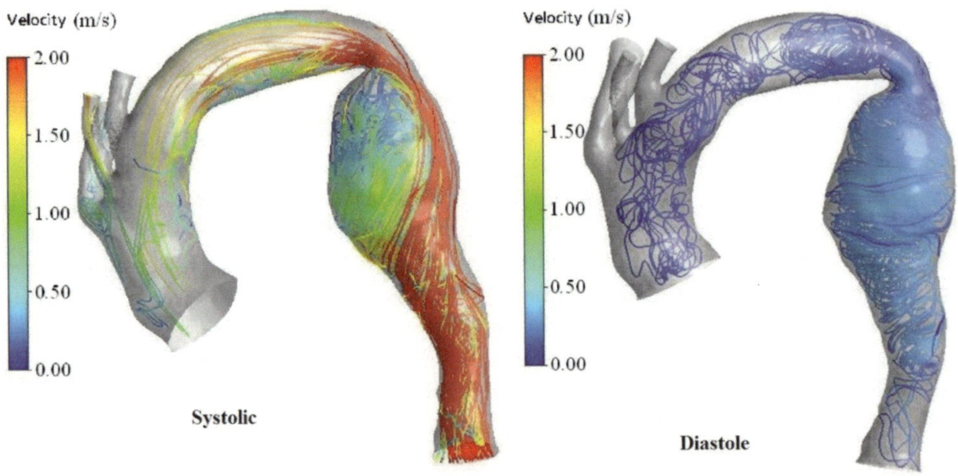

Fig. 6. Streamline of blood flow at systolic and diastole in aortic arch aneurysm

For more realistic simulation of patient-specific thoracic aneurysm blood flow, a real vasclar model containing ascending aorta, aortic arch and descending thoracic aorta was constructed basd on CT images (Qiao et al., 2011). This model also contains the innominat artery, left common carotid artery and left subclavian artery. More importantly, there is a fusiform aneurysm in the descending thoracic aorta. In arch aneurysm model, the velocity vectors illustrate a streamline profile with vortices through the aneurysm. Streamlines in an aortic arch aneurysm model at the decreasing phase of systolic and the phase of diastole are shown in Fig. 6. There was large vortexes in the descending aortic aneurysm cavity. This was the main difference of flow characteristics in the thoracic aorta with aneurysm and without aneurysm. In diastolic flow vortex characteristics were more apparent, and there were several vortices; especially in the latter half of the diastolic phase, there was a large vortex of blood flow in the descending aortic aneurysm. Therefore residence time of blood cells and other particles in the cavity of the aneurysm was increased, and the probability that these particles were deposited on these positions increased too. Those factors would increase the growth of aneurysm.

4.3 Fluid structure interaction simulation in layered aortic arch and aortic aneurysm

Although the exactly relationship between the elastic properties of intima layer and that of media layer hasn't been decided, we can deduce from the Fischer's experiment data (Fischer et al., 2002)that the Young's modulus of intima layer is smaller than that of media layer. In this present study, the Young's modulus of intima layer is assumed three times larger than that of media layer, as same as the adventitia layer:

$$3E_i = E_m = 3E_a \tag{6}$$

where E_i, E_m and E_a are the Young's modulus of intima layer, media layer and adventitia layer, respectively. The mean Young's modulus of vessel wall is same, based on the assumption that the Young's modulus of layer is in inverse proportion to the volume of layer, so:

$$E_i \cdot V_i + E_m \cdot V_m + E_a \cdot V_a = E \cdot V \tag{7}$$

where V_i, V_m, V_a, and V are the volume of intima layer, media layer and adventita layer, respectively. Using the volume equation, Equation 6 becomes:

$$E_i \cdot t_i + E_m \cdot t_m + E_a \cdot t_a = E \cdot t \tag{8}$$

where t_i, t_m, t_a and t are the thickness of intima layer and that of medial layer, respectively.

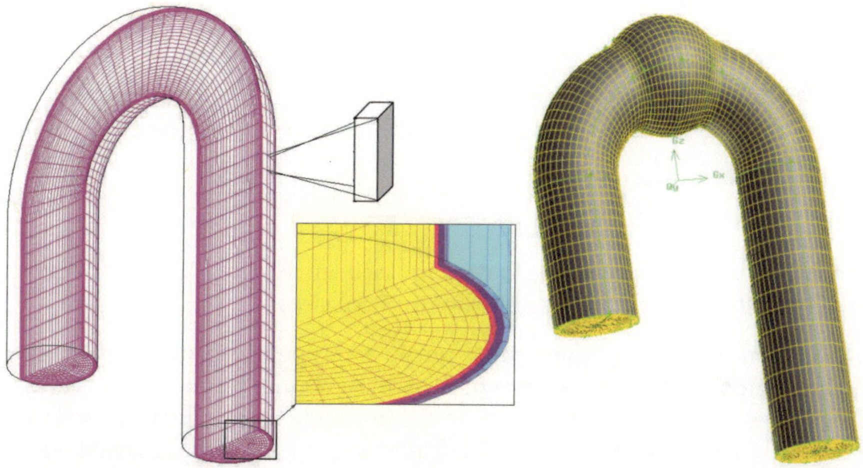

Fig. 7. Three-layered aortic arch model and aneurysm model

In cardiovascular biomechanics one of the major topics today is the simulation and analysis of the fluid-structure interaction of the cardiovascular system using computational methods (Taylor, 1999). Di Martino and colleagues (Di Mrrtino et al., 2001) provided the notion of interaction between solid and fluid domains as it contributes to aneurysm rupture potential. Fluid-structure interaction (FSI) of the domains allows computation of the flow and pressure fields in the aneurysm, simultaneously with the wall stresses.

We performed the fluid structure interaction simulation in three-layered aortic arch model (Gao et al., 2006abc). Fig. 7 shows the three-layered aortic arch model and aneurysm model. The velocity in the entrance region of the ascending aorta is blunted and skewed towards the inner wall of the aortic arch and the values become higher at the side of inner wall. Skewing is more marked in mid ascending portion. Downstream of the top arch, however, skewing of the velocity reverses, and the location of maximum velocity shifted towards the outer wall of aortic arch, which agrees with previous studies (Shahcheraghi et al., 2002).

The variations of stresses along the arch were not uniform, due to the arch structure. The circumferential stress gets first peak at the mid ascending portion and second peak at the mid descending portion and it would be unpredictable by using Laplace's Law. Hence, the shape of the arch and the hemodynamic forces acting on the vessel wall (Liepsch, 2002) may play important roles in aorta mechanics. The longitudinal stress gets its peak values at the entrance to the ascending portion and the top of the arch and the distal end of the arch.

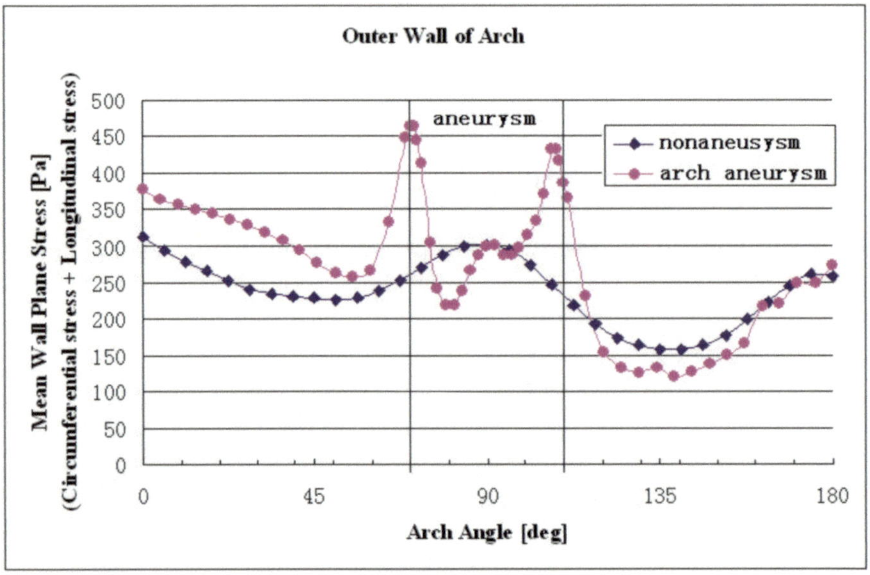

Fig. 8. Comparisons of wall stress distribution in nonaneurysm model and aneurysm model for compose stress (circumferential stress+longitudinal stress).

The FSI simulation was also performed on aortic arch aneurysm model (Gao et al., 2008). Fig. 8 shows composite stress (composition of the circumferential stress vector and the longitudinal stress vector) in aneurysm model comparing with nonaneurysm model. The wall stresses on aneurysm model were indicated to be complexly distributed with large regional variations at inflection points. The wall stresses on nonaneurysm model was relatively low and uniformly distributed. The previous study found that the failure strength of aneurysm wall was lower than that of nonaneurysm wall (Vorp et al., 1996) and the peak wall stress on aneurysm was from 45% to 69% of its failure strength, whereas the peak wall stress of nonaneurysm aorta was less than 10% of its failure strength (Raghavan et al., 2000). The maximum stresses occur at the proximal and distal ends of aneurysm. This result suggests that maximum stresses do not occur at the location of the maximum diameter but at the regions of high curvature that are associated with the proximal and distal ends. It agrees with previous studies (Raghavan et al., 2000; Di Martino et al., 2001; Vorp et al., 1998). Most aneurismal ruptures occur at the posterolateral wall, which correlates to the areas of high stress concentrations (Raghavan et al., 2000; Vorp et al., 1998). Also the actual propensity for rupture for another surface of aneurysm depends on the comparative local value of wall strength, since it was found that the strength of tissue near the neck or undilated ends of aneurysm are greater than that in the midsection, where diameter is maximum.

The arterial stiffness was significantly higher in aneurysm wall compared with healthy aortic wall (Di Martino et al., 2001; Sonesson et al., 1997). It has been suggested that aneurysms develop as a result of an alteration in the connective tissue metabolism and this might change arterial wall stiffness (Sonesson et al., 1997). Our results indicated that wall stiffness in aneurysms increase maximum stresses in inflection points. So wall stiffness in aneurysm might make the stress more increased in aneurysm. Morris et al. (2005) used the photoelastic method to simulate the failures at the proximal end and distal end of aneurysm model. It was also reported that aortic dissection originated in a distal aortic arch aneurysm (Tsukamoto et al., 2003). Arterial stiffness that increased both with age and certain disease may increase cardiovascular risk (Blacher et al., 1999). The main structural alterations at the site of the large artery media account for arterial stiffening (Benetos, 2003). The aortic wall has multi-layered composite structure and stress can not be assumed uniformly distributed through the wall thickness. The non-homogeneous stress distribution through wall thickness was showed (Fig. 9) and stresses are found to be higher in the media and reach a peak value in the media near the adventitia at inflection points and the medial stiffening increased the stress in media and peak value.

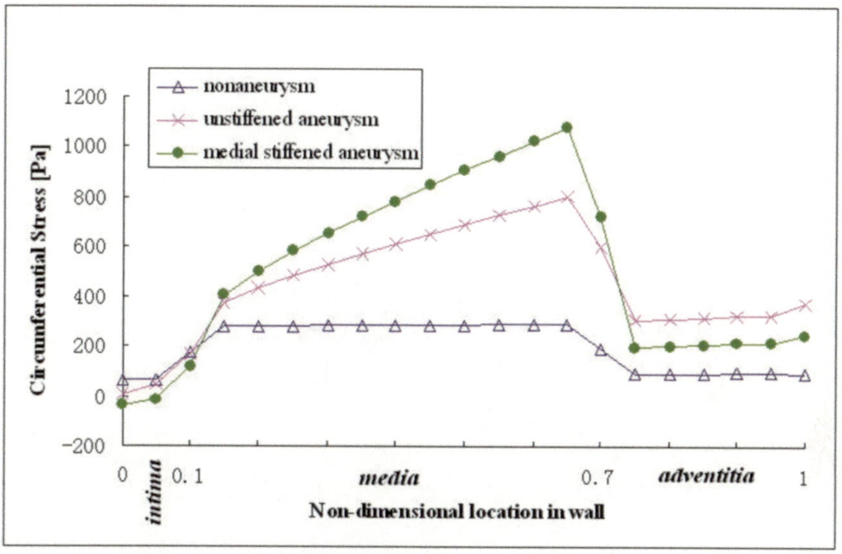

Fig. 9. Comparisons of wall stress distribution across wall for nona neurysm wall, unstiffened aneurysm wall, stiffened aneurysm wall.

4.4 Simulation in stented aortic arch aneurysm

The traditional treatment requires open surgical repair, which involves an incision and exclusion of the diseased aneurysm with a synthetic graft. An alternative treatment is endovascular aneurysm repair. Endovascular stent is commonly used to bridge the aneurysmal orifice since the first trial of Parodi (Parodi et al., 1995). Endovascular aneurysm repair is a minimally invasive technique to treat aneurysms. An endovascular graft is guided from the iliac to the affected aortic segment to shield the aneurysm from blood pressure, eliminate blood circulation in the aneurysm intrasac, and hence prevent aneurysm rupture.

Different numerical studies have focused on the hemodynamic changes in aneurysm with and without a stent-graft. Despite of the expansive investigation in the endovascular stent for aneurysms, studies of hemodynamics simulation of stented aneurysm at the aortic arch with a localized outpouching (bleb) on top of the dome, at which point aneurysms frequently rupture, are relatively rare. The hemodynamics in fully stented aortic arch aneurysms harboring a bleb has been studied on the dome (Fig. 10) (Qiao et al., 2005). The flow near the dome of the aneurysm is more sluggish after stenting, and flow activities deep within the blebs of the stented aneurysm models are significantly diminished, which agree very well with the studies of Aenis et al. (1997), Lieber et al. (2002) and Liou and Liou (2004). Stenting reduces the momentum transfer from the parent vessel to the aneurysm, thus reducing intra-aneurysmal flow, which produces thrombosis formation and subsequent contraction of the dilated aorta. The simulation results showed that the intra-aneurysmal flow in the stented aneurysm was significantly attenuated, and the pressure and WSSs were decreased. A high pressure zone at the dome of the aneurysm prior to stenting decreases after stent implantation, this phenomenon in the simulation also accords with the results of Aenis et al. (1997) and Liou and Liou (2004). The magnitude and pulsatility of the WSSs along the aneurysmal wall were reduced by stenting, specifically in the bleb region. Considering the widely convinced therapeutic mechanism of endovascular stents, we believe that the stent-induced sluggish flow activity, low pressure, low WSS and hence embolization in the aortic arch aneurysmal sacs can facilitate the occlusion of aneurysms. The hemodynamic characteristics allow us to conclude that we can treat aortic arch aneurysm with bare wire-mesh endovasucular stents.

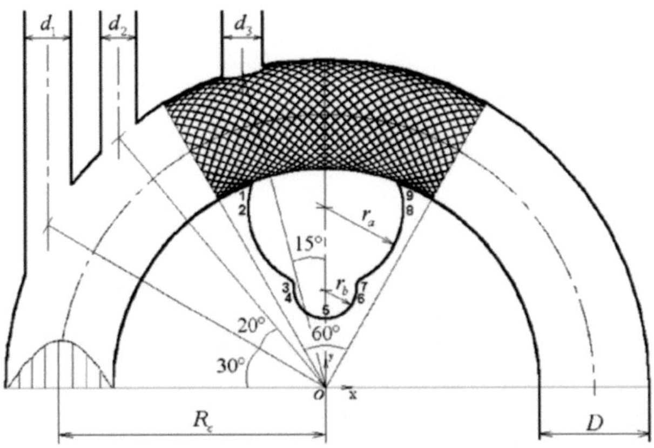

Fig. 10. Geometric models of the stented aortic arch aneurysm harboring a bleb on its dome.

The shape of the stent (e.g., helix-versus mesh-shaped stents) (Liou et al., 2004), the size of the orifice, the porosity of a stent (Rhee et al., 2002) and the stent filament size (Lieber et al., 2002; Bando & Berger, 2003) are important factors that influence the treatment effectiveness of stented aneurysms. The hemodynamics simulations concerning the optimization of all these factors are still open to question. Other prospective approaches, such as stent-graft (Chuter et al., 2003) (covered stent, coated by porous polyurethane) (Ruiz et al., 1995), coiling (Asakura et al., 2003), and multiple overlapping stents (Doerfler et al., 2004), are emerging as therapeutic alternatives to surgery for the treatment of aneurysms, and are under way for clinical trial.

5. Conclusion

The aorta is continuously exposed to high pulsatile pressure and shear stress, making it prone to mechanical injury. Aneurysmal degeneration that occurs in the aortic arch is termed a aortic arch aneurysm. It has higher risk of rupture than other aneurysm.
The computational modeling in aortic arch aneurysm was designed, implemented and evaluated using a series of technologies-based tools. These tools modeled the biomechanical aspects of aortic arch aneurysm. The computational modeling presented in the chapter combined imaging data, geometrical reconstruction, hemodynamics, the interaction between blood flow and aortic wall, and the effect of endovascular stent. The developed modeling will aid research and ensure that medical professionals benefit through the precise information about aortic arch aneurysm. It will also improve the accuracy and efficiency of the medical procedures.

6. References

Abdolrazaghi, M.; NavidBakhsh, M. & Hassani, K. (2008). Abdominal and Thoracic Aortic Aneurysm Modeling. *American Journal of Applied Science* Vol.5(8), pp. 1052-1058.

Aenis, M.; Stancampiano, A.P.; Wakhloo, A.K. & Lieber, B.B. (1997). Modeling of flow in a straight stented and nonstented side wall aneurysm model. *J. Biomech. Eng.* Vol.119, pp.206–212.

Asakura, F.; Tenjin, H.; Sugawa, N.; Kimura, S. & Oki, F. (2003). Evaluation of intra-aneurysmal blood flow by digital subtraction angiography: Blood flow change after coil embolization. *Surg. Neurol.* Vol.59, pp.309–318.

Bando, K. & Berger, S.A. (2003). Research on fluid-dynamic design criterion of stent used for treatment of aneurysms by means of computational simulation. *Comput. Fluid Dyn. J.* Vol.11, pp.527–531.

Benetos, A. (2003). Pulse pressure and arterial stiffness in type 1 diabetic patients. *Journal of Hypertension,* Vol.21, pp.2005-2007.

Bengtsson, H.; Bergqvist, D. (1993). Ruptured abdominal aortic aneurysm: a population-based study. *J Vasc Surg* Vol.18, pp. 74–80.

Blacher, J.; London, G.M. & Safar, M.E. (1999). Influence of age and end-stage renal disease on the stiffness of carotid wall material in hypertension. *J. Hypertens.,* Vol.17, pp.237-244.

Botnar, R.; Rappitsch, G.; Scheidegger, M.B.; Liepsch, D.; Perktold, K. & Boesiger, P. (2000). Hemodynamics in the carotid artery bifurcation: a comparison between numerical simulations and in vitro MRI measurements. *J Biomech.* Vol.33(2), pp.137-44.

Chuter, T.A.M.; Schneider, D.B.; Reilly, L.M.; Lobo, E.P. & Messina, L.M. (2003). Modular branched stent graft for endovascular repair of aortic arch aneurysm and dissection. *J. Vasc. Surg.* Vol.7, 859–863.

Crawford, E.S.; Stowe, C.L.; Crawford, J.L.;Titus, J.L. & Weilbaecher, D.G. (1984). Aortic arch aneurysm. A sentinel of extensive aortic disease requiring subtotal and total aortic replacement. *Ann Surg.* Vol.199(6), pp. 742-52.

Di Martino, E.S.; Guadagni, G.; Fumero, A.; Ballerini, G.; Spirito, R.; Biglioli, P. & Redaelli, A. (2001). Fluid-structure interaction within realistic threedimensional models of the aneurysmatic aorta as a guidance to assess the risk of rupture of the aneurysm. *Medical Engineering and Physics* Vol.23, pp.647-655.

Di Martino, E.S.; Guadagni, G.; Fumero, A.; Ballerini, G.; Spirito, R.; Biglioli, P.; Redaelli, A. (2001). Fluid-structure interaction within realistic three-dimensional models of the aneurysmatic aorta as a guidance to assess the risk of rupture of the aneurysm. *Med. Eng. Phys.*, Vol. 23, pp.647-655.

Doerfler, A.; Wanke, I.; Egelhof, T.; Stolke, D. & Forsting, M. (2004). Double-stent method: therapeutic alternative for small wide-necked aneurysms. Technical note. *J. Neurosurg.* Vol.100, pp.150–154.

Doublin, D.B. & Rovick, A.A. (1969). Influence of vascular smooth muscle on contractile mechanics and elasticity of arteries. *Americal Journal of Physiology,* Vol. 217, pp.1644-1651.

Fischer, E.I.; Armentano, R.L.; Pessana, F.M.; Graf, S.; Romero, L.; Christen, A.I.; Simon, A. & Levenson, J. (2002). Endothelium-dependent arterial wall tone elasticity modulated by blood viscosity, Am. J. Physiol. Heart Circ. Physiol. Vol.282, pp.389-394.

Fu, W. Y.; Qiao, A.K. & Fu, P. (2008) Boundary identification and triangulation of STL model. In: *Proceeding of the first International Conference on Biomedical Engineering and Informatics.* Sanya, pp. 27–30

Gao, F.; Guo, Z.; Sakamoto, M. & Matsuzawa, T. (2006a). Fluid-structure Interaction within a Layered Aortic Arch Model. *Journal of Biological Physics,* Vol.32, pp.435-454.

Gao, F.; Guo, Z.; Watanabe, M. & Matsuzawa, T. (2006b). Loosely Coupled Simulation for Aortic Arch Model under Steady and Pulsatile Flow, *Journal of Biomechanical Science and Engineering,* Vol.1, pp.327-341.

Gao, F.; Watanabe, M. & Matsuzawa, T. (2006c). Stress analysis in a layered aortic arch model under pulsatile blood flow. *BioMedical Engineering OnLine,* Vol.5:25.

Gao, F.; Ohta O. & Matsuzawa, T. (2008). Fluid-structure interaction in layered aortic arch aneurysm model: Assessing the combined influence of arch aneurysm and wall stiffness. *Australas. Phys Eng Sci Med.* Vol. 31, pp.32-41.

Kilner, P.J.; Yang, G.Z.; Mohiaddin, R.H.; Firmin, D.N. & Longmore, D.B. (1993). Helical and retrograde secondary flow patterns in the aortic arch studied by three-directional magnetic resonance velocity mapping. *Circulation.* Vol.88(5 Pt 1), pp.2235-2247.

Knowles, A.C. & Kneeshaw, J.D. (2004). Aortic arch surgery. In: Mackay JH, Arrowsmith JE (Eds). *Core Topics in Cardiac Anaesthesia.* London: Greenwich Medical Media. pp.191-194.

Lieber, B.B.; Livescu, V.; Hopkins, L.N. & Wakhloo, A.K. (2002). Particle image velocimetry assessment of stent design influence on intraaneurysmal flow. *Ann. Biomed. Eng.* Vol.30, pp.768–777.

Liou, T.M. & Liou, S.N. (2004). Pulsatile flows in a lateral aneurysm anchored on a stented and curved parent vessel. *Exp. Mech.* Vol.44, pp.253–260.

Liou, T.M.; Liou, S.N. & Chu, K.L. (2004). Intra-aneurysmal flow with helix and mesh stent placement across side-wall aneurysm pore of a straight parent vessel. *J. Biomech. Eng.* Vol.126, pp.36–43.

Long, A.; Rouet, L. & Bissery, A. (2004). Compliance of abdominal aortic aneurysms: Evaluation of tissue Doppler imaging. *J. Ultrasound in Medical and Biology,* Vol.30, Vol.1099- 1108.

Morris, L.; Delassus, P.; Callanan, A.; Walsh, M.; Wallis., F.; Grace, P & McGloughlin, T. (2005). 3-D numerical simulation of blood flow through models of the human aorta. *J Biomech Eng* Vol.127(5), pp.767—75.

Morris-Stiff, G.; Haynes, M. & Ogunbiyi, S. (2005). Is Assessment of Popliteal Artery Diameter in Patients Undergoing Screening for Abdominal Aortic Aneurysms a Worthwhile Procedure. *European Journal of Vascular and Endovascular Surgery,* Vol.30, pp. 71-74.

Qiao, A.K.; Fu, W.Y. & Liu, Y.J. (2011) Study on hemodynamics in patient-specific thoracic aortic aneurysm, *Theor. Appl. Mech. Lett.* Vol. 1 (1), 014001-1-4

Raghavan, M.L.; Vorp, D.A.; Federle, M.P.; Makaroun, M.S. & M.W. Webster, M.W. (2000) Wall stress distribution on three-dimensionally reconstructed models of human abdominal aortic aneurysm. *J. Vasc. Surg.,* Vol.31, pp.760-769.

Rideout, V.C. (1991). Mathematical and computer modeling of physiological systems. New York: Prentice Hall.

Rupnic, M. & Runvovc, F. (2002). Simulation of steady state and transient phenomena by using the equivalent electronic circuit. *J. Computer Methods and Programs in Biomedici.,* Vol. 67, pp.1-12.

Shahcheraghi, N.; Dwyer, H.A.; Cheer, A.Y.; Barakat, A.I. & Rutaganira, T. (2002). Unsteady and three-dimensional simulation of blood flow in the human aortic arch. *J Biomech Eng* Vol.124(4), pp.378-387.

Sonesson, B.; Hansen, F. & Lanne, T. (1997). Abdominal aortic aneurysm: a general defect in the vasculature with focal manifestations in the abdominal aorta?. *J. Vasc. Surg.,* Vol. 26(2), pp.247-254.

Taylor, C.A. (1999). Predictive medicine: computational techniques in therapeutic decision-making. *Computer Aided Surgery,* 4:231-247, 1999.

Tokuda, Y; Song, M.H.; Ueda, Y.; Usui, A.; Akita, T.; Yoneyama, S. & Maruyama, S. (2008). Eur J , Three-dimensional numerical simulation of blood flow in the aortic arch during cardiopulmonary bypass. *Cardiothorac Surg.* Vol. 33(2), pp.164-7

Tsukamoto, S.; Shindo, S.; Obana, M.; Akiyama, K.; Shiono, M. & Negishi, N. (2003). DeBakey IIIb aortic dissection originating in a distal aortic arch aneurysm. *Ann. Thorac. Cardiovasc. Surg.,*Vol. 9(3):209-211.

Vorp, D.A.; Raghavan, M.L. & Webster, M.W. (1998). Mechanical Wall Stress in Abdominal Aortic Aneurysm: In°uence of Diameter and Asymmetry. *J. Vasc. Surg.,* Vol.27, pp.632-639.

Vorp, D.A.; Raghavan, M.L.; Muluk, S.C.; Makaroun, M.S.; Shapiro, R. & Webster, M.W. (1996). Wall Strength and Sti®ness of Aneurysmal and Nonaneurysmal Abdominal Aorta. *Ann. New York Acad. Sci.,* 800:274-277, 1996.

Xie, J.; Zhou, J. & Fung, Y.C. (1995). Bending of blood vessel wall: stress-strain laws of the intima-media and adventitial layers. J. Biomech. Eng., Vol. 117, pp. 136-145.

Qiao, A.; Liu, Y.; Chang, Y. & Matsuzawa, T. (2005). Computational study of stented aortic arch aneurysms. In: *27th Annual International Conference of the IEEE Engineering in Medicine and Biology Society*. Shanghai, China, September 2005.

Rhee, K.; Han, M.H. & Cha, S.H. (2002). Changes of flow characteristics by stenting in aneurysm models: influence of aneurysm geometry and stent porosity. *Ann. Biomed. Eng.* Vol.30, pp.894–904.

Ruiz, C.E.; Zhang, H.P.; Douglas, J.T.; Zuppan, C.W., & Kean, C.J. (1995). A novel method for treatment of abdominal aortic aneurysms using percutaneous implantation of a newly designed endovascular device. *Circulation* Vol.91, pp.2470–2477.